Assembling Therapeutics

This volume examines the ways in which people engage with therapeutic practices, such as life coaching, mindfulness, complementary and alternative medicine, sex and relationship counselling, spiritual healing and self-tracking. It investigates how human and non-human actors, systems of thought and practice are assembled and interwoven in therapeutic engagements, and traces the situated, material and political dimensions of these engagements. By focusing on lived experiences through ethnographically informed case studies, the book elucidates the diverse forms, meanings and embodied effects of therapeutic engagements in different settings, as well as their potential for both oppressive and subversive social change. In this way, *Assembling Therapeutics* contributes to our understanding of multiple modes of healing, self-knowledge and power in contemporary societies.

Suvi Salmenniemi is Professor of Sociology at the University of Turku, Finland.

Johanna Nurmi is a postdoctoral researcher in Sociology at the University of Turku, Finland.

Inna Perheentupa is currently finalising her doctoral dissertation in Sociology at the University of Turku, Finland.

Harley Bergroth is currently finalising his doctoral dissertation in Sociology at the University of Turku, Finland.

Therapeutic Cultures

Series Editors

Daniel Nehring, East China University of Science and Technology, China
Ole Jacob Madsen, University of Oslo, Norway
Edgar Cabanas, Universidad Camilo José Cela, Spain
China Mills, University of Sheffield, UK
Dylan Kerrigan, University of the West Indies, Trinidad and Tobago

This interdisciplinary series explores the role which therapeutic discourses and practices play in the organisation of social life, critically addressing the two broad questions of how therapeutic knowledge is popularised beyond academia and mental health care, and how it participates in popular culture, and in institutional structures and processes in government, law, education, media, health, work, family life, public and private policies.

Therapeutic Cultures seeks to address the histories of therapeutic culture and engage with its contemporary manifestations, so welcomes books that examine the transnationalisation of therapeutic discourses and practices and their uses in local institutional settings, as well as studies of the ways in which therapeutic discourses and practices participate in the social organisation of power, and how they become ingrained across a wide array of institutions.

Titles in this series

For more information about this series, please visit: https://www.routledge.com/sociology/series/TC

Assembling Therapeutics
Cultures, Politics and Materiality

**Edited by Suvi Salmenniemi,
Johanna Nurmi, Inna Perheentupa
and Harley Bergroth**

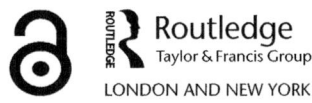

LONDON AND NEW YORK

First published 2020
by Routledge
2 Park Square, Milton Park, Abingdon, Oxon OX14 4RN

and by Routledge
52 Vanderbilt Avenue, New York, NY 10017

Routledge is an imprint of the Taylor & Francis Group, an informa business

British Library Cataloguing-in-Publication Data
A catalogue record for this book is available from the British Library

Library of Congress Cataloging-in-Publication Data
Names: Salmenniemi, Suvi, 1975- editor.
Title: Assembling therapeutics: cultures, politics and materiality/ edited by Suvi Salmenniemi [and three others].
Description: Abingdon, Oxon; New York, NY: Routledge, 2019. | Series: Therapeutic cultures | Includes bibliographical references and index.
Identifiers: LCCN 2019017109 (print) | ISBN 9780815377979 (hbk)
Subjects: LCSH: Applied psychology–Social aspects | Self-help techniques–Social aspects. | Self-care, Health–Social aspects. | Therapeutics–Social aspects.
Classification: LCC BF636 .A757 2019 (print) | LCC BF636 (ebook) | DDC 158–dc23
LC record available at https://lccn.loc.gov/2019017109
LC ebook record available at https://lccn.loc.gov/2019981318

ISBN: 978-0-815-37797-9 (hbk)
ISBN: 978-1-351-23339-2 (ebk)

Typeset in Times New Roman
by Deanta Global Publishing Services, Chennai, India

Printed and bound in Great Britain by
TJ International Ltd, Padstow, Cornwall

Contents

Notes on the contributors

Kia Andell is a doctoral candidate at the University of Turku. Drawing on narratives of uncanny sensory experiences, her dissertation explores the science-public relationship and relations between scientific and experience-based knowledges.

Harley Bergroth is a doctoral candidate in Sociology at the University of Turku. His research interests revolve around cultural studies of technology, science and embodiment. His PhD thesis focuses on data-driven life management and self-monitoring practices in everyday life. He is a board member of the Finnish Society for Science and Technology Studies.

Felix Freigang received a master's degree in social and cultural anthropology from Freie Universität Berlin in 2018 and is currently preparing for a PhD project on the technological imaginaries of Artificial Intelligence and affective computing in the fields of mental health and well-being. Freigang's theoretical interests lie in medical and psychological anthropology, STS and media ethnography as well as affect theory.

Ilpo Helén is Professor of Sociology at the University of Eastern Finland. His studies focus on the politics and economy of new biomedicine, medical genomics and biobanking, and on the biopolitics of healthcare. He has developed an approach to critical analysis of the government of life and related technologies embedded in Foucauldian critical genealogy and in science and technology studies. He has authored several books and articles published in, for example, *Economy and Society*, *Science and Technology Studies*, *Acta Sociologica* and *European Journal of Human Genetics*.

Marja-Liisa Honkasalo, MD, PhD has long-standing experience in cultural studies of health and illness. She has been director of the Center for the Study of Culture and Health at the University of Turku, Finland. She has also worked as Professor of Medical Anthropology at the University of Linköping in Sweden. She is Associate Professor of Sociology at the School of Social Sciences at the University of Helsinki. She is currently a visiting scholar at the University of the Arts, Center for the Study of Artistic Research, Finland.

Joni Jaakola is a PhD student at the University of Turku, Finland. His research interests include science and technology studies, materiality and cultural studies of health as well as sociology of knowledge, social theory and political sociology. His PhD research focuses on the automatisation and robotisation of health care.

Marjo Kolehmainen is a postdoctoral research fellow at the University of Tampere. She works on the research project *Just the Two of Us? Affective inequalities in intimate relationships* funded by the Academy of Finland. Her current research explores the practices of relationship and sex counselling. Her research interests include affect, gender, sexuality and methodology. She has authored articles published in, for example, *Feminist Media Studies*, *Subjectivity*, *Sexualities* and *The Sociological Review*. She is also a co-editor of *Affective Inequalities in Intimate Relationships* (Routledge, 2018).

Ilmari Kortelainen works at the University of Tampere, Finland. His research has focused on bodily skills and methods for professional training in the workplace through body phenomenology and affect theory. He is interested in the ways of conceptualising the mindfulness-based interventions used in the information society. He is also interested in generating alternative, socially responsible utilisation of meditative practices, such as meditation and social enquiry. He is the co-editor of *Mindfulness and Sciences* (2014, in Finnish).

Julia Lerner is senior lecturer at the Department of Sociology and Anthropology, Ben-Gurion University of the Negev, Israel. Her research interests are in the fields of anthropology of knowledge and migration. At the intersection of these fields, she explores experiences of relocation and translation of ideas in post-Soviet Russia and in the Russian-speaking collective in Israel. She has published articles on the adaptation of the therapeutic language in post-Soviet emotional culture in *Slavic Review* and *Sexuality and Culture*.

Johanna Nurmi is a postdoctoral researcher in Sociology at the University of Turku. Her work focuses on the critique of biomedicine expressed from both outside and within the biomedical field. She is currently studying the contestation of vaccination by lay groups and medical professionals, focusing on the practices and politics of vaccine refusal and the negotiation related to vaccination in clinical encounters.

Inna Perheentupa is a doctoral candidate in Sociology at the University of Turku. She is currently finalising her ethnographic study of the politicisation of gender and sexuality in contemporary Russia. Her research interests include gender studies, political sociology and cultural studies.

Virve Peteri is an academy research fellow in sociology at the University of Tampere and a visiting scholar at the Institute for the Study of Science, Technology and Innovation at the University of Edinburgh. She has long-standing expertise in the study of media, technologies, spatial arrangements and materiality.

Suvi Salmenniemi is professor of sociology at the University of Turku, Finland. She has conducted research on therapeutic knowledges and practices in Finland and Russia and is the Principal Investigator of the project *Tracking the therapeutic: Ethnographies of wellbeing, politics and inequality*, funded by the Academy of Finland (2015–2019). Her research interests include therapeutic practices and wellbeing, political sociology, cultural studies and feminist research. Her current research explores the politics of popular psychology, new spiritualities and complementary and alternative medicine in Finland. She is the author of *Democratization and Gender in Contemporary Russia* (Routledge, 2008) and the editor of *Rethinking Class in Russia* (Ashgate, 2012). Her articles have appeared in *The Sociological Review*, *Sociology*, *European Journal of Cultural Studies* and *British Journal of Sociology*.

Steven Stanley is a critical psychologist who has worked in the School of Social Sciences at Cardiff University for the past 15 years. He is interested in the history and philosophy of psychology, therapeutic cultures, and the ethics and politics of mindfulness meditation. He is the Principal Investigator of the *Mapping Mindfulness* project, the first large-scale social study of the UK mindfulness movement, funded by the Leverhulme Trust. Steven has recently co-edited the *Handbook of Ethical Foundations of Mindfulness* (Stanley, Purser & Singh, Springer, 2018).

Elaine Swan is a feminist sociologist and senior lecturer at the University of Sussex Business School, based in the Future of Work Hub. She has three research projects, one of which is an ongoing exploration of the interface between therapy culture and the workplace. She has published a monograph, *Worked Up Selves*, and several articles and chapters. Recent papers explore coaching in relation to gender, race and class, and whiteness and digital multimodal semiotics. Her other projects are studies of foodwork and pedagogies, and critical diversity studies. She is currently completing a book on *Foodwork and Intercultural Organising* based on ethnographic studies of food social enterprises and has co-edited a collection on Food Pedagogies. Recent chapters focus on digital food cultures, food femininities and whiteness.

Tatiana Tiaynen-Qadir is a postdoctoral researcher at the Faculty of Social Sciences, University of Tampere, Finland. Her research focuses on transnational anthropology of the family, religious studies and the culture of therapeutic in modern Russia and Finland. She has published two monographs and a number of articles and chapters in peer-reviewed journals and edited volumes.

Ariel Yankellevich is a PhD candidate in the Department of Sociology and Anthropology at Ben-Gurion University of the Negev, Israel. He holds a BA (Sociology and Psychology) and an MA (Sociology) from the Hebrew University of Jerusalem. His dissertation explores the construction of new forms of therapeutic subjectivity among Israel's 'last republican generation'. His previous research examined the logics and practice of resilience building interventions for potential victims of war and terrorism in Israel. His research interests include the sociology of therapeutic cultures, medical and psychological anthropology and neoliberal subjectivity.

1 From culture to assemblages

An introduction

Suvi Salmenniemi, Harley Bergroth,
Johanna Nurmi and Inna Perheentupa

Therapeutic life management is a billion-dollar business worldwide, woven into the fabric of our daily lives through media culture, workplace activities, technology, healthcare and politics. Reality TV propagates self-improvement through countless makeover shows; schools and kindergartens offer training in emotion management; workers are encouraged to cope with structural stress factors with the help of mindfulness sessions and motivational seminars; and bookstore shelves groan under the weight of popular psychology books promising to unleash one's inner potential and deliver happiness, love and harmony. Therapeutic discourses are also intertwined with processes of digitalisation, which are opening up new avenues for everyday therapeutic engagement through wearable, near-body computing and mobile health applications. The therapeutic, referring to psychological, spiritual and holistic discourses and practices that encourage cultivation, care and transformation of the self, is so ubiquitous in the codes and conduct of contemporary everyday lives that its normalising power often goes unnoticed. However, as a variant of a longstanding cultural-historical injunction to 'know thyself', it significantly shapes the everyday lifeworlds we inhabit.

The seminal role and increasingly global reach of therapeutic discourses and practices in contemporary social formations have been taken up and intensively debated in the social sciences and humanities. Scholars have critically discussed 'the psychologisation of everything'; that is, the dominating role of emotions and psychological vocabularies in making sense of and regulating human life (Rose, 1990; Illouz, 2008). This phenomenon has been captured in the concept of therapeutic culture, which suggests that therapeutic discourses thoroughly permeate the cultures and institutions of the Global North and crucially shape how we understand and relate to ourselves and the social world (Aubry & Travis, 2015; Foster, 2015). Therapeutic culture rests on a particular understanding of selfhood, revolving around ideas of psychic interiority, autonomy, authenticity, self-responsibility and continuous self-invention (Rose, 1998; McGee, 2005).

This book arises from a need to advance our understanding and theorisation of therapeutic cultures in our current political conjuncture. It makes novel empirical and theoretical contributions to existing scholarship in three ways. First, while there is now a wide body of literature on therapeutic discourses and techniques and their role in the government of populations, there is a notable lacuna in understanding of how people engage with these discourses and practices. This book addresses this lacuna and taps into ways in which people incorporate therapeutic practices into their daily lives. It explores how people live with, appropriate, produce, negotiate and transform therapeutic practices, and how these practices shape and are shaped by subjectivities. In zooming into lived experiences through ethnographically informed case studies, this book elucidates the diverse forms, meanings and embodied effects of therapeutic engagements in different settings, as well as their potential for both oppressive and subversive social change.

Second, while the overwhelming majority of previous research on therapeutic cultures has focused on Anglo-American societies (see e.g. Aubry & Travis, 2015; McGee, 2005; Ouellette & Hay, 2008; Furedi, 2004; Cloud, 1998; Foster, 2015, 2016), this book brings in case studies from other countries, including Germany, Russia, Finland and Israel. In this way, it contributes to a growing body of research on therapeutic cultures beyond the Anglo-American purview (see e.g. Matza, 2012; Nehring et al., 2016; Madsen, 2014; Mäkinen, 2014; Hendriks, 2017). Globally, therapeutic practices share many central elements; yet, as this book shows, they also become invested with different meanings and constitutions as they travel to and are adopted and practised within different historical, cultural and geographical contexts.

Third, this book makes a theoretical contribution by introducing the notion of assemblage into discussion of the therapeutic, and by investigating how human and non-human actors, systems of thought and practice are assembled and interwoven in therapeutic engagements. We suggest that, rather than as 'culture', therapeutic practices and discourses can be productively conceptualised as diverse, situated and context-specific 'assemblages' that may be politicising or depoliticising, individualising or collectively oriented, commonly welcomed or shunned by the public imaginary – and, of course, many of these things simultaneously. By engaging with assemblage thinking, the book seeks to decentre the somewhat totalising narratives of therapeutic culture, which tend to depict it as a coherent and unified entity producing similar effects regardless of time and place. The analytical lens of assemblage allows us to bring to the fore the multiplicity of therapeutic configurations in different contexts, and to underscore their material and political dimensions, which have not been studied enough in previous literature.

The chapters of this book thus dive into the complexity of therapeutic assemblages across various areas, including mindfulness and life coaching (Stanley and Kortelainen; Yankellevich), relationship and sex counselling (Kolehmainen), religious and spiritual self-care practices (Lerner; Tiaynen-Qadir), extraordinary experiences as instantiations of care and healing (Andell et al.), complementary and alternative health practices (Salmenniemi et al.), feminist politics (Perheentupa), organisational fun culture (Peteri) and data-driven digital life management (Bergroth and Helén; Freigang). They examine how the 'therapeutic' works in diverse symbolic and material contexts, and ask what makes people's self-cultivation practices 'therapeutic', and how therapeutic assemblages relate to power, politics and the production of social reality. We argue that, rather than 'therapeutic culture' imposing itself on lives anywhere in the world, 'therapeutic' is always assembled into being from a variety of resources, not only by the masses 'out there', but also by the very people who attempt to study it. We thus join scholars who are calling for acknowledgement of the complexity of therapeutic cultures and their capacity to serve many, seemingly incongruous ends (Aubry & Travis, 2015), and for investigation of their diverse manifestations, without *a priori* assumptions about their effects (Illouz, 2008).

We will discuss each of these three contributions in more detail. However, before doing that, we first offer a brief overview of existing research on therapeutic culture.

Mapping therapeutic culture

Self-care and self-betterment are longstanding phenomena dating back to antiquity (Foucault, 1988), and have been part and parcel of many different political, religious and cultural formations (Madsen, 2015; Kelly, 2001; see also Tiaynen-Qadir, and Stanley and Kortelainen in this book). The rise of modern-style therapeutic self-help discourse traces back to American father figure, Benjamin Franklin (1706–1790) who, apart from the Declaration of Independence (US, 1776), produced texts providing simple guidance on how to become wealthy and how to lead a virtuous and happy life, and kept charts monitoring his own virtuousness (Madsen, 2015: 5; Schaupp, 2016: 251). A century later, British publisher and author, Samuel Smiles published *Self-Help* (1859), a pioneering book in the modern self-help genre that popularised rational and utilitarian ideas of self-improvement (Kelly, 2001: 201). Later that century, the New Thought movement gained momentum in the United States, merging psychological and religious discourses in the propagation of positive thinking (Woodstock, 2005). Thus, since its inception, the modern-style therapeutic discourse has been a complex assemblage drawing on religion, spirituality, medicine, psychology, natural science, business management and so on. However, while the phenomenon of self-betterment is old, new to our current moment are its thoroughly naturalised, individual-centred and psychologically infused ontology, and its intensive commodification, digitalisation and global circulation. These aspects are addressed in this book.

Existing scholarship on therapeutic culture can be roughly divided into three strands. The first is a longstanding strand of cultural critique addressing the therapeutic ethos as an emblematic element of late modern 'cultural decline'. On the one hand, the therapeutic ethos is seen as threatening to undermine public morality and political and communal life, promote individualism and narcissism, and deflect political critique by offering psychological solutions to complex structural problems (see e.g. Furedi, 2004; Lasch, 1979; Rieff, 1966; for a comprehensive and critical review, see Lichterman, 1992; Illouz, 2008; Madsen, 2015). This scholarship has tended, to paraphrase Aubry and Travis (2015: 4), to 'excoriate rather than analyze' the therapeutic ethos. On the other hand, proponents of reflexive modernisation (e.g. Giddens, 1992) suggest that proliferation of the therapeutic discourse is connected with the individualisation process and the erosion of the role of traditions and traditional authorities in late modern societies. In this context, therapeutic practices may have a potentially empowering role by providing individuals with cultural resources with which to reflect on and assemble their identities and biographies.

The second approach is grounded in the (post-)Foucauldian governmentality tradition, which links the rise of 'psy' to historically shifting forms of government (Rose, 1990, 1998). Rooted in a genealogical approach, this body of scholarship argues that 'advanced liberal' or 'neoliberal' government is characterised by governing through freedom, choice and responsibility; 'at a distance' rather than through repression and control. Therapeutic knowledges and techniques are seen as crucial ingredients of this art of government, giving rise to self-managing and enterprising subjects (Rose, 1990, 1998; Binkley, 2011; Foster, 2015). In promising liberation of the self, psy governmentalities make the self 'work seamlessly for and within a system of power' (Illouz, 2008: 3). Subjects are obliged to be free and to make life meaningful by searching for happiness and self-realisation (Rose, 1998: 151). Through attachment to various therapeutic technologies of the self, 'we are governed by our active engagement in the search for a form of existence that is at once personally fulfilling and beneficial to our families, our communities and the collective well-being of the nation' (ibid.: 78).

Third, a vast body of empirical analyses on therapeutic discourses and techniques draws on diverse theoretical resources and focuses particularly on popular media culture as an influential transmitter of the therapeutic ethos. These studies have examined, for example, reality TV, makeover shows and talk shows (Ouellette & Hay, 2008; Ringrose & Walkerdine, 2008; Harvey & Gill, 2011; Lerner & Zbenovich, 2013), women's magazines (Gill, 2009; Madsen & Ytre–Arne, 2012) and self-help literature (McGee, 2005; Woodstock, 2005; Hazleden, 2003; Rimke, 2000; Nehring et al., 2016; Salmenniemi & Adamson, 2015; Tiaynen-Qadir & Salmenniemi, 2017). They have identified key ideas, generic conventions and strategies of persuasion in the therapeutic discourse, as well as analysed representations of gender, sexuality and class and how they produce and sustain relationships of power and privilege. In addition to examining media culture, the therapeutic discourse has also been critically interrogated in the context of education, detailing how therapeutic and neoliberal discourses coalesce to construct normative ideas about autonomous, enterprising and competitive students (Ecclestone & Hayes, 2008; Brunila, 2011; Brunila & Siivonen, 2016), and has been applied to management and corporate culture, highlighting the mobilisation of therapeutic practices in managing worker subjectivities (Swan, 2010; Davies, 2015).

As this review elucidates, a lot of important work has been done to interrogate how therapeutic discourses subjectivate and interpellate, and operate as an oppressive ideology or form of governmentality. However, there is still a paucity of research on the lived experience of therapeutic practices, especially outside the Anglo-American context (see, however, Lichterman, 1992; Illouz, 2008; Matza, 2012; Sointu, 2013; Nehring & Kerrigan, 2019; Salmenniemi & Vorona, 2014; Pagis, 2016).

This book addresses this gap through an ethnographic investigation of what inspires people to engage with therapeutic practices and what makes these practices meaningful to them. In the next sections, we flesh out what this entails.

Ethnographies of the therapeutic

Ethnography is particularly well suited to capturing the complexities and nuances of everyday life that may easily slip under the radar of grand social theory and macro-level indicators. For example, while it may seem plausible to claim that we live in a certain 'age' – such as therapeutic or neoliberal – the actual meaning of such 'age' is always interpreted, appropriated, put into effect and challenged in everyday practice. The idea of an overarching 'therapeutic culture' is a case in point: such a concept can take us only so far in understanding the nuanced functionalities and manifestations acquired by various therapeutic life management discourses and strategies in different contexts. This is mainly because the notion of 'culture' tends to invite connotations of a static, monolithic and universal structure of action and thought, and thus overlooks the differences and flexibilities in such structures in personal, national, technological, spatial and historical settings.

Ethnographic sensibility, involving careful contextualisation and attempts to understand other lifeworlds using the self as the instrument of knowing (Ortner, 2006: 42), is thus one of the main threads connecting the contributions of this book. We approach ethnography as an intersubjective practice of 'engaging in, wrestling with, and being committed to the human relationships' in the fields we explore (Campbell & Lassiter, 2015: 4–5). In line with recent anthropological discussions (Hannerz, 2003; Huttunen, 2010), we understand the 'therapeutic' as a field consisting of multiple sites and social relations, as reflected from many different angles and using different types of research materials in this book.

Through the ethnographic approach, we seek to move away from the 'epistemology of suspicion' (Illouz, 2008: 4), which tends to posit therapeutics as politically and culturally dubious and its practitioners as politically reactionary and imprisoned by false consciousness, and to explore how people encounter, engage and live with therapeutic practices. Some chapters examine how people narrate and experience therapeutic practices, while others analyse the practices themselves, such as mindfulness or self-tracking – and many chapters tackle both.

Studies drawing on critical analysis of public discourse have tended to underplay agency and overlook the critical capacities of actors (see Illouz, 2008: 4). They often create an impression of therapeutic practitioners as passive receivers of ideological interpellations. This means that the analytical space between discourse and experience has been neglected. The ethnographic approach adopted in this book allows us to address this space. In addition to ethnography, we also align here with the active audience paradigm of cultural studies, and suggest that therapeutic practitioners are not cultural dopes, but active producers of meaning from within their own cultural contexts (Barker, 2000: 269). Therapeutic discourses carry multiple, and sometimes contradictory, meanings; and how practitioners in different social positions make sense of and work with them is an open empirical

question (see Illouz, 2008: 4; Radway, 1984). As the chapters in this book eluci-
date, practitioners engage with therapeutic practices and discourses in complex
ways, which may both challenge and reproduce ideological formations.

This book's authors use their embodied and sensory experiences to provide rich
and empathetic understandings of the therapeutic worlds mapped in their chapters. While emotional detachment and absence of the researcher's body and affect
have often been adopted in pursuit of objectivity, embodied researcher experiences form a different 'landscape for analytical insight' (Cerwonka & Malkki,
2007). Throughout this book, the authors create these landscapes through sensory
explorations of their field sites and the different therapeutic practices and experiences within them. For instance, Marjo Kolehmainen's chapter on relationship
and sex counselling paints a vivid picture of how the researcher's body relates to
the therapeutic assemblages scrutinised during fieldwork. Her work shows how
examining the researcher's bodily states can strengthen analytical work and help
to capture affective atmospheres as they unfold in therapeutic events. In another
chapter, Tatiana Tiaynen-Qadir describes her ethnographic process of drawing on
her own bodily experiences of Orthodox Christian liturgy to analyse and understand aspects of the sacred and *therapeia* that her participants attempt to put into
words. Throughout her fieldwork, she participated in church services and choir
practices, which gave her an embodied perspective on the sensory experiences
relating to therapeutic and spiritual practices narrated by her participants.

Two other chapters also draw on long-term ethnographic involvement in the
lives of research participants. Julia Lerner has studied women's religious practice
and how it is informed by therapeutic self-management in a transnational context, combining in-depth interviews with ethnographic knowledge of her research
participants' everyday lives. Inna Perheentupa has participated in the activities
of feminist and LGBTQ groups in Russia as part of her fieldwork, and also conducted virtual ethnography on feminist online sites. This has allowed her to gain
deeper insights into the everyday political struggles in which her interlocutors are
engaged and to appreciate the therapeutic dimensions of these struggles.

Sensory and embodied experiences are also an important starting point for the
chapter by Steven Stanley and Ilmari Kortelainen. It uses audiovisual recordings
and Stanley's experience of a mindfulness training event, as well as the authors'
own practices of mindfulness and meditation, to analyse the affective discursive
practices of mindfulness from an 'insider-outsider' position. In a similar vein,
the chapter by Suvi Salmenniemi, Johanna Nurmi and Joni Jaakola makes use of
insights derived from Salmenniemi's participant observation in various therapeutic events and treatments. The chapter by Harley Bergroth and Ilpo Helén, analysing discourses and experiences of self-tracking technologies, is also affected and
shaped by Bergroth's personal experimentation with everyday fitness tracking
devices during the course of the research.

Virve Peteri and Felix Freigang make use of ethnographic methods to understand the role of technologies and spaces in shaping subjectivities and emotional
realms. Peteri examines how new forms of office decoration and spatial planning in the workplace connect with the therapeutic ethos and regulate bodies,

moods and emotions. She describes how her own profoundly embodied sense of uneasiness during fieldwork sensitised and helped her to relate to her interlocutors' experiences of these spaces and the ideological dilemmas with which they wrestled. Freigang's chapter, in turn, traces ways in which mood-tracking applications do or do not work to combat mental illness in the context of inadequate mental health services, and highlights the contradictory effects and reactions to which they may give rise.

Finally, the chapters by Ariel Yankellevich and by Kia Andell, Harley Bergroth and Marja-Liisa Honkasalo, while not rooted in participant observation, adopt an ethnographically inspired approach through comprehensive immersion in their research settings and careful fleshing out of the embodied, sensory and affective experiences emerging in the research materials.

The bottom-up, embodied and sensory research practices used in this book also invite us to rethink notions of participation in ethnographic fieldwork. Conducting interviews and observation using a number of sensory experiences can, in itself, constitute participation (Pink, 2009). As our focus in this book is on plugging gaps in the 'sociology of therapeutic cultures' (Swan, 2010), these rich ethnographic practices help form understandings of people's ways of experiencing and making sense of their worlds and may provide routes to knowledge and memories that would otherwise be hard to reach. Thus, ethnographic perspectives create new ways to understand how and why people choose to engage with various therapeutic practices, and what makes therapeutic practices meaningful for them.

Assembling therapeutics

In addition to advancing an ethnographic approach to therapeutic practices, this book also paves the way for an alternative theorisation of therapeutic engagements through the concept of assemblage. In so doing, it seeks to decentre 'culture' as a deterministic 'force' that is massive, enclosing and sometimes almost invincible. We propose that the therapeutic can be conceptualised as an assemblage of ideas, practices, spaces, objects and bodies yielding multiple, contextually specific and sometimes contradictory effects. This helps to highlight the multifarious and processual nature of the therapeutic, which defies any universalising and totalising effects.

The concept of an assemblage is an open-ended collage of sorts. According to McFarlane (2011: 206), it is usually mobilised to connote 'indeterminacy, emergence, becoming, processuality, turbulence and the sociomateriality of phenomena', and it has become part of the vocabulary of contemporary social theory. For example, French philosophers, Gilles Deleuze and Felix Guattari (1987) approached it as a 'general logic' of thinking about the world as being in perpetual flux, and French sociologist, Michel Callon (2005) has employed it to develop actor–network theoretical accounts of the functioning of sociotechnical systems. However, the French term preferred by such thinkers is *agencement*. While *agencement* is typically translated into English as 'assemblage', the two terms actually come from different etymological roots and mean different things, since the word *assemblage* also exists in the French lexicon. Simply put, *agencement* is a play on words that is sensitive to both the idea of 'an arrangement' (un agencement) and 'agency' (agence). Caliskan and Callon (2010: 9) elaborate that 'agencies and arrangements are not separate. *Agencements* denote socio-technical arrangements when they are considered from the point [of] view of their capacity to act.' *Assemblage* denotes a rather narrower meaning, that of 'a bringing or coming together' (see also Nail, 2017; Hardie & Mackenzie, 2007).

Perhaps owing to these complexities, in the social scientific literature, assemblage has appeared as a protean concept employed in various ways. For example, it has served as a conceptual tool to explore philosophical questions about ontology, existence and agency, and to argue for a rhizomatic understanding of the social, highlighting complex processes of 'becoming' rather than any fixed underlying 'essences' of things (Deleuze & Guattari, 1987; DeLanda, 2006; Introna, 2013). In new materialist social research, it has been widely drawn on to highlight processes of human–technology co-construction; object-oriented accounts of social life and power; and the effects, possibilities, restrictions and (unexpected) consequences imposed by the material and technical worlds on human thought and action when human and non-human entities come together to inter- and intra-act (Coole & Frost, 2010; Bennett, 2010; Latour, 2005; Mol, 2002; Lupton, 2016). Yet others, especially in anthropological research, have employed the concept to highlight the active labour of pulling together and sustaining diverse, sometimes apparently incompatible elements that have no inherent allegiance with one another (see Collier & Ong, 2005; Li, 2007; Zigon, 2011a, 2011b). For example, in their highly influential work, Collier and Ong (2005: 4) examine how 'global forms', such as neoliberalism, science and expert systems, are territorialised in assemblages, defining new material, collective and discursive relationships. They approach assemblages as 'the product of multiple determinations that are not reducible to any single logic' (ibid.: 12).

Assemblage theorisation has also been taken up in the methodological litera-ture, as an idea suggesting that social research and scientific knowledge produc-tion are always situated and contingent – craftwork in themselves – and should acknowledge the pitfalls of overreliance on scientific rationalism (see Law, 2004; Fox & Alldred, 2015). What unites these different ways of working with assem-blage is a sensitivity to *processuality* rather than stability, and a focus on chal-lenging the persistent binaries (such as human/non-human, social/material, order/ chaos, rational/emotional) present in everyday thought.

In this book, we draw insights from these debates on assemblages to ana-lyse and theorise therapeutic practices. The concept of assemblage here denotes not so much a coherent theoretical framework as such, but rather a theoretical-methodological 'lens of inquiry' and a 'style of thought'. On the one hand, the chapters in the book look at the therapeutic as contingent arrangements situated in specific personal, political, material, spatial and discursive contexts. That is to say, 'the therapeutic' is never one but many; it is effectively a different entity with different effects and repercussions in different contexts. On the other hand, we focus on the ongoing work of 'assembling' the therapeutic. This means that we look at the active work conducted by human and non-human beings, technological applications, political ideas and various other actants in making the therapeutic happen in everyday lives. Thus, the chapters in this book also suggest, in various ways, that different kinds of practices, beliefs and everyday arrangements are therapeutic only in the sense that they are made therapeutic.

The specific theoretical contribution of this book to the discussion of therapeutic culture is its approach to the therapeutic as a kind of active craftwork (see McFarlane, 2011) in everyday life. Each chapter looks at how people and other-than-people participate in crafting and maintaining therapeutic assemblages, that is, make sense of and act upon themselves, and make promises, paths and possibilities for a good (or at least better) life to happen. The therapeutic happens through a coming together of many different elements: different technologies, beliefs, programmes, discourses, metaphors and beings, whether 'real' or 'imaginary' (another persistent binary to overcome). This work of 'assembling therapeutics' reveals the multiplicity of the therapeutic, and how the meaning of 'the therapeutic' itself shifts with shifting assemblages. In this spirit of assembling and craftwork, the chapters in this book also combine assemblage thinking with a number of other theoretical resources, including affect theory, metaphor theory, anthropological and sociological study of religion and spirituality, Foucauldian analytics of power, queer theory and Critical Theory, to provide a nuanced understanding of therapeutic practices.

The politics of therapeutic assemblages

The assemblage perspective is a potent theoretical lens through which to deepen our understanding of two themes that run through this book as key analytical threads: *politics* and *materiality*. Although these themes are enmeshed in complex ways – politics being material, and materiality being political – we elaborate on each in the remainder of this Introduction.

We begin by exploring the politics of therapeutic engagements and, more specifically, the types of political imaginaries and actions that these engagements may enable or foreclose. Historically, therapeutic knowledges and practices have been intimately intertwined with social movements, including the countercultural movements of the 1960s and 1970s, such as the women's liberation, New Age and alternative health movements and radical community therapy groups (see Aubry & Travis, 2015; Staub, 2015; Saks, 2003; Bondi & Burman, 2001). The rise of humanistic psychology, which challenges behaviourist models and champions the concepts of 'self-actualisation' and 'inner potential', found particularly strong resonance in countercultural movements that criticised the prevailing capitalist, authoritarian and patriarchal social order. The popularisation of therapeutic discourse, with its focus on trauma and healing, also helped open up new discursive spaces for 'speaking out' about forms of injustice and suffering that have long been silenced in public, such as child abuse and violence against women, and has empowered groups and individuals who were previously marginalised (Stein, 2011; Illouz, 2008).

Despite this deep historical interconnection, the predominant interpretation in therapeutic culture scholarship conceives therapeutic practices as a tool for political domination, diverting attention from structural forms of injustice to empowering the psychologised self. It has been argued that the social critique embodied in countercultural movements has been commodified and merged to reinforce a neoliberal agenda (Höllinger, 2004; Redden, 2002), leading to the dissipation of radical collective action against social injustice (Cloud, 1998). By rendering structural relations of power as personal psychopathologies to be solved by ethical work on the self, the therapeutic ethos has been seen as legitimising middle-class norms, targeting the transformative energy towards the self rather than social structures, and cultivating autonomous, self-sufficient and enterprising subjects capable of and willing to engage in constant self-invention and self-governance (MacNevin, 2003; Skeggs & Wood, 2012; Nehring et al., 2016; Cloud, 1998; Mäkinen, 2014; Madsen, 2015; Foster, 2016).

However, the chapters in this book tell a more complicated story. Therapeutic practices may certainly oppress, depoliticise, manufacture political quietism and cement symbolic and material hierarchies of power, but they may also serve as vehicles for social change and animate political critique (see Salmenniemi, 2019). While proponents of the depoliticisation thesis often conceive politics as 'contentious politics' (e.g. Cloud, 1998), this book adopts a broader stance on politics by delving into the terrain of micropolitics and everyday resistance, which is often overshadowed by the focus on organised forms of political action (Scott, 1989; Bayat, 1997; Lilja & Vinthagen, 2014). Indeed, this book underlines the need to acknowledge the multidimensional nature of political contestation, ranging from confrontational to circumventing, productive to hindering, individual to collective, accommodating to enforcing, and materialistic to virtual (Baaz et al., 2018: 4). Broadening the notion of politics and revealing often individualised, covert and small-scale acts of resistance allows us to appreciate the complexity of power relations within the therapeutic field, and reminds us that political subjectivity should always be analysed in relation to local and ethical conditions that dictate how political agency takes shape (Mahmood, 2005: 9).

In this spirit, Ariel Yankellevich's chapter in this book addresses the popularisation of life coaching among the Israeli (mostly Ashkenazi) middle class. He argues that the field of coaching cannot be adequately grasped by a single logic of individualisation or depoliticisation, but should rather be understood as a particular moral and ethical assemblage that combines individual self-development with collectivist dispositions towards the common good of the nation. Coaching entails not withdrawal from, but a reconfiguration of, social responsibility and political engagement. The chapter shows how coaching's neoliberal therapeutic rationality is assembled with local discourses of the self and the nation, which enable coaches to negotiate their social positions and find new sources of legitimation in the context of shifting social and cultural hierarchies. Julia Lerner's chapter on Russian-speaking migrant women's religious experiences also interrogates the relationship between the therapeutic and neoliberalism. Lerner shows how neoliberal, religious and therapeutic elements intertwine in the narratives of these women, and how, rather than emptying the self of its communal content, this assemblage potentially augments communal attachments. Both chapters highlight the importance of analysing therapeutic engagements through the intersecting categories of class, gender, ethnicity and generation.

While Yankellevich's and Lerner's chapters underline ways in which neoliberal and therapeutic discourses intertwine to support each other, Salmenniemi, Nurmi and Jaakola highlight instead how therapeutic assemblages need not necessarily align with neoliberal governing projects, but may also be mobilised to critique and contest them. Drawing on Critical Theory and analysing therapeutic practitioners' narratives of contemporary working life, they show how therapeutic assemblages operate as forms of everyday resistance to the destructive effects of the neoliberal ethic of work. They highlight how practitioners seek to deal with their deeply embodied sense of alienation by assembling personalised therapeutic packages consisting of diverse practices, objects and forms of knowledge. Rather than optimising and accruing value to themselves, they mobilise therapeutic techniques to pull themselves back to life from the murky waters of burnout and depression. In this sense, these techniques allow them to craft hope and a sense of agency in difficult life circumstances.

In their chapter, Stanley and Kortelainen also critically engage with interpretations of mindfulness as a thoroughly commodified, neoliberal and individualising technology of the self. They suggest that, rather than assuming particular *a priori* effects, one should rather regard them as objects of empirical inquiry, and thus approach mindfulness as a contextually specific practice assembled from different and sometimes contradictory elements.

Virve Peteri's chapter continues the discussion of everyday resistance by analysing the production of playfulness in the workplace. She approaches activity-based office designs as 'therapeutic spaces' seeking to elicit creativity and positive emotions and traces ways in which employees seek to challenge and subvert the new patterns of emotion control introduced by office design. Although the organisation's leadership encourages workers to invest in fleeting sensations and moods as a source of inspiration, and to ignore historically constituted social bonds between them, the workers continue to maintain and invest in long-term friendships and solidarities. Moreover, although they are no longer allowed to have personal spaces, many continue to attach themselves to particular desks and thus refuse to comply with the new culture of mobility and flexibility. In this way, the chapter highlights the centrality of material and spatial arrangements for domination and subversion.

The chapters by Inna Perheentupa and Felix Freigang examine therapeutic practices in the context of collective mobilisation and 'speaking out'. Perheentupa conceptualises feminist activism in Russia as therapeutic politics. She shows how activists come together to deal publicly with their traumatic experiences connected with gendered violence. Holding onto their political agency serves a therapeutic function for the activists in the context of repressive political conditions and a trauma culture. Freigang, for his part, discusses the proliferation of digital mood-tracking applications as a response to inadequate mental health services in

Germany. He shows how the mood-tracking app can facilitate the politicisation of mental health, such as contesting victimisation and stigmatisation relating to mental health problems and inadequate psychotherapeutic care, thus echoing the long tradition of social health movements and patient activism.

As Freigang's chapter elucidates, some chapters in this book engage in readings of politics inspired by new materialism and actor–network theory. Viewed from these perspectives, politics is neither exclusively, nor even primarily, a human domain of action and decision making, but is heavily influenced and directed by the material world (Latour, 2005; Bennett, 2010). This sensitises us to exploring the contingencies and specificities of power and resistance in particular arrangements of human and non-human actors (Law & Singleton, 2013). In this spirit, some chapters empirically explore how human and non-human actors come together to create and restrict avenues of political, socially transformative action. For example, Bergroth and Helén delve into the data-driven, digital milieu of contemporary body-tracking. They show how the sociotechnical domain of tracking one's bodily functions brings together bodies, therapeutic discourses of holistic health, political discourses of 'personalised medicine' and citizen activation policies, and the dividualising, fragmentary logic of algorithmic self-monitoring technologies. This creates regimes of perpetual self-control within which 'the point of self-tracking is to educate people not on their daily step counts or heart rates during sleep *per se*, but mainly on caring for and managing personal "vitality"'. The chapter highlights how self-tracking becomes an everyday political and therapeutic regime for both managing and performing activeness and good health.

Drawing on a unique set of autobiographical narratives on uncanny (i.e. 'supernatural') experiences, Andell, Bergroth and Honkasalo elaborate how experiences of being in touch with mysterious beings, voices, visions and other extraordinary things often interact with pervasive technoscientific-rationalist discourses that reduce such experiences to mental 'errors' or 'disturbances'. As such, these experiences may be both 'sickening' and healing, but are nevertheless crucial actants in people's therapeutic and political assemblages, as they prescribe care for the self, care for others and desires to work on the world.

Materiality: spaces, affects and bodies

As the previous section highlighted, materiality is important for understanding therapeutics as an assemblage. Much of the social scientific literature on therapeutic culture has tended to overlook material culture and embodiment as crucial building blocks for the therapeutic to function in everyday contexts. However, therapeutic culture is not just out there, but functions and is mediated through the mundane material contexts with which human and non-human beings interact. Chapters in this book examine how our mundane material surroundings – objects, gadgets, spaces and bodies – put forward or 'prescribe' (Latour, 1992) the therapeutic in people's everyday lives, and how the therapeutic is embodied in and through the physical realm. They analyse the emergence and transformation of therapeutic practices in complex networks of human and non-human actors and highlight the centrality of affective attachments to how therapeutic practices work in and through bodies.

Both Julia Lerner and Tatiana Tiaynen-Qadir explore the embodied relationship between religion and the therapeutic in a transnational context. Underlining the importance of embodied and material practices of religion, Tiaynen-Qadir underscores how therapeutic engagements are deeply embodied and irreducible to cognition and reason. She examines Orthodox Christian practitioners' embodied and sensory experiences of religion and healing. In response to the 'therapeutic turn' in society, Finnish Orthodoxy has emphasised the therapeutic effects of its practices, although this has been done mainly by reviving the notion of *therapeia* – the ancient Orthodox cure of soul and body – rather than by secularising psychological narratives of the self. Tiaynen-Qadir shows how, in religious practices, glocal therapeutic assemblages are produced in complex and historically situated interactions between human and non-human actors, and how divine intervention is channelled through materiality of sound, archaic texts, iconic art and holy objects. Lerner, for her part, explores how women who were raised in the Soviet Union and migrated to Israel and Europe narrate their religious experiences in therapeutic terms. They emphasise the role of religion in overcoming personal difficulty, gaining control, embodying responsibility and discovering the 'true self' in new and challenging life situations. The women's narratives, imbued with powerful embodied and emotional registers, reveal how religion operates in their everyday lives, and how it has transformed the ways in which they perceive themselves, their personal histories and their social relations.

Embodiment and material culture are also discussed by Bergroth and Helén. They theorise how, through digital-tracking practices, the human body is divided into and presented in the form of ever-extending trajectories based on the body's own movements and beats. Self-tracking prescribes conceptions of selves as 'data derivatives' (Amoore, 2011) that focus not on what the self is, but on what it could (and should) be, producing affective and sustaining engagement with the act and technology of self-tracking. Andell, Bergroth and Honkasalo, for their part, show how uncanny beings and sensations become 'real' actants by participating in people's therapeutic knowledge production. Uncanny experiences are often made sense of through the concrete effects and emotions that they induce in the world. The authors thus approach uncanny phenomena as active agents, and uncanny experiences as social practices and 'therapeutic events' that shape and actualise one's relationship with oneself and with the surrounding world. The uncanny also intertwines with materialities. For example, people's narratives on uncanny encounters shed light on how personal relationships and care relations (are made to) transgress the apparently impenetrable boundary between life and death, by and through everyday technologies such as lamps and candles. Furthermore, embodiment and the emotional sphere are narrated in many ways as crucial to actualising knowledge of – and care for – either the self or, for example, a person who is no longer visibly present in this world. Overall, the authors build an argument that uncanny experiences should not be understood as therapy-in-a-time-of-crisis, in a functionalist sense, but rather as part of active assemblages of knowledge production.

Marjo Kolehmainen prepares new ground for theorising therapeutics by delving into atmospheres as affective assemblages. She proposes that atmospheres offer a novel lens through which to interrogate therapeutic engagements, as they enable a move away from human-centred notions of the therapeutic and the self, and foreground how situational and material therapeutic practices operate in and through both human and non-human bodies. Her chapter traces how 'different objects and bodies come together in situated experiences of registering, engineering or sustaining an atmosphere' in relationship and sex-counselling events. She suggests that part of the appeal of therapeutic engagements is likely to be connected specifically with affective atmospheres rather than with the actual content or advice delivered in counselling. She also makes an important observation regarding the affective dynamics of inclusion and exclusion: 'To register an atmosphere is to sense a connection, which may feel therapeutic in itself; and to fail to catch it may intensify feelings of non-belonging, rendering one more vulnerable'.

Continuing the discussion on affect, the chapter by Stanley and Kortelainen draws on Wetherell's (2013) seminal work on affective practices. This allows a study of meaning-making that does not draw sharp divisions between bodies, discourses, affects and emotions. Stanley and Kortelainen analyse how mindful bodies are assembled in a professional mindfulness training event. They focus on the practical conduct of mindfulness as an assemblage of affective practices, looking into the production of mindfulness meditation, the space, and the practitioners' bodies. The assemblage perspective allows them to foreground mindfulness as a situated and embodied practice that is not 'the same thing' in different settings. Their analysis also shows how mindfulness may be experienced as a 'post-secular' sacralising space.

Freigang explores the affective intensities of a mood-tracking app. In dialogue with Lupton (2014), he suggests that mood-tracking apps can be viewed as sociocultural artefacts into which different aspirations, circuits of societal discourses, economic interests and meanings are inscribed. He coins the concept of 'therapeutic companion' to capture ways in which mood-tracking apps operate in users' everyday lives. The chapter shows how mood-tracking apps may become both empowering and contested, engendering both excitement and disappointment.

Virve Peteri's chapter foregrounds the need to appreciate space as an active agent in shaping and transforming experiences, emotions and subjectivities. She shows how 'fun culture' in organisations can be viewed as an assemblage of bodies, materials and spaces that aim to generate happier, more playful, creative, agile and mobile worker subjectivities. This has profoundly gendered implications, as the ideal subject inhabiting the new playful office space appears to be a young man interested in PlayStation games and relaxing on a beanbag.

Perheentupa adopts another angle on discussions of space and emotion. She shows how feminism in Russia is understood and produced as a therapeutic space, a 'shelter' in which activists can momentarily shield themselves from a society in which they feel unsafe. Moreover, she shows how feminist activism revolving around cultural trauma translates experiences of psychic injury and painful memories into collective action that provides a shared forum for healing.

Conclusion: reassembling the therapeutic

This and subsequent chapters underline the need to understand and appreciate therapeutic practices as part of our everyday symbolic and material landscape. In a similar vein to critical scholarship, which has problematised the idea of neoliberalism as 'an economic tsunami that is gathering force across the planet, pummelling each country in its path and sweeping away old structures of power' (Ong, 2007: 3), this book calls attention to the therapeutic not as a 'tsunami', but as situated and contingent assemblages without predetermined outcomes and effects. Indeed, the chapters in this book challenge the notion of a singular therapeutic culture and testify that therapeutic engagements cannot be tamed under any one narrative, whether it be neoliberal governmentality, depoliticisation or individualisation (see also Illouz, 2008). Combining a bottom-up ethnographic approach with assemblage thinking may, we hope, advance critical understanding of how we live with and assemble our 'therapeutic companions'.

Acknowledgements

This book has been supported by two research projects: *Tracking the Therapeutic: Ethnographies of Wellbeing, Politics and Inequality*, funded by the Academy of Finland (grant number 289004) and *The Puzzle of the Psyche*, funded by Kone Foundation (grant number 46-8917). We would like to thank Daniel Nehring and the contributors to this book for helpful comments on this Introduction.

References

Amoore, L. 2011. Data derivatives: On the emergence of a security risk calculus for our times. *Theory, Culture & Society 28*:6, 24–43.

Aubry, T. & Travis, T. 2015. What is therapeutic culture, and why do we need to 'rethink it'? In *Rethinking Therapeutic Culture*, edited by T. Aubry & T. Travis. Chicago, IL: University of Chicago Press, 1–23.

Baaz, M., Lilja, M. & Vinthagen, S. 2018. *Researching Resistance and Social Change: A Critical Approach to Theory and Practice*. London: Rowman & Littlefield International.

Barker, C. 2000. *Cultural Studies: Theory and Practice*. London: SAGE.

Bayat, A. 1997. Un-civil society: The politics of the 'informal people'. *Third World Quarterly 18*:1, 53–72.

Bennett, J. 2010. *Vibrant Matter: A Political Ecology of Things*. Durham, NC: Duke University Press.

Binkley, S. 2011. Psychological life as enterprise: Social practice and the government of neo-liberal interiority. *History of the Human Sciences 24*:3, 83–102.

Bondi, L. & Burman, E. 2001. Women and mental health: A feminist review. *Feminist Review 68*:1, 6–33.

Brunila, K. 2011. The projectisation, marketisation and therapisation of education. *European Educational Research Journal 10*, 425–437.

Brunila, K. & Siivonen, P. 2016. Preoccupied with the self: Towards self-responsible, enterprising, flexible and self-centred subjectivity in education. *Discourse: Studies in the Cultural Politics of Education 7*:1, 56–69.

Caliskan, K. & Callon, M. 2010. Economization, part 2: A research program for the study of markets. *Economy and Society 39*:1, 1–32.

Callon, M. 2005. Why virtualism paves the way to political impotence: A reply to Daniel Miller's critique of "The laws of the market". *Economic Sociology: European Electronic Newsletter 6*:2, 3–20.

Campbell, E. & Lassiter, L. E. 2015. *Doing Ethnography Today*. Chichester: Wiley-Blackwell.

Cerwonka, A. & Malkki, L. H. 2007. *Improvising Theory: Process and Temporality in Ethnographic Fieldwork*. Chicago, IL: University of Chicago Press.

Cloud, D. 1998. *Control and Consolation in American Culture and Politics: Rhetoric of Therapy*. Thousand Oaks, CA: SAGE.

Collier, S. & Ong, A. 2005. Global assemblages, anthropological problems. In *Global Assemblages: Technology, Politics, and Ethics as Anthropological Problems*, edited by A. Ong & S. Collier. Malden, MA: Blackwell Publishing, 3–22.

Coole, D. H. & Frost, S. (eds) 2010. *New Materialisms: Ontology, Agency and Politics*. Durham, NC: Duke University Press.

Davies, W. 2015. *The Happiness Industry*. London: Verso.

DeLanda, M. 2006. *A New Philosophy of Society: Assemblage Theory and Social Complexity*. London: Continuum.

Deleuze, G. & Guattari, F. 1987. *A Thousand Plateaus: Capitalism and Schitzophrenia*. Minneapolis, MN: University of Minnesota Press.

Ecclestone, K. & Hayes, D. 2008. *The Dangerous Rise of Therapeutic Education*. London: Routledge.

Foster, R. 2015. The therapeutic spirit of neoliberalism. *Political Theory 44*:1, 82–105.

Foster, R. 2016. Therapeutic culture, authenticity and neoliberalism. *History of the Human Sciences 29*:1, 99–116.

Foucault, M. 1988. *The History of Sexuality, Vol. 3: The Care of the Self*. New York, NY: Vintage Books.

Fox, N. J. & Alldred, P. 2015. New materialist social inquiry: Designs, methods and the research-assemblage. *International Journal of Social Research Methodology 18*:4, 399–414.

Furedi, F. 2004. *Therapy Culture: Cultivating Vulnerability in an Uncertain Age*. London: Routledge.

Giddens, A. 1992. *The Transformation of Intimacy: Sexuality, Love & Eroticism in Modern Societies*. Cambridge: Polity Press.

Gill, R. 2009. Mediated intimacy and postfeminism: A discourse analytic examination of sex and relationships advice in a women's magazine. *Discourse & Communication 3*:4, 345–369.

Hannerz, U. 2003. Being there… and there… and there! Reflections on multi-site ethnography. *Ethnography 4*:2, 201–216.

Hardie, I. & Mackenzie, D. 2007. Assembling an economic actor: The agencement of a hedge fund. *The Sociological Review 55*:1, 57–80.

Harvey, L. & Gill, R. 2011. The sex inspectors: Self-help, makeover and mediated sex. In *Handbook on Gender, Sexualities and Media*, edited by K. Ross. Oxford: Blackwell.

Hazleden, R. 2003. Love yourself: The relationship of the self with itself in popular self-help texts. *Journal of Sociology 39*:4, 413–428.

Hendriks, E. C. 2017. *Life Advice from Below: The Public Role of Self-Help Coaches in Germany and China*. Leiden: Brill.

Höllinger, F. 2004. Does the counter-cultural character of New Age persist? Investigating social and political attitudes of New Age followers. *Journal of Contemporary Religion* *19*:3, 289–309.

Huttunen, L. 2010. Tiheä kontekstointi: Haastattelu osana etnografista tutkimusta. In *Haastattelun Analyysi*, edited by J. Ruusuvuori, P. Nikander & M. Hyvärinen. Tampere: Vastapaino, 39–63.

Illouz, E. 2008. *Saving the Modern Soul: Therapy, Emotions, and the Culture of Self-Help.* Berkeley, CA: University of California Press.

Introna, L. D. 2013. Epilogue: Performativity and the becoming of sociomaterial assemblages. In *Materiality and Space: Technology, Work and Globalization*, edited by N. Mitev & F.-X. de Vaujany. London: Palgrave Macmillan.

Kelly, C. 2001. *Refining Russia: Advice Literature, Polite Culture, and Gender from Catherine to Yeltsin.* Oxford: Oxford University Press.

Lasch, C. 1979. *The Culture of Narcissism.* London: W.W. Norton.

Latour, B. 1992. Where are the missing masses? The sociology of a few mundane artifacts. In *Shaping Technology – Building Society: Studies in Sociotechnical Change*, edited by W. Bijker & J. Law. Cambridge, MA: MIT Press, 225–259.

Latour, B. 2005. *Reassembling the Social: An Introduction to Actor–Network Theory.* Oxford: Oxford University Press.

Law, J. 2004. *After Method: Mess in Social Science Research.* London: Routledge.

Law, J. & Singleton, V. 2013. ANT and politics: Working in and on the world. *Qualitative Sociology 36*:4, 485–502.

Lerner, J. & Zbenovich, C. 2013. Adapting the therapeutic discourse to post-Soviet media culture: The case of Modnyi Prigovor. *Slavic Review 72*:4, 828–849.

Li, T. M. 2007. Practices of assemblage and community forest management. *Economy and Society 36*:2, 263–293.

Lichterman, P. 1992. Self-help reading as a thin culture. *Media, Culture & Society 14*:3, 421–447.

Lilja, M. & Vinthagen, S. 2014. Sovereign power, disciplinary power and biopower: Resisting what power with what resistance? *Journal of Political Power 7*:1, 107–126.

Lupton, D. 2014. Apps as artefacts: Towards a critical perspective on mobile health and medical apps. *Societies 4*, 606–622.

Lupton, D. 2016. Digital companion species and eating data: Implications for theorising digital data–human assemblages. *Big Data & Society 3*:1, 1–5.

MacNevin, A. 2003. Remaining audible to the self: Women and holistic health. *Atlantis 27*:2, 16–23.

McFarlane, C. 2011. Assemblage and critical urbanism. *City 15*:2, 204–224.

McGee, M. 2005. *Self-Help, Inc.: Makeover Culture in American Life.* Oxford: Oxford University Press.

Madsen, O. J. 2014. *The Therapeutic Turn.* London: Routledge.

Madsen, O. J. 2015. *Optimizing the Self: Social Representations of Self-Help.* London: Routledge.

Madsen, O. J. & Ytre-Arne, B. 2012. Me at my best: Therapeutic ideals in Norwegian women's magazines. *Communication, Culture & Critique 5*:1, 20–37.

Mahmood, S. 2005. *Politics of Piety: The Islamic Revival and the Feminist Subject.* Princeton, NJ: Princeton University Press.

Mäkinen, K. 2014. The individualization of class: A case of working life coaching. *The Sociological Review 62*:4, 821–842.

Matza, T. 2012. 'Good individualism'? Psychology, ethics, and neoliberalism in postsocialist Russia. *American Ethnologist 39*:4, 804–818.

Mol, A. 2002. *The Body Multiple: Ontology in Medical Practice*. Durham, NC: Duke University Press.

Nail, T. 2017. What is an assemblage? *SubStance 46*:1, 21–37.

Nehring, D., Alvarado, E., Hendriks, E. C. & Kerrigan, D. 2016. *Transnational Popular Psychology and the Global Self-Help Industry*. London: Palgrave.

Nehring, D. & Kerrigan, D. 2019. *Therapeutic Worlds: Popular Psychology and the Socio-Cultural Organisation of Intimate Life*. London: Routledge.

Ong, A. 2007. Neoliberalism as a mobile technology. *Transactions of the Institute of British Geographers 32*, 3–8.

Ortner, S. B. 2006. *Anthropology and Social Theory: Culture, Power and the Acting Subject*. Durham, NC: Duke University Press.

Ouellette, L. & Hay, J. 2008. *Better Living through Reality TV*. Oxford: Wiley-Blackwell.

Pagis, M. 2016. Fashioning futures: Life coaching and the self-made identity paradox. *Sociological Forum 31*:4, 1083–1103.

Pink, S. 2009. *Doing Sensory Ethnography*. London: SAGE.

Radway, J. 1984. *Reading the Romance: Women, Patriarchy and Popular Literature*. Chapel Hill, NC: University of North Carolina Press.

Redden, G. 2002. The new agents: Personal transfigurations and radical privatization in New Age. *Journal of Consumer Culture 2*:1, 33–52.

Rieff, P. 1966. *The Triumph of the Therapeutic*. London: Chatto & Windus.

Rimke, H. M. 2000. Governing citizens through self-help literature. *Cultural Studies 14*:1, 61–78.

Ringrose, J. & Walkerdine, V. 2008. Regulating the abject: The TV make-over as site of neoliberal reinvention toward bourgeois femininity. *Feminist Media Studies 8*:3, 227–246.

Rose, N. 1990. *Governing the Soul: The Shaping of the Private Self*. London: Routledge.

Rose, N. 1998. *Inventing Our Selves: Psychology, Power and Personhood*. Cambridge: Cambridge University Press.

Saks, M. 2003. *Orthodox and Alternative Medicine*. London: SAGE.

Salmenniemi, S. 2017. 'We can't live without beliefs': Self and society in therapeutic engagements. *The Sociological Review 65*:4, 611–627.

Salmenniemi, S. 2019. Therapeutic politics: Critique and contestation in the post-political conjuncture. *Social Movement Studies 18*:4, 408–424.

Salmenniemi, S. & Adamson, M. 2015. New heroines of labour: Domesticating postfeminism and neoliberal capitalism in Russia. *Sociology 49*:1, 88–105.

Salmenniemi, S. & Vorona, M. 2014. Reading self-help literature in Russia: Governmentality, psychology and subjectivity. *British Journal of Sociology 69*:1, 43–63.

Schaupp, S. 2016. Measuring the entrepreneur of himself: Gendered quantification in the self-tracking discourse. In *Lifelogging: Digital Self-Tracking and Lifelogging*, edited by S. Selke. New York, NY: Springer, 249–266.

Scott, J. C. 1989. Everyday forms of resistance. *Copenhagen Papers 4*, 33–62.

Skeggs, B. & Wood, H. 2012. *Reacting to Reality Television: Performance, Audience, Value*. London: Routledge.

Sointu, E. 2013. *Theorizing Complementary and Alternative Medicines: Wellbeing, Self, Gender, Class*. Basingstoke: Palgrave Macmillan.

Staub, M. 2015. Radical. In *Rethinking Therapeutic Culture*, edited by T. Aubry & T. Travis. Chicago, IL: University of Chicago Press, 96–107.

Stein, A. 2011. The forum: Therapeutic politics – An oxymoron? *Sociological Forum 26*:1, 187–193.

Swan, E. 2010. *Worked Up Selves: Personal Development Workers, Self-Work and Therapeutic Cultures*. Basingstoke: Palgrave Macmillan.

Tiaynen-Qadir, T. & Salmenniemi, S. 2017. Self-help as a glocalised therapeutic assemblage. *European Journal of Cultural Studies 20*:4, 381–396.

Wetherell, M. 2013. *Affect and Emotion: A New Social Science Understanding*. London: SAGE.

Woodstock, L. 2005. Vying constructions of reality: Religion, science, and 'positive thinking' in self-help literature. *Journal of Media and Religion 4*:3, 155–178.

Wright, K. 2008. Theorizing therapeutic culture: Past influences, future directions. *Journal of Sociology 44*:4, 321–336.

Zigon, J. 2011a. A moral and ethical assemblage in Russian Orthodox drug rehabilitation. *Ethos 39*:1, 30–50.

Zigon, J. 2011b. *'HIV Is God's Blessing': Rehabilitating Morality in Neoliberal Russia*. Berkeley, CA: University of California Press.

2 Assembling mindful bodies

Mindfulness as a universal 'laboratory of practice'

Steven Stanley and Ilmari Kortelainen

This chapter explores how mindful bodies are assembled within mindfulness-based therapies. Our objective is to investigate the intersubjective dynamics taking place within mindfulness-based training, especially the interactions between expert-level mindfulness teachers and the attendees of mindfulness courses, who are sometimes also themselves teachers and trainers of mindfulness. We analyse the specific ways in which mindful bodies are assembled by one particularly influential mindfulness teacher during a professional training event. We pay close attention to the sociality of mindful bodies and the group-based practices of mindfulness teaching in action. We focus our analysis upon the 'affective-discursive' practices (Wetherell, 2013) that are used to make bodies mindful. We find that the mind-body of the mindfulness practitioner, along with the space of meditation practice, are put together using diverse and potentially contradictory resources. We argue on the basis of our analysis that it is precisely the sheer multiplicity of the assemblage of mindfulness which makes it so portable, transferable and potent.

There is arguably insufficient attention given to the practical conduct of mindfulness-based therapeutics, within both the mainstream psychological literatures, which engage in measurement and experimentation, and in the humanities and social sciences literatures, which tend to comprise cultural and textual analyses (Arthington, 2016; Barker, 2014; Eklöf, 2017). The study reported in this chapter builds upon the growing ethnographic literature on mindfulness, especially in anthropology, by analysing mindfulness as an assemblage of affective-practices. We will show how the study of mindfulness may, in turn, contribute to much broader transdisciplinary investigations of self-governance, therapeutic culture and religion/secularity (Illouz, 2008; McGee, 2012).

Wetherell (2013) argues that a focus on affective practices allows researchers to study social meaning-making without making sharp divides between bodies, discourse, affects and emotions. 'The concept of affective-practice … encompasses the movement of signs but it also tries to explain how affect is embodied, is situated and operates psychologically' (Wetherell, 2013:159). This theoretical framework is a good fit for studies of mindfulness, because the practice of mindfulness involves bodily routines where discourse, bodily knowledge and silence are commonly interspersed. In accordance with our focus on affective-practices,

we argue that studies of mindfulness, as well as other related mind-body therapies, would benefit from unpacking the practices actually involved in therapeutic
cultures by giving special attention to social action, metaphor and embodiment,
materiality and spatiality.

By analysing the affective-discursive practices which make up the assemblage
of mindfulness, we show how one particular mindfulness teacher draws upon a
variety of conceptual, historical, metaphorical, material and bodily resources to
assemble mindfulness. Mindfulness is discursively imagined to be a universal
'laboratory' for self-healing. Embedded within this overarching metaphorical
framework are practices of visualising, technologising and naturalising mindfulness. We further find that the spatial metaphors of mindfulness, in which the
mind-body are 'seen' within a 'laboratory' of practice, are also subtly challenged
by the teacher and some participants, who sacralise the space of mindfulness.
We show how the presence of 'post-secular' themes in mindfulness training may
problematise making sharp divides between psychotherapy, religion and spirituality (Madsen, 2014; Lerner, Salmenniemi et al., and Tiaynen-Qadir, this book).

In the sections that follow, we summarise the historical background of mindfulness and current research informing our study; discuss our methodology and
methods; present our analysis; before finally making some concluding remarks.

Assembling mindfulness

Since the late nineteenth century, people of Anglo-American and Nordic countries
have adopted Asian mind-body training regimes as therapeutic ways of living with
industrial capitalism (Williams, 2014). Along with yoga, Tai Chi and Transcendental
Meditation, mindfulness – Buddhist *sati*, insight meditation, or *vipassanā* – illustrates this trend. Emerging out of complex cross-cultural encounters, most notably
early twentieth-century British colonial expansion in Southeast Asia and the 1960s
countercultural movement, mindfulness has now become a predominant feature of
the globalised self-help industry (Nehring et al., 2016; Madsen, 2015).

Humanities scholars have shown how Buddhist disciplines such as mindfulness have been transformed as they move across time and place. Mindfulness has
been made compatible with empirical science and turned into a secular psychological therapy for the purpose of self-healing (McMahan, 2008; Sharf, 1995).
Many clinical psychologists, medics and neuroscientists now suggest mindfulness, when applied in standardised eight-week courses of Mindfulness-Based
Stress Reduction (MBSR) and Mindfulness-Based Cognitive Therapy (MBCT)
can be effective for the relief of chronic pain, stress, anxiety and depression.

The mass expansion of mindfulness provision in the past twenty years, particularly in the United States, has led some commentators to describe a 'mindfulness
movement' (Wilson, 2014). Interest in mindfulness has grown markedly during
times of rapid socio-economic and technological change and political uncertainty.

Today, mindfulness is being implemented across the UK at an astonishing
rate, within an ever-expanding array of sectors and for a multitude of purposes.
While predominantly applied as MBCT (Segal et al., 2013) for the treatment of

depression, in recent years mindfulness has moved out of the clinic and into the public sphere. As well as the National Health Service (NHS) mindfulness can now also be found in the Westminster, Welsh, Scottish and Northern Ireland governments and parliaments; schools, colleges and universities; private, public and third-sector workplaces; and even smartphone 'apps'. Mindfulness is being employed ever more readily, as a way to ensure national well-being, happiness and 'flourishing' (Davies, 2015); productivity, performance and efficiency (Cederström & Spicer, 2015); and sustainability, creativity and activism (Rowe, 2016). Mindfulness has become professionalised and institutionalised in the UK to such an extent that this nation may represent the vanguard of mindfulness practice globally.

To date, academic and popular debate on mindfulness has been characterised by polemics, starkly polarised between proponents and critics of mindfulness. Advocates promote mindfulness as a panacea for world peace (Tan, 2012), while critics expose 'McMindfulness' as a corporate capitalist bandwagon (Purser & Loy, 2013; Purser, 2019).

On the one hand, of the almost 3,000 psychology and neuroscience articles published since 2010, the overwhelming majority present positive evaluations of mindfulness as being an effective therapeutic tool (Valerio, 2016). MBCT has been recommended by the National Institute for Clinical and Health Excellence and has been made available on the UK NHS for the treatment of relapsing depression since 2004. The evidence-base did not initially result in the 'roll-out' of provision in the UK, so in 2014, a Mindfulness All-Party Parliamentary Group (MAPPG) was established. Mindfulness was taught to 130 parliamentarians and 220 Westminster government staff, aiming to build on the momentum of the 'grass-roots' mindfulness community, and lobby politicians to roll-out mindfulness *en masse* across diverse civil society sectors of health, education, workplace and criminal justice. The authors of the 2015 MAPPG report seek to turn the UK into a 'Mindful Nation' (MAPPG, 2015; see also Cook, 2016).

On the other hand, the somewhat evangelical promotion of mindfulness as a universal *panacea* has given way to a backlash, with critics arguing mindfulness has been 'over-sold' (Brazier, 2013). Mindfulness, as the latest incarnation of popular Western Buddhism, is arguably becoming established as 'the hegemonic ideology of global capitalism', its meditative 'awareness' stance being 'the most efficient way, for us, to fully participate in the capitalist dynamic while retaining the appearance of mental sanity' (Žižek, 2001: 12–13). Asian religious traditions are framed psychologically as 'spiritualities' and meditative practices are commodified for consumers, contradicting their socially radical origins (Carrette & King, 2005). Critics suggest mindfulness is being presented as a neoliberal 'self-technology' which medicalises, psychologises and individualises well-being and suffering as being the sole responsibilities of the autonomous individual (Arthington, 2016; Purser, 2019). This critique of mindfulness mirrors the canonical theoretical critique of therapeutic culture, made since the 1960s, as illustrating a widespread cultural decline (see Salmenniemi et al. in this book).

Yet, it has also been suggested, based on recent qualitative research, that mindfulness may pose a challenge to the ideal of self-contained individualism, thereby exposing the limits of neoliberalism (Carvalho, 2014; Cook, 2016; Mamberg & Bassarear, 2015). While mindfulness teachers may present mindfulness as merely a secular 'technique' of self-improvement, they may also present mindfulness as a spiritual or sacred practice and encourage self-transcendence among their students. Recent ethnographic and discourse analytic research on mindfulness has investigated the ethico-moral and embodied-discursive ways in which mindfulness teachers and students practically constitute and construct meanings of mindfulness in practice. They demonstrate how both mindfulness, and the self-identities of mindfulness teachers, are socially produced in complex and contradictory ways, which are contextually specific (Arat, 2017; Drage, 2018a, 2018b; Stanley & Longden, 2016; Vogel, 2017; Wheater, 2017). So, rather than assuming *a priori* that mindfulness automatically represents a de-politicising and individualising practice of self-governance, we can instead ask what kinds of social and cultural worlds are being imagined through movements towards mindfulness (Illouz, 2008; Thomson, 2006). We can be mindful of the cultural, ethical and political contexts and consequences of mindfulness, understood as a social, as well as a psychological, phenomenon (Kirmayer, 2015; Purser, Forbes & Burke, 2016; Stanley, Purser & Singh, 2018).

Mindfulness is commonly framed as an internal psychological state or trait and accompanied by a universalising rhetoric. Teachers and psychologists often describe mindfulness as a basic human capacity, similar to capacities for attention and consciousness, shared by all people, and as being a universally applicable therapeutic intervention. The creator of the Stress Reduction Clinic at the University of Massachusetts Medical Centre and MBSR programme Jon Kabat-Zinn (1994) provides an operational definition of mindfulness as a conscious awareness that arises when we 'pay attention on purpose, in the present moment and non-judgmentally' (ibid.: 4). While mindfulness is often presented as a merely secular therapeutic technique, it is also often suggested to be a spiritual or sacred practice, or indeed a 'universal dharma' being skillfully taught in secular settings ('dharma' is sometimes translated as 'Buddhist teachings', or the 'truths' taught by the Buddha). Williams and Kabat-Zinn (2011) argue that mindfulness-based interventions such as MBSR and MBCT are 'Dharma-based portals' (ibid.: 12) which contain a 'universal dharma' taught in secular settings (Kabat-Zinn, 2011: 301). Kabat-Zinn (2017) has recently described MBSR as a 'skillful means' of mainstreaming and making available to course participants the 'universal essence of dharma' (ibid.: 1130), which is implicitly (rather than explicitly) transmitted to them through the embodiment and 'authentic presence' (ibid.: 1134; endnote 15) of the mindfulness teacher. Mindfulness is often presented as a universal capacity – sometimes suggested to be equivalent to consciousness, awareness and attention – in both its secularised and sacralised manifestations. The notion that 'the mind' is universal, as well as the idea of mindful awareness itself being potentially curative and liberative, have historical precedents in psychology, medicine and Buddhism, as well as in the counter-cultural turn to spirituality, suggestively illustrated by

The Doors in their song 'Universal Mind' (1970): 'I was doin' time in the universal mind, I was feelin' fine, I was turnin' keys, I was settin' people free, I was doin' alright, … I'm the freedom man'.

A situated perspective for researching therapeutic cultures suggests mindfulness might not be the same thing in different settings (for example, secular or religious). Meanings of mindfulness multiply across different environments, and vary between cultures, such as between the UK, Nordic region and Germany. We find that the place of mindfulness in healthcare, for example, differs greatly between the US, UK, Danish, Swedish and Finnish contexts (Hickey, 2010, Kortelainen et al., 2017; Plank, 2010). We therefore need to pay careful attention to specific versions of 'mindfulness', rather than assuming a coherent totality prior to empirical investigation. We should instead study the specific spaces and places through which mindfulness is made manifest and lived.

Mindfulness, metaphor and assemblage

To practice mindfulness, people must learn how to 'be mindful', and it is how mindfulness is practically realised through concrete teaching and training encounters that we are interested in examining. To recognise an inner state, practice or event as illustrating 'mindfulness' (or otherwise), there must be public criteria which make it recognisable as 'mindfulness' (Wittgenstein, 1958). In order to 'be mindful', people must (among other things) learn how to use a conceptual vocabulary of mindfulness, which along with much of our language for 'inner' psychological life, is pervasively metaphorical (Danziger, 1997; Mamberg & Bassarear, 2015; Varra, Drossel & Hayes, 2009). Yet there have been few studies of the metaphorical construction of mindfulness.

Lakoff and Johnson (1980) describe a metaphor as involving one conceptual domain being chosen to refer to another conceptual domain. According to metaphor theories, metaphors are ways to conceptualise and modify human experience, and hence they can influence how a practitioner of mindfulness recognises, experiences and interprets mindfulness. Ricœur (1991), one of the developers of modern metaphor theory, suggests that contradictions on the level of ordinary use of language are a site where human beings can change their interpretations of objects, since such contradictions are semantically ambiguous and leave the meaning unresolved. Such metaphors can reflect cultural assumptions that mindfulness teachers articulate, as well as ideals of body and mind that are carried over from the history of psychology. As such, in the metaphors employed in MBCT, as we shall explore here, the conceptual domain may be borrowed from various cultural, social or psychological spheres. Even before this choice is made, before the metaphor is imbued with detailed content, the idea of what constitutes mindfulness becomes mixed with cultural images and other creative ways of imagining what meditation involves. Old conceptual connections can be suspended and new ones that attempt to capture how our minds and bodies actually experience mindfulness can be created (Kortelainen, 2013: 158). In addition, we suggest through our analysis that metaphors and especially particular networks of bodily metaphor that are used within mindfulness training discourse could potentially mould and transform the corporeal experience of participants in mindfulness training courses.

In turn, such ideas about metaphor can be applied to the concept of 'assemblage', which is itself metaphorical. The verb 'assemble' suggests practices of putting together, making, constructing or building. To create an assemblage may involve arranging, laying out or putting together (Wetherell, 2013). Or, alternatively, we might speak of practices of 'composing' political and economic worlds (Higgins & Larner, 2017). In making bodies mindful, we suggest, practitioners of mindfulness pull together diverse resources, producing themselves and the space of mindfulness practice, to create a recognisable whole. We may also find occasions where the forms of order created through assembling are momentarily broken and we can study such breaks in the flow of meaning-making.

A day of mindfulness practice

The material which forms the primary basis of our analysis is a five-hour audiovisual recording of 'A Day of Mindfulness Practice and Dialogue' (DoP) taught by Mark Williams, which took place in the middle of the international Mindfulness in Society (2015) conference organised by the Centre for Mindfulness Research and Practice (CMRP) (School of Psychology, Bangor University, Wales). Mark Williams is a Professor of Clinical Psychology, founder of the CMRP and the Oxford Mindfulness Centre (Oxford University), and co-founder of MBCT. The CMRP conference was held at the Crowne Plaza Hotel in Chester, England, a corporate-style hotel that hosts academic and business conferences, as well as hosting a series of other CMRP conferences. A pharmaceutical conference had just been held prior to this mindfulness conference. The DoP took place in the hotel's 'Kings Suite' – a large ballroom with rows of chairs, two screens for projecting PowerPoint presentations and a disco ball on the ceiling (see Figure 2.1). The video recording of the DoP was downloaded from the publically available CMRP website for the cost of £35. As a source of mindfulness instruction in the early twenty-first century, the internet provides a way for people to learn mindfulness through computer screens, smartphones, tablets or wearable devices (see, Bergroth and Helén, Freigang in this book). Our analysis points to this broader milieu of therapeutic self-tracking and how mindfulness teachers and trainers may themselves receive expert mindfulness instruction online (Eklöf, 2017).

While being a professional practitioner conference in a corporate hotel conference centre, the DoP also resembles a retreat taking place within a secular setting. The event displays hybrid themes of conference/retreat (Tresch, 2011). The social organisation of the DoP broadly mirrors a Buddhist silent retreat in the insight meditation or *vipassanā* traditions (Pagis, 2009). The teacher sits at the front, sometimes on a raised platform, facing a group of students sitting in rows on chairs, cushions or stools. (The spatial arrangement of Zen Buddhist retreats is often quite different, Preston, 1998.) Williams wore a formal, white dress shirt and black trousers, with a pen in his top pocket and a lapel microphone; he also sat on a meditation bench, on a mat, on a podium raised above the audience of mostly seated practitioners. Bathed in a bright white light, with large bunches of flowers on either side, routinely chiming bells, Williams came across through his physical presence and teaching discourse as simultaneously a professional scientist, evidence-based therapist, paternalistic 'father figure' and a kind of religious priest, spiritual guru or healer.

For around three-quarters of the time, attendees are instructed how to 'look within' their mind-bodies, alternately sitting in silence with their eyes closed (or downcast), or engaging in walking meditation. For the remainder of the time, they are invited by Williams to 'share' together in pairs their 'experience' of practising mindfulness, before discussing these experiences in front of the whole group. 'Sharing experiences' of meditation in group settings is a remarkable feature of mindfulness courses, which distinguishes them from Buddhist retreats, many of which are held in silence. The practice of public group confession, which makes up the 'dialogue' and 'inquiry' periods of mindfulness courses, is perhaps likely to have been inherited from Christian religious groups, who influenced the development of confession in lay psychotherapy in the early twentieth century (Falby, 2003).

As well as analysing the video of the DoP, we also selectively present analysis of the popular self-help title *Mindfulness: Finding Peace in a Frantic World* (Williams & Penman, 2011). This book presents a modified version of the MBCT programme, contains an accompanying CD of guided meditations and informs the teaching of mindfulness in the Westminster UK government, the NHS, as well as school-based mindfulness programmes. As such, this book deserves careful and close scrutiny, but has yet to be the focus of empirical investigation.

We conduct a philosophically and historically informed conceptual analysis of mindfulness-based therapeutics in action, synthesising metaphor theory and discourse analysis. Our aim is to analyse materials that are produced largely without the intervention of researchers. We are interested in what happens in mindfulness training and practice. Our study is inspired by studies of discourse and interaction, as well as ethnography, which attempt to retrospectively study life as it is lived, rather than relying upon experiments, questionnaires or interviews. Our analysis draws on a number of other resources, which befits the cross-sectional fluidity of our topic of study, including sociological studies of attention, ethnomethodology, conversation analysis, Foucault-inspired post-structuralism, body phenomenology, rhetorical and discursive psychology (for further detail, see Stanley & Crane, 2016).

We take the experiential and agentic aspects of mindfulness as an embodied practice seriously and therefore have focussed this analysis upon affective-discursive practices. While analysing the affective-discursive practices which 'make up' mindfulness, we became particularly interested in the metaphorical vocabularies employed by mindfulness teachers and their students, and the ways in which these vocabularies are practically taken up, or resisted, during the ongoing flow of mindfulness training.

Our analytic sensitivity has been cultivated through our personal histories of practice and teaching of mindfulness, meditation and related contemplative,

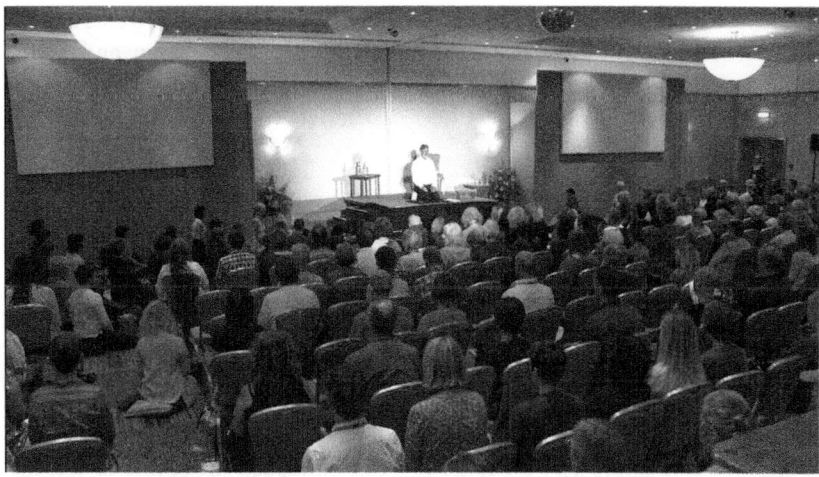

Figure 2.1 Mark Williams (MW) teaching 'A Day of Mindfulness Practice and Dialogue' (DoP).

movement and body-based practices. While our study is not an ethnographic one, we share an ethnographic sensibility and interest in the social and phenomenological aspects of the lived experience of mindfulness meditation, while at the same time bringing analytic attention to reports of 'experience' as forms of social action. The first author attended the DoP as a practitioner-researcher and he is pictured sitting in the audience to the top right of Figure 2.1. Our 'insider-outsider' position, or position as 'sympathetic-critics', is common in the broader field of studies of mindfulness and research on related complementary and alternative therapies.

'So the Seeing was the Release': visualising mindfulness

We are interested in how mindfulness is presented and articulated through discourse practices. In this and the following sections, we analyse how mindfulness is spatialised as a 'laboratory of practice' and visualised as 'seeing' the mindbody; how the person is technologised as an information processing machine; and naturalised as being subject to weather patterns and gravity. Together, such hybrid and potentially contradictory affective-discursive practices contribute to the universalising and standardising of mindfulness meditation practice. However, this secularising of mindfulness does not go unchallenged. We show how some participants subtly resist the idea of mindfulness as like a 'laboratory' by sacralising the space of mindfulness practice.

The parallel made previously between the social situation of mindfulness training and the Buddhist 'insight' meditation tradition of retreat is additionally emphasised through the repeated use of the metaphor of mindfulness as involving an inward 'gaze'. The optic metaphor of mind, such as in the notion of a 'mind's eye', is commonly found in modern Buddhist literature, as well as being the object of much critical debate in philosophy of mind, psychology and cognitive science (Clegg, 2013; Rorty, 1979; Zerubavel, 1997). The metaphor is nicely illustrated by Nyanaponika Thera (1954) in *The Heart of Buddhist Meditation* when he writes that:

> Western humanity, in particular, will have to learn from the East to keep the mind longer and more frequently in a receptive, but keenly observing state – a mental attitude which is cultivated by the scientist and the research worker, but should increasingly become common property. This attitude of Bare Attention will, by persistent practice, prove to be a rich source of knowledge and inspiration. (p. 36)

Examples of optic metaphors taken from Mark Williams' teaching discourse on the DoP, which illustrate how the mind is 'seen', include: 'the ability to see, the mind'; 'important observation'; 'to look to see if unpleasantness comes up … what is there to be held (.) what is offering itself up to us to be gazed at'; 'just observing the breath and somehow being drawn in to notice its quality in some way'; 'so you were able to see more clearly "ah this is my inner critic" … so the seeing was the release'. It is assumed in some modern Buddhist literature, as well as in certain psychological studies of consciousness, that the mind can 'watch' or 'observe' its own workings and functions (Varela & Shear, 1999; for a critique of this assumption from an enactivist cognitive science perspective, see Thompson, 2017).

The optic metaphor of mindfulness goes hand-in-hand with imagining the DoP, and mindfulness meditation practice itself, as a scientific 'laboratory'. The person learning to be mindful 'observes' their mind-body within the 'laboratory' of their meditation practice. By 'seeing' patterns of mind and body, practitioners of mindfulness potentially release themselves from cycles of 'suffering'. Williams comes across as a kind of scientist-therapist, who teaches people how to 'heal' themselves by taking notice of what is happening in each moment. The quality of this attention, which is described as an 'instrument' in need of training, is considered to be part of every human being. The act of paying attention itself is considered to be similar to the measuring qualities of an instrument, although there is sometimes ambiguity about whether this is a scientific or musical instrument. Williams equates mindfulness with 'tuning the instrument of our practice', 'discovery' and noticing the 'quality of each breath'. This way of describing meditation as a laboratory, and mindfulness as similar to scientific observation, is common within discourses of 'scientific Buddhism', well illustrated in the mid-twentieth century book *An Experiment in Mindfulness* (Shattuck, 1958; see also Lopez, 2012).

An interesting feature of the training is how the optic metaphor of 'the mind' relates to 'the body'. Attention to bodily experience is emphasised in MBCT, unlike in Cognitive Behavioural Therapy (CBT), where the focus is changing patterns of thinking. Yet, there is some ambiguity in MBCT discourse about whether the attention is more in 'the mind' of the practitioner, or if it is part of a more holistic entity called the 'mind-body' (for example). An arguably more nuanced description of bodily knowledge, as found for example in phenomenology, or even wider cognitive science ('embodied cognition', Varela, Thompson, and Rosch, 1991) is rarely evident in MBCT, even though Williams might be aware of theories which speak of the 'mind-body' as a 'joined' or even 'extended' process.

'Just like a computer': technologising mindfulness

Mindfulness is often promoted as a way for people to regain control and agency, making 'choices', in the face of increasing automation, thus reclaiming their humanity within an expanding 'digital capitalism' (King, 2016). At the same time, mindfulness itself is often explained using metaphors taken from science and technology. We found that technoscientific metaphors are frequently used in the popular book *Mindfulness: Finding Peace in a Frantic World* (Williams & Penman, 2011). Mindfulness, and the meditating person, are described using technoscientific and communicational terms, such as microphone, radio, radar, tuning, cinema, amplifier and barometer. In particular, mindfulness is a way of releasing people from what psychologists call 'automatic pilot'. For example, Williams and Penman (2011) use a simile to compare the mind of the person reading their book to a multi-tasking computer, which may 'crash' due to being on 'autopilot'. As is standard in popular self-help, they address the reader personally and directly ('you'), using a somewhat dramatic example.

> Very soon the autopilot can become overloaded with too many thoughts, memories, anxieties and tasks – just like a computer with too many windows left open. Your mind slows down. You may become exhausted, anxious, frantic and chronically dissatisfied with life. And again, just like a computer, you may freeze – or even crash. (ibid.: 86)

Many of the descriptions of mindfulness practice involve a distinctly disembodied language of computation and information processing, such as 'autopilot', 'mode', 'system' and 'feedback' which are common to cognitive psychology and cybernetics. Mindfulness is framed, for example, as a way to help people notice when they are in a 'doing mode' of mind, such as automatically reacting to experiences. Mindfulness is claimed to help people to 'switch' into a 'being mode' of mind, in which they gently notice and respond kindly to what is happening.

The 'being mode' of mindfulness is commonly considered to be in opposition to 'mind wandering' (Morrison et al., 2019; Mrazek et al., 2013). But the conference programme (see Figure 2.2) illustrates some of the conceptual and moral complexity in narrating 'mind wandering' within the context of a mindfulness training event. By writing 'we need mind-wandering in our practice' Williams

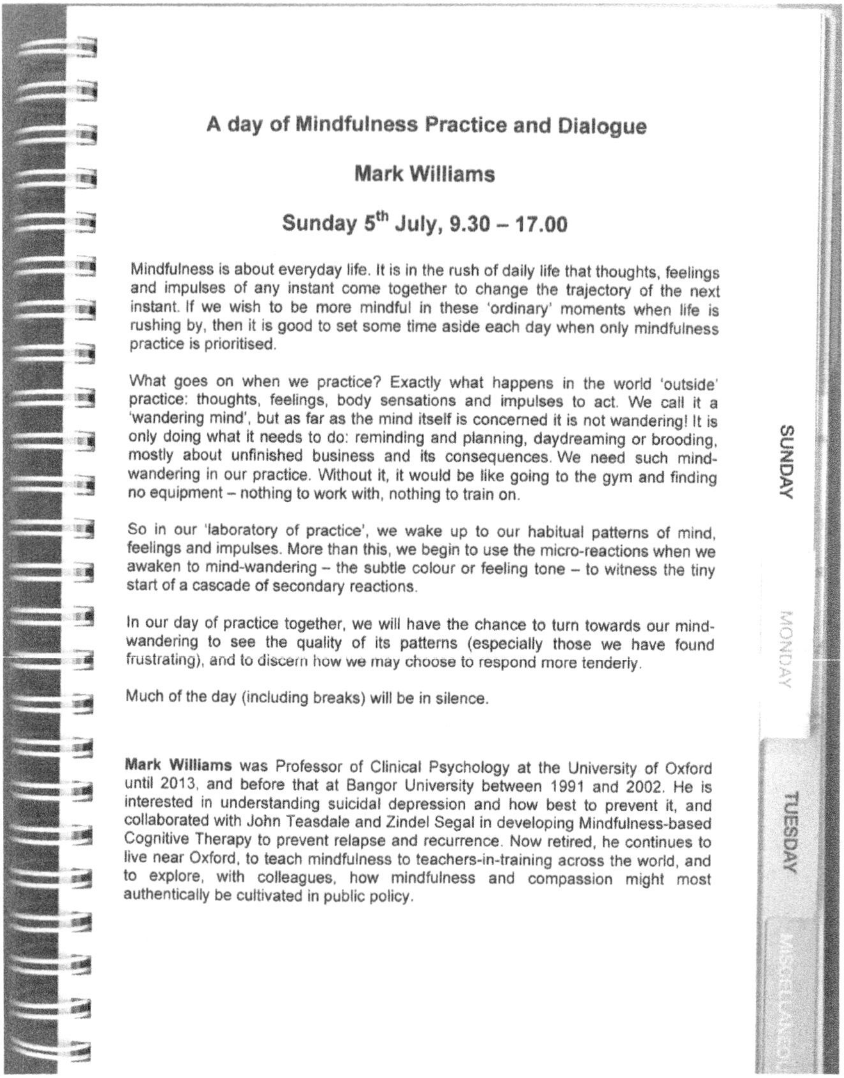

A day of Mindfulness Practice and Dialogue

Mark Williams

Sunday 5th July, 9.30 – 17.00

Mindfulness is about everyday life. It is in the rush of daily life that thoughts, feelings and impulses of any instant come together to change the trajectory of the next instant. If we wish to be more mindful in these 'ordinary' moments when life is rushing by, then it is good to set some time aside each day when only mindfulness practice is prioritised.

What goes on when we practice? Exactly what happens in the world 'outside' practice: thoughts, feelings, body sensations and impulses to act. We call it a 'wandering mind', but as far as the mind itself is concerned it is not wandering! It is only doing what it needs to do: reminding and planning, daydreaming or brooding, mostly about unfinished business and its consequences. We need such mind-wandering in our practice. Without it, it would be like going to the gym and finding no equipment – nothing to work with, nothing to train on.

So in our 'laboratory of practice', we wake up to our habitual patterns of mind, feelings and impulses. More than this, we begin to use the micro-reactions when we awaken to mind-wandering – the subtle colour or feeling tone – to witness the tiny start of a cascade of secondary reactions.

In our day of practice together, we will have the chance to turn towards our mind-wandering to see the quality of its patterns (especially those we have found frustrating), and to discern how we may choose to respond more tenderly.

Much of the day (including breaks) will be in silence.

Mark Williams was Professor of Clinical Psychology at the University of Oxford until 2013, and before that at Bangor University between 1991 and 2002. He is interested in understanding suicidal depression and how best to prevent it, and collaborated with John Teasdale and Zindel Segal in developing Mindfulness-based Cognitive Therapy to prevent relapse and recurrence. Now retired, he continues to live near Oxford, to teach mindfulness to teachers-in-training across the world, and to explore, with colleagues, how mindfulness and compassion might most authentically be cultivated in public policy.

SUNDAY

MONDAY

TUESDAY

MISCELLANEOUS

Figure 2.2 'A Day of Mindfulness Practice and Dialogue' conference programme.

implicitly defends against the idea that mindfulness is incompatible with mind wandering. Mindfulness without mind wandering is considered to be similar to a 'gym' without 'equipment'.

'The gym' is first used as a simile for the space of 'practice', before Williams employs a metaphor of mindfulness training as a 'laboratory of practice'. This 'laboratory' is simultaneously imagined as both scientific and therapeutic. The person 'awakens' inside the laboratory of practice, 'turning towards' mind wandering and thereby witnessing the 'cascade of secondary reactions'. While not explicitly describing mindfulness practice as a 'laboratory' during the DoP itself, Williams nevertheless routinely describes mindfulness using keywords from this metaphorical thesaurus (seeing, discovery, observation). During the DoP, Williams suggests 'testing this out with experiments' on the 'workbench' of the mind. Mindfulness practice is presented primarily as a scientific experiment with therapeutic effects, rather than as a religious or spiritual enterprise.

When functioning together, the use of optic and technoscientific metaphors may be an attempt by mindfulness teachers to universalise and standardise mind and body. This is similar to the attempts by early psychologists, who were 'observers' of their own experiences, to train their inwardly directed attentions through introspection, thus turning themselves into reliable scientific instruments (Coon, 1993). 'Objective' ways to collect data became typical of the mid-twentieth century psychology of behaviourism, although 'behaviour' referred to physical movement, observed from the outside. The body was construed physically through a mechanical and sterile objectivity (Stam, 1998). This served the science of the time in producing measurable knowledge of a human organism, understood as a machine. The body as envisaged by behaviourism is not a fluid, processual, unsure or flowing body. The potential lack of nuance of behaviourist language for describing the human body has been called into question in, for example, affect theory (Blackman, 2012). We are similarly using the concept of affective-practice to analyse and subtly problematise some of the assumptions made in the discourse of expert mindfulness training.

The mechanical mindset of behaviourism still haunts the account of mindfulness within MBCT, and Williams' standpoint perhaps shows some influence of the early psychology of introspection too (see above). Williams also builds upon these influences with cognitive and experiential – humanistic and phenomenological – forms of understanding through his emphasis on the importance of 'sharing' subjective experience in pairs and with the larger group. In the following section we will show how Williams also applies naturalistic and organic metaphors, when advising how people should pay attention to the present moment.

'Ah, Gravity': naturalising mindfulness

The use of technoscientific metaphors is balanced with natural and organic ways of describing mindful (and unmindful) bodies (cloud, river, stream, waterfall, avalanche, garden, tree, seeds, spider's web). Naturalistic imagery such as landscapes, beaches and deserts are commonly found in the popular representation of mindfulness and Buddhist meditation, for example, on the front cover of the TIME magazine edition on 'The Mindfulness Revolution' (Mitchell, 2014). In the following example, Williams uses a metaphor of 'weather' as a way of describing the emotional experience of a 'bad mood'. By using this metaphor, he suggests practitioners' experience resembles impersonal forces of nature, which are not subject to their direct influence and control.

Extract 1: Weather Pattern

Mark Williams (MW)	You've done what exactly what you have to do which is actually just notice the sense of the feeling tone and I think this sense of the overall? Weather pattern? And then little micro-climates within it … yeah? That can just some- and sometimes the overall weather pattern's very stormy and then the- the interesting thing is to discover is the micro-climate still stormy or are there some things which are really curious because in the midst of all this thing my bad mood for example I'm- 'oh that was a moment of pleasantness' 'well that can't be right' (laughs)
Group	(laughter)
MW	So it's just a sense of discovery, of what's of what's here and er I- you know I love the equation thing but I think I- you came back to just say 'okay so what actually is here now'

Williams' use of the metaphor 'weather pattern' involves a management of agency. While he suggests the mindful person is not solely responsible for their 'bad mood', which may change like the weather, they can nevertheless decide to 'observe' this weather (see also Williams and Penman, 2011: 87). The practice of mindfulness is equated with the act of 'discovery'. A mindfulness practitioner is like a naturalist conducting a field observation. This is a subtly different style of observation, and positioning of the observer, to the laboratory experimentation discussed earlier. Patterns of 'mood' resemble weather patterns and the job of the mindfulness practitioner is to neutrally 'notice' their distinctive nuances and changing character. Williams does not explicitly say 'weather pattern' is a metaphor, implying this represents real experience. The wild and lively mind-body of the practitioner is naturalised as an impersonal force. This is similarly illustrated by Kabat-Zinn (1994) who remarks: 'You can't stop the waves, but you can learn to surf'.

In the following extract, Williams uses 'gravity' as a simile, managing accountability for feelings of resentment and anger, and normalising the 'egos' of mindfulness teachers.

Extract 2: Gravity

MW	The ability to see, the mind, especially when it goes off on one when we feel resentment or, angry and we realise that what's happened is somebody has affronted us in some way or you know wid- 'p-people haven't treated us with respect' you know 'that bus driver spoke badly to me' and 'don't they know who I am?' you know 'I've got a senior citizen bus pass'
Group	(laughter)
MW	er so 'I have rights on this bus' you know this sort've thing where the ego gets involved, and and then we can feel really bad cos we're a mindfulness teacher we shouldn't be like this my God, an- an- see if it's possible to see the ego and all of its works as like gravity it's it's just a force of nature and we have to take it into account like we have to take gravity into account and we can use it for things but it's always there (turns to group) we're not gonna get rid of our egos sorry

Group	(laughter)
MW	we're not gonna get rid of our egos so we have to learn to live with them live alongside them just as you say learn to respect to treat them with gra- and see it as gravity so that next time you get angry you can sort've say to yoursel- 'ah gravity'
Group	(laughter)
MW	'there it goes, gravity' yeah 'gravity' just a force yeah

By 'taking the ego into account', 'like gravity', Williams encourages mindfulness teachers to conduct their own natural science-like observations and experiments in everyday life situations. He normalises the experience of feeling resentful and angry at being affronted by a bus driver, employing a personal story, thereby humanising himself as a teacher. 'Seeing' the mind is prescribed as a morally and therapeutically efficacious course of action, which may be in conflict with an internalised stereotype of a mindfulness teacher who 'shouldn't be like this my God'. We have to learn to live with 'ego' in mindfulness training, a similar point to 'needing' mind wandering. Seeing the ego as being like gravity, just a force of nature, involves naturalising the self and emotions. Williams attempts to bring an objective and neutral model of the body as a natural organism into the participants' self-observation. Images of gravity, along with weather patterns, might become part of practitioners' subjective meditative experience. After all, the act of *seeing* the mind-body as a powerful force of nature, and not always subject to individual control, is itself implied to be therapeutic. Mindfulness practitioners are being trained to imagine themselves as a natural scientist who heals herself through self-observation.

Describing 'mood' and 'ego' as natural phenomena does not necessarily contradict the technoscientific language discussed previously. Both metaphors involve imagining an objective realm, commonly shared by all people, which can potentially be observed (or even measured) experientially through a kind of 'inner empiricism'. Naturalising mindfulness is therefore closely intertwined with technologising mindfulness, as both practices are potentially involved in making mindfulness universal and its training standardised. While Williams introduces his audience to multiple descriptions of what happens during mindfulness practice, the quality of paying attention is assumed to be fundamentally the same, or at least very similar, among different people. By using natural science rhetoric, Williams renders the observational capacity of mindfulness as compatible with empirical science, thus making mindfulness appear trustworthy and reliable. If mindfulness practice is equivalent, or similar, to conducting a natural scientific observation or experiment, then it can produce observable, and potentially replicable, objective results.

'Like a doorway opening': sacralising mindfulness

So far, we have discussed constructions of mindfulness which are decidedly secular-sounding. Mindfulness training involves taking a scientific approach, such as a naturalistic observation, and/or a kind of laboratory experimentation. Ocular metaphors of 'seeing' the mind reinforce the orientation of a scientist who, by watching their experience, heals themselves. Yet, in addition to this secularising of mindfulness, the dialogue between Williams and the attendees of the DoP goes further. This is evident in the sharing of experiences that extend beyond breathing which subtly challenges a sole emphasis in meditation on attending to physical sensations of the body alone.

Extract 3: Doorway (I)

Participant 2	It really struck me in that moment that the ah opening to the quality of the breath is like a doorway into the immediacy of of this whole experience erm so it's not just the quality of the breath … you know that instruction it's like a kind of a doorway inta- err opening to this as opposed to being caught in reflection er erm yeah
MW	What is it a can you say more about the that shift, it sounds like a really interesting shift between erm … just observing the breath and somehow being drawn into notice its quality in some way? What is it about that that draws you in do you think

This participant subtly challenges what we have described above as a technoscientific interpretative frame, that is, mindfulness as a purely objective scientific pursuit. Participant 2 uses a simile – 'it's like a kind of a doorway' – and suggests that the instruction of 'opening' to the quality of the breath is a potential 'doorway' to 'this'. The use of the indexical 'this' points to this as yet unnamed experience. Later on, following the sequence reported in this extract, Participant 2 further describes, with some apparent difficulty, where the doorway opens onto: 'this experience as it is'; 'rich vividness of this'; 'vital immediacy'; 'the richness of this'. However, Williams keeps returning to the feeling of the breath as the focus of discussion, as he does in Extract 3, proceeding to make a contrast between 'ideas' and 'life' and how practitioners can inadvertently 'put the breath on automatic … pilot'. Williams later encourages paying attention 'inside the texture of the breath' in 'this moment'.

While in one sense, people who practice mindfulness have authority over their own so-called 'first-person' experience, and 'share' this during spoken dialogue, in another sense the elicited confessions of 'experience' of meditation are also monitored and regulated by external authorities, such as mindfulness teachers, spiritual gurus and contemplative scientists (Pagis, 2009; Tresch, 2011). We find that mindfulness teachers tend to balance their position as being liberal, 'open-minded', 'neutral' and 'permissive' figures while also exerting (sometimes very subtly) the strict regulation, control and disciplined prescription of authority figures (Crane et al., 2015; Stanley & Longden, 2016). This balancing act, which involves the negotiation of contrary themes of equality and expertise, can be described as a 'permissive prescription' (cf. Billig et al., 1988; see also Peteri in this book). By redirecting the topic of dialogue back to the feeling of breathing, Williams displays a subtle resistance to the participants' attempt to discuss the 'doorway' opened through the instruction, as well as what might be beyond the doorway.

Soon after this sequence of interaction, however, Williams takes up an invitation from another participant to explore the 'doorway opening'.

Extract 4: Doorway (II)

Participant 3	So as you're saying that erm sometimes one can be quite distant an an we talk about compassion for ourselves and so on but actually actually having that emotional response to the feeling of the breath or or being with it or that that doorway opening which is a which is an emotion that's actually quite difficult to talk about?
MW	mmm (nods head) mmm it's difficult to talk about yeah that's what wonderful about it
Group	(some 'mmm' acknowledgements)
MW	We come to the edge of words and are called into silence the and and intimacy with what is most most real for us and it's like we suddenly realise that we don't need more information we need- we're being called to yield to what we already know in our hearts whereas when we sit we're often thinkin' 'with just a bit more information I'll be the perfect meditator'
Group	(laughter)
MW	erm rather than in those moments of intimacy yielding to what we already know erm when we've reached the edge of words or inner language hmm thank you

In these moments of dialogue, the discursive aspects of practice are (somewhat paradoxically) de-emphasised, and instead emphasis is given to 'doorways' to experiences, which seemingly cannot be easily captured or expressed through language alone. Stillness, silence and the arising of what might be termed 'religious' or 'spiritual' experiences may make their discursive inscription a challenge, perhaps necessarily so. Indeed, difficulty 'talking about' certain experiences, such as emotions and doorways, can attest to the limits of language. Williams does not say who, or what – if anyone – is 'calling' us into silence in these moments. He does not use words such as religious or spiritual or sacred (Williams and Penman, 2011 do acknowledge 'heart' and 'soul'). Yet, he describes 'moments of intimacy', 'yielding' to 'what we already know in our hearts'.

Recent research on mindfulness has suggested, rather than representing distinctly secular, religious or spiritual discourse alone, that some varieties of mindfulness teaching are instead better captured by the idea of 'post-secularity', in which secular spaces are sacralised and enchanted (Arat, 2017; McMahan, 2012). This idea is supported by our materials. There is little explicit discussion of religion or spirituality during the DoP, and yet the discourse is not simply secular. The discussion of 'doorways' and being 'called into silence' could be interpreted as deriving from discourses of religion, such as contemplative strands of Christianity, or forms of spirituality in which ineffable psychological and emotional 'experience' is foregrounded (Drage, 2018a, 2018b; James, 1902).

Williams and Participant 3 collaboratively produce an account in which the space of mindfulness is sacralised and imagined to be a kind of 'post-secular' laboratory, which potentially transcends words and physical materiality. Williams appears to undermine, or at least put a limit on, the usefulness of the central metaphor of cognitive science – information – when he says 'we don't need more information'. He suggests that mindfulness practice itself, especially its silent dimensions, may provide a different – equivalent or superior – form of knowledge to science. A wordless knowledge.

The somehow 'difficult' or 'beautiful' experiences encountered among the mindfulness practitioners, as seen in breathing as a 'doorway' to some other understanding, along with much more profoundly disturbing experiences, are claimed to be more commonplace than popular and professional discourse about mindfulness courses might imply (Ellis, 1984; Farias et al., 2016: 1012; Shapiro, 1992). Lindahl and others have pointed out that such experiences are seldom investigated within the mindfulness field, since the 'positive' therapeutic benefits of training have been emphasised (Lindahl et al., 2014: 2; Lindahl, 2017; Kornfield, 1979). The unusual affects and body-consciousness related experiences mostly remain hidden, or at least downplayed, in the materials we have studied so far.

Conclusion

In this chapter, we have problematised the idea of mindfulness as a 'free-floating' and universal *panacea*. By situating mindfulness within a specific training environment, we have implicitly criticised the idea that mindfulness is a totalising discourse, producing the same effects everywhere it goes – such as individualisation or self-governance. We have shown how, rather than being a singular and coherent totality, the therapeutic culture of mindfulness can be understood as an assemblage.

When we look at what happens during specific occasions of mindfulness teaching in action, we find a complex reality which cannot be easily accounted for by notions of an amorphous 'therapy culture' (Furedi, 2004). Our analysis has given special attention to the multiple affective-discursive practices, which are put together to 'make up' mindful bodies – visualising, technologising and naturalising. Such metaphors and similes are used within an overarching framework in which mindfulness, within the specific context we have studied, is spatialised as a 'laboratory of practice'. Yet, even this framework of meaning was subtly challenged by some participants who attempted to transcend the boundaries of the self-healing laboratory, opening up a 'doorway' into a realm which we described as involving a 'post-secular' sacralising of space.

Our analysis illustrates how the affective-discursive practices making up mindfulness training may possess multiple functions with potentially contradictory effects. Mindfulness-based therapies humanise cognitive-behaviourism, bringing humanistic and Asian-inspired practices into the heartland of 'evidence-based' clinical psychology and medicine (Dryden & Still, 2006). By importing the body, meditation and emotional awareness into evidence-based psychotherapy, MBCT pushes against the boundaries of cognitive science. Mindfulness potentially softens the rigid boundaries of experimentalism, allowing a sense of 'beauty', 'wonder' and 'the sacred' to be drawn into the matrix of the 'psychological complex' (Rose, 1985). Yet, at the same time, meditation itself is being imagined as a simultaneously organic and technoscientific hybrid. The logic of scientific observation, experimentation and discovery are possibly being distributed into the body politic through mindfulness training courses, similarly to how medical ideas are being spread through the mindfulness movement (Barker, 2014).

Mark Williams, the innovative co-founder of MBCT, offers multiple perspectives on the meditative experience. His expert teaching of mindfulness allows for various interpretations of what a 'mindful' experience can be like. He makes available a diversity of resources, such that people can make 'choices' about how they practice mindfulness. This open-endedness of self-care practices allows mindfulness to become a potentially never-ending pursuit of self-improvement and healing (Barker, 2014; Vogel, 2017). The training we have analysed creates new norms for embodied healthcare which have historical precedents and the multiplicity of the mindfulness assemblage serves the open-endedness of its techniques.

Yet, there are limits to this multiplicity. The rigorous training involved in mindfulness practice potentially produces a standardising of theory and practice, which parallels early attempts in psychology to apply introspection as a scientific method (Coon, 1993). Within the mindfulness training session we analysed, the mindful bodies that are being co-produced by the expert teacher and his students are not explicitly marked by social difference or diversity. The mind-body of the mindfulness practitioner, at least within this DoP, is presented as being able-bodied and implied to be genderless, sexless, raceless and classless. That is, no explicit topicalising of sex, gender, sexuality, race, ethnicity or class takes place within this MBCT training event, although the ageing body is implicitly acknowledged in the 'bus pass' anecdote. In this sense, mindful bodies are implied to be universal and transcendent of society, culture and history (Drage, 2018a, 2018b). Being mindful is also suggested to be independent of religious or political belief. Mindfulness is made to be a universally accessible technique, applicable to all people at all times, and in principle inclusive of everyone's experience.

Paradoxically, this universalising is being done by a seemingly homogenous group of people. In common with Anglo-American 'convert' Buddhist groups, the population of mindfulness teachers and trainers have anecdotally been reported as being relatively homogenous – mostly white and middle-class – and course attendees tend to be white, middle-aged, and highly educated females (Wilson, 2014; see also Figure 2.1). American Buddhist meditation is advertised to young, white, middle-class, female city-dwellers (Mitchell, 2014). Yet, the founders of MBSR and MBCT are commonly identified as white, male, Anglo-American scientists and clinical psychologists, with especially female and Asian founders often being forgotten within historical accounts. Feminist philosophers of science have challenged the ideal of the 'objective observer' in science and exposed the assumptions made in behaviourist and cognitivist theories of the body. In her essay 'Loving the computer: cognition, embodiment and the influencing machine', philosopher Elizabeth Wilson suggests that 'at the heart of cognitive theories we find the body of the thinking man' (Wilson, 1996: 557).

We found mindfulness-based therapeutics to be a complex milieu and domain of practice, distinguished by multiplicity and paradox. Indeed, it is arguably the variety of influences, paradoxical tensions and contradictory functions of the mindfulness assemblage which contribute to its productive power. In our view, the productive power of mindfulness, and its potentially curative properties, are principally the result of the contradictory practices which make up this community of practice. Assemblage thinking and affective-discursive practice analysis, when combined together, help to illustrate how tensions and contradictions can be productive of knowledge. In our study, we have not interviewed participants of mindfulness courses to find out about their experiences of mindfulness, yet our analysis suggests how future studies might investigate the ways meditation is learned and experienced by participants, and how teachers and students of mindfulness manage tensions and contradictions of mindfulness practice. It will be interesting also to discover in future investigations how the multiple meanings of mindfulness, which make it so transferable and portable, are interpreted by diverse social actors, across a broader range of institutional and geographical contexts and situations. MBSR and MBCT are now being exported from Anglo-American contexts to North Western and Eastern Europe and even to Asian countries, under the banner of 'global mental health'. Future social studies of mindfulness might investigate how such practices are being received in the places where they allegedly originated.

References

Arat, A. 2017. 'What it means to be truly human': The postsecular hack of mindfulness. *Social Compass 64*:2, 167–179.

Arthington, P. 2016. Mindfulness: A critical perspective. *Community Psychology in Global Perspective 2*:1, 87–104.

Barker, K.K. 2014. Mindfulness meditation: Do-it-yourself medicalization of every moment. *Social Science & Medicine 106*, 168–176.

Billig, M., Condor, S., Edwards, D., Gane, M., Middleton, D., & Radley, A. 1988. *Ideological Dilemmas*. London: Sage.

Blackman, L. 2012. *Immaterial Bodies. Affect, Embodiment, Mediation*. London: Sage.

Brazier, D. 2013. Mindfulness reconsidered. *European Journal of Psychotherapy & Counselling 15*:2, 116–126.

Carrette, J., & King, R. 2005. *Selling Spirituality: The Silent Takeover of Religion*. London: Routledge.

Carvalho, A. 2014. Subjectivity, ecology, and meditation – performing interconnectedness. *Subjectivity 7*:2, 131–150.

Cederström, C., & Spicer, A. 2015. *The Wellness Syndrome*. Cambridge: Polity Press.

Clegg, J.W. (Ed.). 2013. *Self-Observation in the Social Sciences*. London: Transaction.

Cook, J. 2016. Mindful in Westminster: The politics of meditation and the limits of neoliberal critique. *HAU: Journal of Ethnographic Theory 6*:1, 141–161.

Coon, D.J. 1993. Standardizing the subject: Experimental psychologists, introspection, and the quest for a technoscientific ideal. *Technology & Culture 34*:4, 757–783.

Crane, R.S., Stanley, S., Rooney, M., Bartley, T., Cooper, L., & Mardula, J. 2015. Disciplined improvisation: Characteristics of inquiry in mindfulness-based teaching. *Mindfulness 6*:5, 1104–1114.

Danziger, K. 1997. *Naming the Mind*. London: Sage.

Davies, W. 2015. *The Happiness Industry*. London: Verso.

Drage, M. 2018a. *'Universal Dharma': Authority, Experience and Metaphysics in the Transmission of Mindfulness-Based Stress Reduction.* Unpublished PhD Thesis, University of Cambridge.

Drage, M. 2018b. Of mountains, lakes and essences: John Teasdale and the transmission of mindfulness. *History of the Human Sciences 31*:4, 107–130.

Dryden, W., & Still, A. 2006. Historical aspects of mindfulness and self-acceptance in psychotherapy. *Journal of Rational-Emotive and Cognitive-Behaviour Therapy 24*:1, 3–28.

Eklöf, J. 2017. Neurodharma self-help: Personalized science communication as brain management. *Journal of Medical Humanities 38*:3, 303–317.

Ellis, A. 1984. The place of meditation in cognitive-behaviour therapy and rational-emotive therapy. In *Meditation: Classic and Contemporary Perspectives*, edited by D.H. Shapiro, & R.N. Walsh. New York: Aldine, 671–673.

Falby, A. 2003. The modern confessional: Anglo-American religious groups and the emergence of lay psychotherapy. *Journal of History of the Behavioural Sciences 39*:3, 251–267.

Farias, M., Wikholm, C., & Delmonte, R. 2016. What is mindfulness-based therapy good for? Evidence, limitations and controversies. *The Lancet 3*:11, 1012–1013.

Furedi, F. 2004. *Therapy Culture: Cultivating Vulnerability in an Uncertain Age.* London: Routledge.

Harrington, A. 2008. *The Cure Within: A History of Mind-Body Medicine.* London: WW Norton & Co.

Harrington, A., & Dunne, J. 2015. When mindfulness is therapy: Ethical qualms, historical perspectives. *American Psychologist 70*:7, 621–631.

Hickey, W.S. 2010. Meditation as medicine: A critique. *CrossCurrents 60*:2, 168–184.

Higgins, V., & W. Larner. (Eds.). 2017. *Assembling Neoliberalism: Expertise, Practices, Subjects.* Basingstoke: Palgrave MacMillan.

Illouz, E. 2008. *Saving the Modern Soul: Therapy, Emotions, and the Culture of Self-Help.* London: University of California Press.

James, W. 1902. *The Varieties of Religious Experience.* London: Routledge.

Kabat-Zinn, J. 1994. *Wherever You Go, There You Are.* London: Piatkus.

Kabat-Zinn, J. 2011. Some reflections on the origins of MBSR, skillful means, and the trouble with maps. *Contemporary Buddhism 12*:1, 281–306.

Kabat-Zinn, J. 2017. Too early to tell: The potential impact and challenges—ethical and otherwise—inherent in the mainstreaming of dharma in an increasingly dystopian world. *Mindfulness 8*:5, 1125–1135.

Kerr, C.E., Sachett, M.D., Lazar, S.W., Moore, C.I., & Jones, S.R. 2013. Mindfulness starts with the body: Somatosensory attention and topdown modulation of cortical alpharhythms in mindfulness meditation. *Frontiers in Human Neuroscience 7*:12, 1–15.

King, R. 2016. 'Paying attention' in a digital economy: Reflections on the role of analysis and judgement within contemporary discourses of mindfulness and comparisons with classical Buddhist accounts of sati. In *Handbook of Mindfulness: Culture, Context, and Social Engagement*, edited by R. Purser, D. Forbes, & A. Burke. New York: Springer, 27–46.

Kirmayer, L.J. 2015. Mindfulness in cultural context. *Transcultural Psychiatry 52*:4, 447–469.

Kornfield, J. 1979. Intensive insight meditation: A phenomenological study. *Journal of Transpersonal Psychology 11*, 45–58.

Kortelainen, I. 2013. *Interpretation and Analysis: Conceptions of the Philosophical Method in Paul Ricoeur's Hermeneutics*. Acta Universitatis Tamperensis: 1852. Tampere: Tampere University Press.

Kortelainen, I., Omaheimo, J., Saari, A., & Ranki, K. 2017. Läsnäolon kokemus ja politiikka. [Politics of being present]. *Niin&näin* 2/2017, 61–62.

Lakoff, G., & Johnson, M. 1980. *Metaphors We Live By*. London: University of Chicago Press.

Lindahl, J. 2017. The varieties of contemplative experience: A mixed-methods study of meditation-related challenges in Western Buddhists. *PLOS ONE*. http://journals.plos.org/plosone/article?id=10.1371/journal.pone.0176239 (accessed 10 April 2018).

Lindahl, J., Kaplan, C.T., Winget, E.M., & Britton, W.B. 2014. A phenomenology of meditation-induced light experiences: Traditional Buddhist and neurobiological perspectives. *Front Psychol 4*, 973.

Lopez, D.S. Jr. 2012. *The Scientific Buddha: His Short and Happy Life*. London: Yale University Press.

Madsen, O.J. 2014. *The Therapeutic Turn*. London: Routledge.

Madsen, O.J. 2015. *Optimizing the Self*. London: Routledge.

Mamberg, M.H., & Bassarear, T. 2015. From reified self to being mindful: A dialogical analysis of the MBSR voice. *International Journal for Dialogical Science 9*:1, 11–37.

McGee, M. 2012. From makeover media to remaking culture: Four directions for the critical study of self-help culture. *Sociology Compass 6*:9, 685–693.

McMahan, D.L. 2008. *The Making of Buddhist Modernism*. Oxford: Oxford University Press.

McMahan, D.L. 2012. The enchanted secular: Buddhism and the emergence of transtraditional 'spirituality'. *The Eastern Buddhist 43*:1–2, 205–223.

Mindfulness All-Party Parliamentary Group. 2015. *Mindful Nation UK*. The Mindfulness Initiative, October. http://themindfulnessinitiative.org.uk/images/reports/Mindfulness-APPG-Report_Mindful-Nation-UK_Oct2015.pdf (accessed 10 April 2018).

Mitchell, S.A. 2014. The tranquil meditator: Representing Buddhism and Buddhists in US popular media. *Religion Compass 8*:3, 81–89.

Morrison, H., McBriar, S., Powell, H., Proudfoot, J., Stanley, S., Fitzgerald, D., & Callard, F. (2019). What is a psychological task? The operational pliability of 'task' in psychological laboratory experimentation. *Engaging Science, Technology & Society 5*: 61–85.

Mrazek, M.D., Franklin, M.S., Phillips, D.T., Baird, B., & Schooler, J.W. 2013. Mindfulness training improves working memory capacity and GRE performance while reducing mind wandering. *Psychological Science 24*:5, 776–781.

Nehring, D., Alvarado, E., Hendriks, E., & Kerrigan, D. 2017. *Transnational Popular Psychology and the Global Self-Help Industry: The Politics of Contemporary Social Change*. Basingstoke: Palgrave MacMillan.

Pagis, M. 2009. Embodied self-reflexivity. *Social Psychology Quarterly 72*:3, 265–283.

Plank, K. 2010. Mindful medicine: The growing trend of mindfulness-based therapies in the Swedish health care system. *Finnish Journal of Ethnicity and Migration 5*:2, 47–55.

Preston, D. 1998. *The Social Organization of Zen Practice*. Cambridge: Cambridge University Press.

Purser, R. 2019. *McMindfulness: How Mindfulness Became the New Capitalist Spirituality*. London: Repeater.

Purser, R., Forbes, D., & Burke, A. 2016. *Handbook of Mindfulness: Culture, Context, and Social Engagement*. New York: Springer.

Purser, R., & Loy, D. 2013. Beyond McMindfulness. *Huffington Post*. http://www. huffingtonpost.com/ron-purser/beyond-mcmindfulness_b_3519289.html (accessed 17 March 2017).

Reveley, J. 2016. Neoliberal meditations: How mindfulness training medicalises education and responsibilizes young people. *Policy Futures in Education 14*:4, 497–511.

Ricœur, P. 1991. *A Ricœur Reader: Reflection and Imagination*, edited by M.J. Valdés. New York: Harvester-Wheatsheaf.

Ricœur, P. 2008/1975. *The Rule of Metaphor: Multi-Disciplinary Studies of the Creation of Meaning in Language*, edited by R. Czerny with K. McLaughlin, & J. Costello. London: Routledge & Kegan Paul.

Rorty, R. 1979. *Philosophy and the Mirror of Nature*. Oxford: Princeton University Press.

Rose, N. 1985. *The Psychological Complex*. London: Routledge & Kegan Paul.

Rowe, J.K. 2016. Micropolitics and collective liberation: Mind/body practice and left social movements. *New Political Science 38*:2, 206–225.

Segal, Z.V.J., Williams, J.M.G., & Teasdale, J.D. 2013. *Mindfulness-Based Cognitive Therapy for Depression* (2nd Edition). New York: Guilford Press.

Shapiro, D.H. 1992. Adverse effects of meditation: A preliminary investigation of long-term meditators. *International Journal of Psychosomatics 39*, 62–67.

Sharf, R.F. 1995. Buddhist modernism and the rhetoric of meditative experience. *Numen 42*:3, 228–283.

Shattuck, E.H. 1958. *An Experiment in Mindfulness*. New York: Samuel Weiser.

Stam, H.J. 1998. *The Body and Psychology*. London: Sage.

Stanley, S., & Crane, R. 2015. Discourse analysis of naturally occurring data: The relational development of mindfulness. *SAGE Research Methods Datasets*. http://methods. sagepub.com/dataset/discourse-analysis-mindfulness.

Stanley, S., & Longden, C. 2016. Constructing the mindful subject: Reformulating experience through affective-discursive practice in mindfulness-based stress reduction. In *Handbook of Mindfulness: Culture, Context and Social Engagement*, edited by R. Purser, D. Forbes, & A. Burke. New York: Springer, 305–322.

Stanley, S., Purser, R., & Singh, N. (Eds.). 2018. *Handbook of Ethical Foundations of Mindfulness*. New York: Springer.

Tan, C.-M. 2012. *Search Inside Yourself: The Unexpected Path to Achieving Success, Happiness (and World Peace)*. New York: HarperCollins.

Thera, N. 1954. *The Heart of Buddhist Meditation*. Sri Lanka: Buddhist Publication Society.

Thompson, E. 2017. Looping effects and the cognitive science of mindfulness. In *Meditation, Buddhism, and Science*, edited by D.L. McMahan, & E. Braun. Oxford: Oxford University Press, 47–61.

Thomson, M. 2006. *Psychological Subjects: Identity, Culture and Health in Twentieth-Century Britain*. Oxford: Oxford University Press.

Tresch, J. 2011. Experimental ethics and the science of the meditating brain. In *Neurocultures: Glimpses Into an Expanding Universe*, edited by F. Ortega, & F. Vidal. Frankfurt: Peter Lang, 49–68.

Valerio, A. 2016. Owning mindfulness: A bibliometric analysis of mindfulness literature trends within and outside of Buddhist contexts. *Contemporary Buddhism 17*:1, 157–183.

Varela, F., & Shear, J. (Eds.). 1999. *The View From Within: First-Person Approaches to the Study of Consciousness*. Thorverton, UK: Imprint Academic.

Varela, F., Thompson, E., & Rosch, E. 1991. *The Embodied Mind*. London: MIT Press.

Varra, A.A., Drossel, C., & Hayes, S.C. 2009. The use of metaphor to establish acceptance and mindfulness. In *Clinical Handbook of Mindfulness*, edited by F. Didonna. New York: Springer, 111–123.

Vogel, E. 2017. Hungers that need feeding: On the normativity of mindful nourishment. *Anthropology & Medicine 24*:2, 159–173.

Wetherell, M. 2013. *Affect and Emotion: A New Social Science Understanding*. London: Sage.

Wheater, K. 2017. *Once More to the Body: An Ethnography of Mindfulness Practitioners in the United Kingdom*. Unpublished PhD Thesis, Oxford University.

Williams, R.J. 2014. *The Buddha in the Machine*. London: Yale University Press.

Williams, J.M.G., & Kabat-Zinn, J. 2011. Mindfulness: Diverse perspectives on its meaning, origins, and multiple applications at the intersection of science and dharma. *Contemporary Buddhism 12,* 1–18.

Williams, M., & Penman, D. 2011. *Mindfulness: Finding Peace in a Frantic World*. London: Piatkus.

Wilson, E. 1996. 'Loving the computer': Cognition, embodiment, and the influencing machine. *Theory & Psychology 6*:4, 577–599.

Wilson, J. 2014. *Mindful America: The Mutual Transformation of Buddhist Meditation and American Culture*. Cambridge: Cambridge University Press.

Wittgenstein, L. 1958. *Philosophical Investigations*. London: Wiley-Blackwell.

Žižek, S. 2001. *On Belief*. London: Routledge.

Zerubavel, E. 1997. *Social Mindscapes: An Invitation to Cognitive Sociology*. London: Harvard University Press.

3   Affective assemblages

Atmospheres and therapeutic knowledge production in/through the researcher-body

Marjo Kolehmainen

'We did something in a different manner, and the whole atmosphere changed'. Thus concluded one of the speakers at a relationship enhancement seminar after having encouraged participants to shake hands with somebody previously unknown to them and to thank them for being there. However, although experts in (or organisers of) relationship and sex counselling occasionally address the importance of sustaining a sound atmosphere at home in order to maintain a good couple relationship, it is relatively rare to hear them comment on the atmosphere of an ongoing event. Graham[1] was an exception with his comment about the relationship enhancement seminar. He was one of the experts who spoke at the seminar, and he invested a great deal in activating his audience, using various means from urging couples to hug to making people jump up and down. These efforts seemed to aim for the co-production – intensively performed by both Graham and his participants – of an affective atmosphere, which speaks to his recognition that an appropriate atmosphere was essential to the organisation of a successful relationship enhancement seminar. It also highlights how atmospheres, although individually felt, belong to collective situations and reach beyond individual, autonomous subjects (Anderson, 2009; Seyfert, 2012). Whether acknowledged or not, atmospheres are a significant part of human experience. In what follows, I propose that affective atmospheres are important for understanding therapeutic cultures, especially in collective events that concentrate on relationship and sexual issues.

This chapter engages with the issue of affective atmospheres in therapeutic cultures by drawing upon a detailed study of relationship and sex counselling in Finland. I first became interested in atmospheres because of the ambivalences I encountered during my on-site participant observations as a feminist scholar. During those observations, I from time to time found the relationship or sex advice being given at some events personally or professionally problematic but this did not necessarily prevent me from experiencing the atmospheres of the events in question as warm, entertaining or safe. For instance, I encountered disruptive moments because of a firm reliance on gendered stereotypes, such as the idea that men are sexually active and women sexually passive, or a persistent renewal of heteronormative values, such as the equation of intimate relationships with heterosexual marriage (see Kolehmainen, 2018). I have also had an academic interest in the study of atmospheres and moods since working on a research project on affective inequalities in intimate relationships, which aimed to develop and work with methodologies that provide better access to affect as an embodied experience (see Kolehmainen and Juvonen, 2018).[2] I assumed that by paying attention to my own bodily states, I might be able to better work with affect in its embodied form. Here I seek to elaborate on these ambivalences by analysing them and other personal experiences of atmospheres during fieldwork, thereby giving them status within the affective processes of knowledge production.

The theoretical premises of this chapter are rooted in assemblage theory, which highlights the connectivities between objects and bodies. Assemblage theory is a way of mapping how things come together and what the assembled relations enable to become or block from becoming (Ringrose and Renold, 2014: 774; De Landa, 2006). As I focus on a certain kind of assemblage – that of an atmosphere – the concept of affect is fruitful for mapping how different objects and bodies come together in situated experiences of registering, engineering or sustaining an atmosphere. The concept of affect offers a means to explore relations between different kinds of bodies – human, non-human, organic, non-organic, artificial and imaginary (e.g. Kolehmainen and Juvonen, 2018; Lahti, 2018; Seyfert, 2012) – that play an essential role in affective atmospheres. Further, affect foregrounds bodies' capacities to affect and become affected (see also Deleuze and Guattari, 2004; Massumi, 2004). Indeed, it is bodily in/capacities that make atmospheres possible in the first place. Hence, rather than being located within individual human bodies, the processes of affecting and becoming affected emerge in and through encounters between bodies and things (Kolehmainen and Juvonen, 2018). The fact that we are capable of sensing an atmosphere indicates that we become affected by other bodies. However, we also contribute to the affecting of other bodies, no matter whether this is through conscious effort or not.

Focusing on affective atmospheres, this chapter attempts to move away from human-centred notions of the therapeutic which manifest themselves, for instance, in a reliance on the concept of the self. Previously, the self has been placed at the core of the analysis of therapeutic cultures, which promote an orientation towards the self and employ psychological discourses as resources for selfhood (Furedi, 2006; Illouz, 2008; Madsen and Ytre-Arne, 2012). The growth of therapeutic cultures has further been linked to the cultural tendency towards individualisation, which gives prominence to lifestyle gurus and personal advisers, who act as the new cultural intermediaries of the self (McRobbie, 2009; Wood and Skeggs, 2004). This has been seen as overlapping with neoliberal tendencies, which emphasise the ability to self-monitor, self-regulate, self-diagnose, make choices and transform oneself (e.g. Oullette and Wilson, 2011; Swan, 2008). While these perspectives have captured several essential features of contemporary Western society and its inclination towards the psychologisation of everyday life, therapeutic cultures nevertheless entail elements that are not best grasped by this kind of framework. In this chapter I approach atmospheres from the perspective of new materialist ontology, which shifts the focus of analysis from the feelings of individualised subjects to impersonal flows of affect through assemblages (see Youdell and Armstrong, 2011: 145). In particular, I mobilise a non-human-centred concept of atmosphere that does not start with an 'I' but invites us to pay attention to the transpersonal, the intercorporeal and the more-than-only-human. The chapter aims to use the lens of affective atmospheres to map how situational and material therapeutic practices operate in/through both human and non-human bodies.

Feeling (with) the field: ethnography in the study of affective atmospheres

In what follows, I will use my own embodied sensations and affective experiences to analyse the experiences of soaking up atmospheres, moving in/out of affective atmospheres, feeling the limits of collective belonging, and failing to 'get' the atmosphere when conducting fieldwork. However, rather than understanding my orientation as a form of autoethnography, I see it as an attempt to open up new insights into relations within assemblages, as my ultimate interest is not in the self. Yet even though atmospheres are best understood from a relational perspective that does not privilege the human subject, they cannot be academically addressed without some sort of rooting in the human body. As Robert Seyfert (2012) points out, affects are conventionally seen as located within an individual subject or body, or else they are seen as atmospheric forces that operate externally to the body. On the one hand, if we believe that affects are individual, we fail to account for their collective and trans-subjective nature. On the other, if we think that people are simply caught by atmospheres, we risk seeing individuals as passive objects with very little agency. Nor do conceptualisations of this kind explain why different people can experience the 'same' atmosphere in different ways – not every individual body is always affected in the same way. The way forwards, then, is to think of affect as the effect of the interactions and encounters of individual human and non-human bodies (ibid.). Of course, some definitions of atmosphere (such as 'transpersonal intensity' or 'the transmission of the other's feeling') emphasise human presence, whereas others (such as 'a sense of place or environment') put more weight on non-human actors or elements. However, atmospheres should be seen neither as residing outside human bodies nor as simply human-made.

For the purposes of this chapter, I draw upon my study on relationship and sex counselling practices in Finland. I consider my study as an affective ethnography, a term which refers to the style of research rather than to a mechanistic method (see Gherardi, 2018). In particular, I focus on analysing my fieldwork notes from 40 events (2015–2017) that ranged from relationship enhancement seminars to a tantric workshop and from events catering to the recently separated to variously themed lectures by experts. These events were collective, public or semi-public occasions whose venues ranged from public libraries to fairs and from religious gatherings to hotel facilities. The events I attended varied a great deal: some were organised by national organisations and employed counselling professionals from psychotherapists to certified couple counsellors as experts; others were part of spiritual, religious or commercial activities and often relied on lay experts. Several events catered to couples who wished to nurture their relationships; others, for instance, targeted those who were recently separated, those who were interested in well-being in general, or those who worked with relationship or sexual issues in their day-to-day professions. It was common to all the events that they did not address particular issues faced by single clients or specific couples, in contrast to private counselling sessions. This conforms to a wider shift in widespread therapeutic cultures: it is no longer just 'sick' selves but also 'healthy' selves who are addressed as potential clients or customers (Ouellette and Wilson, 2011; Swan, 2008). In relationship and sex counselling, this is manifested in the shift from divorce prevention to the nurture and care of relationships (Maksimainen, 2014), which makes it possible to address collectives and groups – and further facilitates atmosphere as a part of therapeutic culture.

Affective ethnography is especially suitable for the exploration of affective atmospheres, as it allows using affect as a resource – enacted through the researcher's embodiment – in the research practice (Gherardi, 2018). Moreover, participant observation allows the researcher to sense, experience and read atmospheres on-site. Social-scientific studies on atmospheres have been relatively scarce, and exploring atmospheres poses a huge challenge to social-scientific enquiry, as atmospheres are often fleeting and barely perceptible (Bille et al., 2015). Of course, from a methodological point of view, the task of investigating atmospheres (or perhaps, investigating *with(in) them*) is challenging. However, participant observation allows us to shift the locus of knowledge production from after-the-event narratives to 'the social as it happens', in a way that makes it possible to explore the atmospheres themselves rather than their descriptions. Atmospheres cannot be felt in retrospect, so they need to become registered in the field. Feeling (with) the field shifts the focus from ethnographic 'knowing' to relating and experiencing, thereby departing from the dissociated and objectifying gaze of the knower in modern science (see Bryld and Lykke, 2000; Coleman and Ringrose, 2013; Law, 2004; Stewart, 2017). Atmospheres can become 'known' through the personal sensation of feeling them, rather than through the distanced gaze of a researcher. Hence, the study of atmospheres makes it evident that researchers are always already part of the assemblages they seek to study (e.g. Fox and Alldred, 2015: 400, 2017: 20). Since there is no binary between a bodiless atmosphere and a body (Seyfert, 2012), the researcher is never outside an atmosphere, regardless of how they feel or whether they register the atmosphere. Hence, to explore atmospheres is to reject binaries of subject/object, researcher/researched and knower/known in a very concrete way.

In practice, I have chosen to experiment by using my own researcher-body as a site of research, as a means to address affective atmospheres. As Lisa Blackman (2015) writes, affect is disclosed in atmospheres. However, affect is not an entity that can be captured as an *it* or a thing; thus, no method can straightforwardly prove or provide evidence for what affect is (ibid.). The methodological question then remains: how can we work methodologically with the concept of affect and actually 'operationalise' it to find ways of understanding how affect works in the social

(Ringrose and Renold, 2014: 773)? One way affect works in the social is through atmospheres: atmospheres highlight how affect operates on us in divergent ways, rather than being external to human subjects (Colebrook, 2002: 39; Seyfert, 2012). In order to analyse such operations, I have integrated my own researcher-body into the research practice. By using my own researcher-body as a site of research, I have been able to produce embodied-affective data (see also Knudsen and Stage, 2015). Embodied-affective data refers to data that foregrounds the embodied experiences of affecting and being affected. It is indexically linked to the bodies 'in' affect – the researcher and participants (Kinnunen and Kolehmainen, 2019; Knudsen and Stage, 2015; Walkerdine, 2010). Here, embodied-affective data refers to data that is produced by my researcher-body as the latter is affected by atmospheres – and of course also affects them through my on-site participation. My reflections of having a body 'in' affect do not, of course, limit themselves to conscious reflections or field-work notes. However, I rely here on my fieldwork notes, which document affects in several ways, from accounts of personal feelings to sensing shifts in atmosphere, and from shifts in textual styles to reflections regarding affects and the interpretations given to them by experts, participants or me.

When bodies are conceptualised as trans-subjective, intercorporeal and capable of both affecting and being affected by other bodies – rather than as singular, autonomous and human-only – the exploration of a researcher-body may help to produce knowledge of affective relations within and of assemblages, rather than of subjective experiences. In this way, foregrounding a researcher-body is not a means to re-centre 'I' or human subjectivity, but is one way of providing an alternative viewpoint from which to consider situatedness within assemblages (see also Fox and Alldred, 2015: 409). Indeed, affects are not a lens onto 'truth' or reality, and this also holds true when we consider the researcher's bodily states (see also Hemmings, 2012; Pedwell and Whitehead, 2012). Researchers have different capacities for 'reading' atmospheres, as indicated in instances when researchers guess wrongly what other people are feeling or are otherwise incompetent in interpreting how other people experience atmospheres (see Wetherell, 2012: 146). Different bodies can also become affected in different ways in the same situation (Seyfert, 2012). Hence, I also attempt here to implicate myself (as a researcher) within the research process and to analytically explore my own affective investments in the subject under investigation (see Blackman, 2015: 25–26). Taking situatedness within assemblages into account opens up possibilities for exploring the power relations inherent to atmospheres. From the perspective of situatedness, then, it becomes possible to attune to how social inclusion and exclusion become orchestrated through atmospheres (Bille et al., 2015: 36), and how these processes get entangled with social differences, among other issues.

Creating an affective atmosphere: on collective belonging

The first occasion when I paid attention to atmosphere was right at the beginning of my study when I attended a tantric workshop, not quite knowing what to expect (see also Kolehmainen, 2018). When I heard that the workshop entailed active participation, including the task of touching strangers, I felt a little reserved. Still, I soon found myself dancing to the rhythm of the music and giving hugs to other attendees. To my surprise, it was rather fun, and I soon started to find the atmosphere humorous and relaxed:

> The tutor says that we can read in books what tantra is and explore self-help guides; however, now we are going to do things and get out of our comfort zones – she tells us how we are going to proceed, how we are going to touch ourselves and other people (oh no! don't want to!) and how different music is going to affect us.
>
> Then we dance. The atmosphere is relaxed, unconstrained and jolly. (Field notes: tantric workshop, 2015)

As I recall the event, the production of a certain kind of atmosphere was key. It appears as if attending the workshop and soaking up a certain kind of atmosphere would be meaningful in their own right, instead of getting straightforward advice or focusing on intentional self-transformation. However, the atmosphere was not there waiting for participants to enter and feel it (see Wetherell, 2012). Rather, the instructor – a woman named Lily – pulled the right strings again and again: she was energetic and actively activated us. She had chosen a playlist and the workshop design made us participants mingle. At first, we started walking hand in hand. At that point Lily commented 'I can see that our auras are uniting', which can be seen as indicating an attempt to create a collective mood. This was followed by some hugging and dancing. In other words, the atmosphere was created step by step, starting with relatively mundane activities that were followed by increasing contact and proximity between bodies. We can see how the (actual, desired or imagined) atmosphere was intensified through the creation of patterns of affective imitation and the mobilisation of several senses: in addition to the movement, there was the music, the touching, the eye contact.

I was caught in the atmosphere most of the time, until the instructor started to talk about how women should not feel ashamed when men looked at their 'boobs and bottoms'. I felt irritated by her words, and my irritation articulated a rupture in the atmosphere as I felt it and resulted in a moment of feeling temporarily out of place. In any case, I could not help finding Lily's words problematic, and thus rather than soaking up the collective atmosphere, I became aware of my position as a feminist (scholar) and adopted an evaluative stance towards the way the workshop was now being conducted:

> The first group is assigned a task to dance in a sexy way. The second group is assigned to look at the first group dancing. My first reaction is irritation, I immediately think this is a way to teach women how to become objects of the male gaze. Nevertheless, my irritation does not rule out the return of good vibes. [–] A woman seeks intense eye contact with me and dances in a flirtatious way in front of me. (Field notes: tantric workshop, 2015)

This example also demonstrates how atmospheres are 'regulated' by moving (individual or collective) bodies and by organising the practices of proximity/distance. During the workshop, the attendees were actively made into a collective, as our personal boundaries were somewhat blurred by our being made to move in the space and make contact with others. However, when we were divided into two groups, the instructor's words now suggested the emergence of gendered and sexualised bodies rather than of an atmospheric collective, in contrast to the beginning when she had talked about uniting auras. Of course, we were still groups of 'women' and 'men' (despite the fact that these two groups were not formed in terms of 'being' any particular gender but rather of 'performing'). If atmospheres are invoked by environments that 'prime and cook affect' so as to prepare and induce bodies to perform in certain ways (Thrift, 2009: 88), we might think that here the bodies were quite literally being made to perform in certain ways, from activities such as hugging to gendering and sexualising processes.

However, the good vibes did return, and later the experience of attending this workshop inspired me to rethink the reasons why people invest in certain therapeutic events. For instance, despite the framework which stressed heterosexuality and binary gender roles, a 'queer' situation in which a woman approached me in a flirtatious way still took place (see also Kolehmainen, 2018). This in turn made me ponder to what extent people 'consume' experiences, atmospheres included, rather than advice, for example. Perhaps the workshop points to the ways in which collective experiences can be experienced *as* therapeutic in themselves, as they may provide welcome feelings or offer a means of social bonding, for instance. It would be reasonable to assume that people look for affective experiences when attending collective forms of the therapeutic realm such as the various events described in this chapter. Indeed, the experience of affect – rather than specific products – has become an important selling point in Western societies (Skeggs, 2005: 971), and this kind of experience is surely part of the allure of forms of therapeutic culture that are about collective events and favour the emergence of affective atmospheres.

Soaking up an atmosphere: atmospheres as therapeutic

Another example of getting caught in the atmosphere comes from an event that was very different from the tantric workshop, as it addressed separation and featured 'experts by experience' as its speakers. Of course, as a sensitive theme, separation is different from the playful tantric workshop. Atmospheres are about norms – about what *should* be felt (Bille et al., 2015) – and appropriate atmospheres differ in different situations such as these two events. Nevertheless, it is still possible to acknowledge here that the intimate atmosphere was intensified through various means and that it caught me despite the way I felt at the beginning of the event. On the morning of that day I had heard about the sudden death of a friend and long-term colleague, and I was saddened by the news. I had made plans to participate in the event, but I really did not feel like going after receiving this news. However, I had been in contact with the organisers beforehand and felt obliged to show up. I still remember the feeling of not wanting to go there. Perhaps not surprisingly, at first I felt out of place and irritated:

> Feeling irritated. [–] My head is congested and a little achy. (Field notes: event targeted at parents who are divorced or separated, 2016)

My remarks in my field notes are quite sour. I made critical comments about how the organisers presented their organisation and related activities, such as 'they just advertise their own organisation all the time', and as demonstrated above, I was not feeling well. However, I started to forget my frustration when the first lay expert shared their personal story. When the next experts by experience started to talk, I became so caught in the atmosphere that it felt inappropriate to make notes, and this highlights the challenges the study of atmospheres can pose for a researcher. It might feel intimidating to observe or make notes, as is demonstrated in the following example, a situation where Miriam (a mother) and Jenny (her daughter) gave a talk on divorce:

> Mother and daughter [–] are already in front (of us). They sit in armchairs next to each other; the chairs are closer to the audience than before the break. The situation is intimate, so I make hardly any notes but just write things down in retrospect from memory. (Field notes: event targeted at parents who are divorced or separated, 2016)

There were elements which created a sense of intimacy, such as the impression of confidential openness. Miriam and Jenny spoke about their personal experiences of divorce, Miriam from the perspective of a recent divorcee and Jenny from the perspective of a daughter of divorced parents. Miriam mentioned a few times in passing that she was 'certain that the right people are here'. In so doing, she actively addressed us as friends, allies or confidants. Atmospheres (also) come to matter through discourse (see Bille et al., 2015: 36), and the references to the 'right people' addressed the audience as a collective in a positive light. Hence, Miriam strongly contributed to the manufacturing of an intimate and warm atmosphere. Both physical and psychological proximity were created as Miriam seemed to talk as if the audience were full of close friends and acquaintances, and she was fairly close to the listeners, as remarked in my field notes. All these elements produced the impression of authenticity, which perhaps made the speakers appear 'genuine' people – and genuineness and authenticity are desired features in the assessment of atmospheres (see Bille et al., 2015).

Furthermore, Miriam and Jenny were sitting in armchairs – furniture usually found in living rooms or other cosy environments – which contributed to the making of a certain kind of atmosphere. Practices from interior design, landscape gardening and architecture, such as arranging light and sound, circumscribe atmospheres (Anderson, 2009). Here the armchairs undermined any obvious traces of authority, reaching beyond dichotomies of speaker/listener and expert/layperson. Furthermore, Miriam and Jenny sat next to each other and obviously had a close relationship, as they were able to talk about intimate family issues openly as mother and child. Unlike many of the expert speakers at the events I attended, they did not make a PowerPoint presentation, which further contributed to the unmaking of the distance between them and their audience. Although Miriam browsed her phone at least once in order to check the topics they had planned to speak about, all the self-evident symbols of a formal presentation were absent.

However, even though organisers and speakers engineer atmospheres in many ways, they themselves may also become affected by the atmosphere. In this case, Miriam and her husband had divorced less than a year before, after a long marriage, and Miriam was visibly moved, as I could see tears in her eyes. This highlights how bodies are located in a circuit of feeling and response (Hemmings, 2005: 551), capable of both being affected and affecting other bodies. The tears indicated a body 'in affect', being already affected – yet they also continued to affect other bodies and to produce a certain kind of atmosphere. Also, the way in which Miriam addressed 'the right people' can be seen as an indicator that atmosphere was important for her, raising the issue of how atmospheres matter not only from the perspective of participants but also from the perspective of experts. Even though Miriam and Jenny's personal motives were not known, the question of whether it is personally rewarding for lay experts to share their insights is still relevant.

Bodily in/capacities: limits of collective belonging?

Although I was very much caught in the intimate atmosphere described above, I faced the limits of collective belonging at another event targeting the divorced or separated. At the latter event there were two couple therapists acting as experts. It emerged from the questions posed to the therapists that there were people at this event who had just undergone break-ups and who were in great pain. I noticed that I too felt a little sad and occasionally had tears in my eyes. I cannot know whether this was due to some sort of affective resonance among us all, or my embodied attempts to fit in, or my being touched by the therapists' talk. However, when we moved on to a breathing practice, I noticed that my embodied experience was different compared with that of the participants who were undergoing a break-up process:

> We all stand up. One of the therapists jokingly says that we do not have to touch each other or anything like that. She says this is similar to a mindfulness or yoga exercise, not exactly like either of them, but this exercise borrows elements from that kind of practice. We close our eyes and breathe deeply. The situation reminds me of yoga and my breathing is effortless. [–] I am slightly amused by the fact that this mindfulness and belief in breathing and the like, this is now so widespread that even therapists rely on it. However, when the therapist asks us how we felt, a woman in front of me replies – to my surprise, perhaps – that a pressing feeling had emerged around her chest or neck, and another woman echoes her. I understand that those of us who are recently divorced or separated felt in a different way than I did,

and that their breathing wasn't as easy as mine. (Field notes: event targeted at the divorced or separated, 2016)

Despite the way I interpreted the situation in my field notes, I cannot know for sure how the actual embodied responses differed, or whether my own experience was really shaped by my not being in the midst of a separation project (perhaps it was about my association with yoga practice, which does not have much to do with the arrangement of intimate relationships). In any case, I remained unmarked by a pressing feeling. Affects can both draw us together and force us apart, and can signal a lack of any intersubjective connection (Hemmings, 2012; Juvonen and Kolehmainen, 2016; Seigworth and Gregg, 2010); here my lack of a certain embodied feeling appeared to mark the limits of shared mood or atmosphere. It was not about different meanings given to our breathing or to our embodied responses; our bodies became affected in different ways in this situation.

Further, this example illustrates how a body's in/capacities to affect and to become affected are the result of relations – not only of relations here and now, but also of past relations and relations to the past. I was able to relate to embodied feelings of break-up pain through my past experiences, but I remained untouched by any pressing feeling. In this way, my personal history became part of the affective assemblage and knowledge production, highlighting the temporal dimensions of affective assemblages and how they are constantly in flux. The affective relations within an assemblage may also comprise traces of the past and should not be understood in ways that exclude embodied, psychic and intangible experiences. This example also shows that human accounts – field notes included – can tell us about situatedness within assemblages rather than about individual reactions (see also Youdell and Armstrong, 2011: 145; Fox and Alldred, 2015: 409). The differences in bodily states indicate that the human bodies that participated in the breathing exercise were situated differently in the assemblage. Further, this exemplifies how similarities and differences are made, unmade and remade through affective atmospheres. Rather than seeing difference/similarity as a question of predefined, fixed and stable subject positions, we can understand difference and similarity as temporal products of shifting relations.

However, regardless of the differences in how I and some other people felt, I was still a part of the production of a situational affective atmosphere, doing the breathing exercise and trying to comply. Especially as this was an event that focused on separation, it felt ethically sound and respectful to those undergoing the process of separation to sense the atmosphere and be wary of causing any discomfort. My fieldwork indeed points to the myriad ways in which researchers participate in the co-production of atmospheres, from participating in activities that are designed to engineer a certain kind of atmosphere to simply being present.

Failing to feel it: on attempts to manipulate affect

On some other occasions when the atmosphere has not caught me, I have associated my not soaking it up with the way the particular event has been organised. For instance, while attending a seminar on well-being which also addressed relationships and sexuality, I became awkwardly aware of the commercial aspect of the event. There were two keynote speakers, introduced by a host – a man named Larry – whose presentation did not feel 'natural' to me, one reason for this being his use of language that I interpreted as being (overly) formal. Larry also introduced the two speakers, who entered the stage and started to discuss and debate different topics linked to the theme. However, I soon started to get the impression that the situation was highly scripted:

> Their lines sound memorised and play-acted. Somehow this situation feels pretty lame. (Field notes: seminar on well-being, 2017)

This experience offers an example of the ways in which 'authentic' and 'genuine' atmospheres are valued. Atmosphere is often thought of as being about something genuine or authentic, in contrast to staging, which is seen as artificial or simulated – even though people's experiences of environments are actually manipulated in many ways (Bille et al., 2015). Here my 'lame' feelings stemmed from a judgement concerning what I assumed was a staged situation, since the debate did not sound like a real debate but rather like a well-rehearsed play. Whereas the examples discussed above of getting caught in atmospheres point to intimacy, closeness and proximity, here the apparent staging highlighted the distance and hierarchy between the speakers and the audience and worked to distract me.

Further, this seminar is an example of how affective labour is invested in creating atmospheres. Whereas earlier capitalist production processes were connected to the production of material objects, contemporary commodities increasingly take the form of information, services, care, communication and affect, which all play central roles in new forms of labour (Hardt, 1999; Hardt and Negri, 2000, 2005; Lazzarato, 2004). In other words, the creation and manipulation of affects are forms of immaterial labour (Hardt, 1999), and this is what human investments in creating atmospheres are all about. Nevertheless, engineering atmospheres is an essential form of capitalisation upon affects. From the perspective of affective labour, then, it seems that affective labour which becomes 'too' visible produces the effect of inauthenticity, which in turn makes the situation appear staged. It was perhaps too obvious that the organisers had made preparations to produce an entertaining event, and their labour was 'revealed' as if they were trying to manipulate an atmosphere too forcefully.

My interpretation of the situation resulted in a distanced evaluation, which perhaps also made it challenging for me to let my body become affected. This illustrates how analysis emerges over time, and not only after fieldwork: before research begins, during live research encounters, and afterwards (Ringrose and Renold, 2014). Here my interpretation of the atmosphere at the time itself became an important part of the experience, which emphasises how atmospheres also challenge the dichotomy of experience/interpretation. It is essential to understand that atmospheres work in/through us, and this highlights that data can be viewed as alive – as active matter with which researchers may engage in open-ended ways (MacLure, 2013; Dernikos, 2018), even though data is often mistakenly regarded as stable, passive and raw (see also St Pierre et al., 2016). Even though my analysis has centred on the ways organisers and experts invest in creating atmospheres by various means, such as by organising practices of proximity/distance and intimacy/detachment, atmospheres cannot be reduced to being human-made, and nor can they be endlessly manipulated, as experiences of failing to get caught in an atmosphere indicate.

Conclusion

In this chapter, I have engaged with the issue of affective atmospheres in therapeutic engagements by drawing upon a study of relationship and sex counselling in Finland. Using my own researcher-body as a site of research, I analysed the experiences of soaking up atmospheres, moving in/out of affective atmospheres, feeling the limits of collective belonging, and failing to 'get' the atmosphere when conducting fieldwork at various events. By drawing upon assemblage theory and new materialist ontology, I have proposed that the exploration of atmospheres offers novel insights into therapeutic cultures, as it makes it possible to move away from human-centred notions of the therapeutic, such as the preoccupation with the self. Affective atmospheres stress how situational and material therapeutic practices operate in/through both human and non-human bodies. Further, therapeutics in itself can be seen as an ever-becoming, vital assemblage of a variety of situational and material practices, objects and things – an aspect that has been much ignored in previous studies. In the majority of studies on therapeutics, the focus has been on top-down approaches which stress how therapeutic discourses are mobilised to govern populations (Salmenniemi, 2017; Kolehmainen, 2018). Approaches of this kind do not acknowledge the lived, networked, relational and embodied experiences that therapeutics are about. The investigation of atmospheres shifts the focus from the self to the collective, from advice-giving to experience, and from governmentality to lived experience.

Therapeutic cultures have been criticised for severing the self from communal relations and fostering an atomistic individualism where the self is cut away from meaningful social and political content (see Illouz, 2008). However, my analysis of affective atmospheres at various events related to relationship and sex counselling speaks to the importance of understanding the therapeutic realm through collective experiences too (see also Perheentupa in this book). The therapeutic ethos does not only manifest itself in the blossoming of psychological discourses as resources for making the self, in the popularity of private counselling sessions, or in the growth of self-help technologies; many kinds of collective or public events also form an essential part of the therapeutic realm. In this way – and even when they employ individualistic discourses – such events also provide concrete arenas for collective experience. To register an atmosphere is to sense a connection, which may feel therapeutic in itself; and to fail to catch it may intensify feelings of non-belonging, rendering one more vulnerable. I hope that future studies will elaborate further on how collective atmospheres contribute to the therapeutic.

Notes

1 All the names in this chapter are pseudonyms.
2 This work was funded by the Academy of Finland project *Just the two of us? Affective Inequalities in Intimate Relationships* (grant number 287983).

References

Anderson, B. 2009. Affective atmospheres. *Emotion, Space and Society 2*, 77–81.

Bille, M., P. Bjerregaard and T. Flohr Sørensen. 2015. Staging atmospheres: Materiality, culture, and the texture of the inbetween. *Emotion, Space and Society 15*, 31–38.

Blackman, L. 2015. Researching affect and embodied hauntologies: Exploring an analytics of experimentation. In B.T. Knudsen and C. Stage (eds), *Affective Methodologies*. Basingstoke: Palgrave Macmillan, 25–43.

Bryld, M. and N. Lykke. 2000. *Cosmodolphins: Feminist Cultural Studies of Technology, Animals and the Sacred*. London: Zed Books.

Colebrook, C. 2002. *Gilles Deleuze*. London: Routledge.

Coleman, R. and J. Ringrose. 2013. Introduction: Deleuze and research methodologies. In R. Coleman and J. Ringrose (eds), *Deleuze and Research Methodologies*. Edinburgh: Edinburgh University Press, 1–22.

De Landa, M. 2006. *A New Philosophy of Society: Assemblage Theory and Social Complexity*. London: Continuum.

Deleuze, G. and F. Guattari. 2004. *A Thousand Plateaus: Capitalism and Schizophrenia*. London: Continuum.

Dernikos, B.P. 2018. Reviving ghostly bodies: Student-teacher intimacies as affective hauntings. In T. Juvonen and M. Kolehmainen (eds), *Affective Inequalities in Intimate Relationships*. London: Routledge, 218–230.

Fox, N.J. and P. Alldred. 2015. New materialist social inquiry: Designs, methods and the research-assemblage. *International Journal of Social Research Methodology 18*:4, 399–414.

Fox, N.J. and P. Alldred. 2017. *Sociology and the New Materialism: Theory, Research, Action*. London and New York: Sage.

Furedi, F. 2006. *Therapy Culture: Cultivating Vulnerability in an Uncertain Time*. London: Routledge.

Gherardi, S. 2018. Theorizing affective ethnography for organization studies. *Organization* (OnlineFirst). https://doi.org/10.1177/1350508418805285.

Hardt, M. 1999. Affective labor. *Boundary 26*:2, 89–100.

Hardt, M. and A. Negri. 2000. *Empire*. Cambridge, MA: University of Harvard Press.

Hardt, M. and A. Negri. 2005. *Multitude*. London: Hamish Hamilton.

Hemmings, C. 2005. Invoking affect: Cultural theory and the ontological turn. *Cultural Studies 19*:5, 548–567.

Hemmings, C. 2012. Affective solidarity: Feminist reflexivity and political transformation. *Feminist Theory 13*:2, 147–161.

Illouz, E. 2008. *Saving the Modern Soul: Therapy, Emotions, and the Culture of Self-Help*. Berkeley: California University Press.

Juvonen, T. and M. Kolehmainen. 2016. Seeing the colors of the rainbows: Affective politics of queer belonging. *SQS Journal 10*:1–2, vi–x.

Kinnunen, T. and M. Kolehmainen. 2019. Touch and affect: Analysing the archive of touch biographies. *Body and Society 25*:1, 29–56.

Knudsen, B.T. and C. Stage. 2015. Introduction: Affective methodologies. In B.T. Knudsen and C. Stage (eds), *Affective Methodologies*. Basingstoke: Palgrave Macmillan, 1–22.

Kolehmainen, M. 2018. Mapping affective capacities: Gender and sexuality in relationship and sex counselling practices. In T. Juvonen and M. Kolehmainen (eds), *Affective Inequalities in Intimate Relationships*. London: Routledge, 63–78.

Kolehmainen, M. and T. Juvonen. 2018. Introduction: Thinking with and through affective inequalities. In T. Juvonen and M. Kolehmainen (eds), *Affective Inequalities in Intimate Relationships*. London: Routledge, 1–16.

Lahti, A. 2018. Listening to old tapes: Affective intensities and gendered power in bisexual women's and ex-partners' relationship assemblages. In T. Juvonen and M. Kolehmainen (eds), *Affective Inequalities in Intimate Relationships*. London: Routledge, 49–62.

Law, J. 2004. *After Method: Mess in Social Science Research*. London: Routledge.

Lazzarato, M. 2004. From capital-labour to capital-life. *Ephemera 43*:3, 187–208.

MacLure, M. 2013. Classification or wonder? Coding as an analytic practice in qualitative research. In B. Coleman and J. Ringrose (eds), *Deleuze and Research Methodologies*. Edinburgh: Edinburgh University Press, 164–183.

McRobbie, A. 2009. *The Aftermath of Feminism: Gender, Culture and Social Change*. London: Sage.

Madsen, O.J. and B. Ytre-Arne. 2012. Me at my best: Therapeutic ideals in Norwegian women's magazines. *Communication, Culture and Critique 5*:1, 20–37.

Maksimainen, J. 2014. Avioliiton pelastamisesta parisuhteen hoitamiseen: Muodosta sisältöön [From saving marriages to taking care of relationships: Moving from form to content]. *Sosiologia 51*:2, 123–138.

Massumi, B. 2004. Notes on the translation and acknowledgements. In G. Deleuze and F. Guattari (eds), *A Thousand Plateaus*. Minneapolis: University of Minnesota Press, ix–xvi.

Ouellette, L. and J. Wilson. 2011. Women's work: Affective labour and convergence culture. *Cultural Studies 25*:4–5, 548–565.

Pedwell, C. and A. Whitehead. 2012. Affecting feminism: Questions of feeling in feminist theory. *Feminist Theory 13*:2, 115–129.

Ringrose, E. and J. Renold. 2014. 'F**k rape!' Exploring affective intensities in a feminist research assemblage. *Qualitative Inquiry 20*:6, 772–780.

Salmenniemi, S. 2017. 'We can't live without beliefs': Self and society in therapeutic engagements. *Sociological Review 65*:4, 611–627.

Seigworth, G.J. and M. Gregg. 2010. An inventory of shimmers. In G.J. Seigworth and M. Gregg (eds), *Affect Theory Reader*. Durham and London: Duke University Press, 1–25.

Seyfert, R. 2012. Beyond personal feelings and collective emotions: Towards a theory of social affect. *Theory, Culture and Society 29*:6, 27–46.

Skeggs, B. 2005. The making of class and gender through visualizing moral subject formation. *Sociology 39*:5, 965–982.

Stewart, K. 2017. In the world that affect proposed. *Cultural Anthropology 32*:2, 192–198.

St Pierre, E.A., A.Y. Jackson and L. Mazzei. 2016. New empiricisms and new materialisms: Conditions for new inquiry. *Cultural Studies ↔ Critical Methodologies 16*:2, 99–110.

Swan, E. 2008. Therapeutic cultures and the contagion of femininity. *Gender, Work and Organization 15*:1, 88–107.

Thrift, N. 2009. Understanding the affective spaces of political performances. In M. Smith, J. Davidson, L. Cameron and L. Bondi (eds), *Emotion, Place and Culture*. Farnham: Ashgate, 79–95.

Walkerdine, V. 2010. Communal beingness and affect: An exploration of trauma in an ex-industrial community. *Body and Society 16*:1, 91–116.

Wetherell, M. 2012. *Affect and Emotion: A New Social Science Understanding*. London: Sage.

Wood, H. and B. Skeggs. 2004. Notes on ethical scenarios of self on British reality television. *Feminist Media Studies 4*:2, 205–208.

Youdell, D. and F. Armstrong. 2011. A politics beyond subjects: The affective choreographies and smooth spaces of schooling. *Emotion, Space and Society 4*:3, 144–150.

4 Therapeutic and *therapeia* within Orthodox Christianity

Tatiana Tiaynen-Qadir

Significant scholarship has illustrated that the modern self-help and therapeutic ethos originates in Protestant Christianity (Illouz, 2008; Woodstock, 2005; Nehring, et al. 2016).[1] For instance, the prolific American self-help genre with its positive thinking can be traced back to late 19th century religious manuals, in which readers were encouraged to control and direct their thoughts so that they 'mirrored' the intentions of God (Woodstock, 2005: 157). In the 1950s, the self-help genre's God was 'generous' and 'full of sweetness' only to disappear from 1990s self-help books altogether (Woodstock, 2005: 165, 175). Referring to the US context of the 1970s, Lasch famously noted that the American cultural climate was no longer religious but deeply therapeutic, producing self-centered and self-absorbed individuals unmindful of salvation (Lasch, 1991: 7). Some research on the Nordic context shows that self-help may also form a kind of alliance with Protestant religion to meet the needs of modern individuals (Madsen, 2012; Ratinen, 2017). Madsen argues that the therapeutic turn has altered Western Christianity, in which God is increasingly ascribed a supportive role of therapist and as a remedy for promoting people's well-being (Madsen, 2012, 2014).

Yet there has been little research on other branches of Christianity with different historical and cultural trajectories and where therapy as a cure of soul and body has also been a vital component for centuries. What kind of therapeutic do we find there? Do we observe similar taming of religion by the therapeutic ethos or perhaps more complex interplay between traditional religious cure and the modern therapeutic (see also Lerner in this book). In this chapter, I explore this important yet under-researched theme by focusing on therapeutic knowledge and practices within Finnish Orthodoxy. Has Finnish Orthodoxy transformed in the face of the therapeutic turn, and if so, how?

I approach both religion and therapeutic knowledge and practices through the lens of *glocalization* that addresses 'the ways in which homogenizing and heterogenizing tendencies are mutually implicative' and historically constituted (Robertson, 1995: 27). Self-help worlds are shaped through the multidirectional processes, in which global and local cultural forms merge, interact and transform (Nehring et al., 2016). Similarly, Finnish Orthodoxy can be seen as a *glocal religion* that developed as a result of concrete historical processes involving a fusion between religious universalism and local particularism (Roudometof, 2014). On the one hand, in its structure, rituals, and theology it is linked to global Orthodox space and histories, on the other hand, it evolved as a particular glocal version of Orthodox Christianity, which combines Finnish, Karelian, Russian, and Byzantine elements (Tiaynen-Qadir, 2017). It is a national church in Finland with a strong national identity, but it also generates a transnational space that incorporates migrants from different cultural and linguistic backgrounds.

I suggest that therapeutic knowledge and practices within Finnish Orthodoxy are best understood through the concept of *glocalized therapeutic assemblage*. This captures the glocal process whereby a diverse set of therapeutic and self-help discursive practices –irreducible to a singular logic –is assembled and entwined (Tiaynen-Qadir and Salmenniemi, 2017). This concept combines the glocalization perspective (as discussed above) with sociological theorizing on assemblages (Collier and Ong, 2005; Zigon, 2010, 2011). However, the sociological lens does not preclude the possibility, indeed the need, of understanding the importance of embodied practices of religion and material religion: sensations, feelings, rhythms, the unspoken, something that lies beyond the realm of cognition (Morgan, 2005; Meyer and Verrips, 2008; Opas and Haapalainen, 2017). Glocal therapeutic assemblage is produced and embedded in complex and historically situated interaction of human and non-human actors, in which the body emerges as the matrix of human experiences.

This chapter is an anthropological investigation of such an assemblage within Finnish Orthodoxy. It draws on my long-term ethnographic fieldwork in one of the parishes of the Orthodox Church of Finland (OCF), which serves as a dynamic site of multicultural and multilinguistic interaction. The main argument presented here is that people's experiences and narratives paint a picture of the therapeutic as a glocalized assemblage that merges various elements together, but in which age-old Orthodox cure of soul and body, *therapeia*, continues to serve as a grounding and constitutive frame. Some practitioners activate psychologizing narratives to articulate some benefits of Orthodox practices for mental health. However, these are minor compared with the varieties of narration techniques, and poetic, spiritual, and religious terms used by individuals to talk about their lived and embodied experiences of religion. In these narratives, the therapeutic does not necessarily figure as the telos of religious practices, but rather, as one of my interlocutors puts it, as their 'by-product'. For Orthodox, therapeutic is more than merely psychologizing well-being discourse, and is closely intertwined with *therapeia*, which has long roots in this religious tradition.

Finnish Orthodoxy and therapeutic turn

Orthodoxy in Finland dates back to the eleventh century: it was indigenized in the region of Karelia under the influence of Novgorodians, who adopted this religion from the Byzantines through Kiev at the end of the 10th century (Martikainen and Laitila, 2014: 153). Throughout history, Orthodox Christianity remained a minority religion in Finland with culturally and historically dominant Lutheranism.

The histories of Finnish Orthodoxy embraced numerous people's dislocations, resettlements, enforced and voluntary moves, as well as alleged tensions between Karelian and Russian Orthodox identities (for detailed historical accounts of these histories see Martikainen and Laitila, 2014). After Finland gained independence from Russia in 1917, OCF became an autonomous Finnish Orthodox archdiocese of the Patriarchate of Constantinople in 1923.

As I have illustrated elsewhere, Finnish Orthodoxy can be seen as a glocal religion that incorporates national and transnational histories and elements (Tiaynen-Qadir, 2017). On the one hand, OCF went through intense nationalization in the 20th century, and has become a national church of a religious minority, amounting to approximately 1.1 per cent of the total population in Finland. On the other hand, starting from the 1990s it has gone through a dynamic process of transnationalization, incorporating migrants from the Eastern European heartlands of Orthodoxy, especially Russian-speakers. Although Finnish is the main liturgical language, church services are also held in Church Slavonic, Ancient Greek, Romanian, Serbian, and English. In its aesthetics – church architecture and interior, icons, and music –OCF variably integrates Byzantine, Russian, and Karelian features (Hanka, 2008; Husso, 2011; Seppälä, 2013; Virolainen, 2013). The Finnish liturgy continues to follow the Russian Orthodox tradition of multivocal choir singing, rather than the Byzantine single-voice. Hymns and chants sung during liturgy include old Valaam, Byzantine, and Slavic chants, as well as compositions by Finnish and Russian composers. In its glocal manifestation, OCF is rather unique in contrast to other Orthodox churches in the world, which are either organized as national or diasporic churches.

In many ways, the aesthetic side of Orthodox rites and materiality also stood for its growing popularity in the 'Romantic movement' starting in the 1970s that appreciated the Byzantine art of icons. The archaic beauty of Orthodoxy was acclaimed among some Finnish intellectuals and artists. At the same time, the church became more liberal in incorporating its members, and more active in ecumenical activity and cooperation with the Evangelical Lutheran Church of Finland. OCF also started to emphasize more pronouncedly therapeutic sides of Orthodoxy, offering 'silence retreats', open to anyone whether a member of the church or not. The New Valaam Monastery in Heinävesi and the Sofia Cultural Center in Helsinki organize a variety of courses, ranging from 'icon clinics' to those that combine Orthodox mysticism, psychical exercises in nature, and 'personal spiritual guidance' (Ortodoksiviesti, 2016: 45). Some Finnish theologians emphasize the 'healing' qualities of the church (*parantava kirkko*) and church service (*parantava liturgia*), metaphorically equating the church with a 'spiritual clinic' (Hakkarainen, 2016). Others underline the therapeutic effect of divine beauty as the 'language of God' (Seppälä, 2010).

Such an articulated emphasis on the therapeutic within official church rhetoric and theology in Finland can doubtless be seen as a response to the therapeutic turn. It emerges as a reaction to the growing industry of happiness and self-help in Finland (Salmenniemi, 2016). Yet the glocal nature of this reaction is also evident in the frequent references of the Finnish theologians of the Orthodox psychotherapy – Jarmo Hakkarainen and Pentti Hakkarainen – to the Greek Metropolitan Hierotheos of Nafpaktos, known for his formulation of Orthodox Christianity as 'therapeutic method' and 'therapeutic science' (Hierotheos, 1993; Hierotheos, 1994; see also Stanley and Kortelainen in this book).

However, this reaction is not so much about the integration of psychology into the modern Orthodox theology, but more about reviving *therapeia* (from Greek θεραπεία, healing and service to God), based on patristic tradition and texts. In Eastern Christianity, there is an age-old tradition of writing spiritual guidance texts. Many of them are still in use and read by contemporary practitioners, for instance Abba Dorotheos's 'Direction of Spiritual Teaching'. The healing powers and attributes of Jesus, 'physician of our souls and bodies', Mary, and many saints also figure in liturgical texts and daily prayers, which again originate in ancient texts. In fact, the very formulation of the Orthodox psychotherapeutic method can be interpreted as a reaction to the global legitimizing of professional psychology and the spread of popular psychology, and the emphasis on *therapeia* is an attempt to strengthen the Orthodox vision of the self, different from a 'psychology without a soul' (Hierotheos, 1993: 46). In this sense, Orthodox *therapeia* resonates with some self-help, esoteric, and New Age strands that challenge secular psychologies (Hanegraaf, 1999; Heelas, 2009; Stanley and Kortelainen in this book).

The metaphysics of the ontological architecture of the cosmos, and the symbolic architecture of the self in Orthodoxy are complex and theosophical in their nature. Unavoidably resorting to simplification, one can say that the triadic dimension of the self, which includes mind, body, and *soul*, lies at the core of the Orthodox understanding of the self. In Orthodox theology, the soul is created in the image of God, and the *nous* is 'the eye of the soul', its 'essence' and 'heart' (Hierotheos, 1994: 119–120). According to Orthodox psychotherapy, the illness of the soul is in the darkening of the *nous,* which was caused by the rebellion of reason against the *nous,* signifying the Fall of Man. This darkness can ultimately be cured by the reconnection with God or the attainment of *theosis,* identified with *theoria,* the vision of God (Hierotheos, 1993: 46). *Noetic hesychia,* translated as stillness and silence from Ancient Greek, is a ceaseless and contemplative prayer, a certain state of being and perceiving the world, and a practice that enables entering into theoria. Following 14th century Gregory Palamas, Mary is portrayed as an epitome of *hesychia,* who is in his words: 'finds holy *hesychia* her guide: silencing the mind, the world standing still, things below forgotten, sharing of the secrets above, laying aside conceptual images for what is better' (Hierotheos, 1994: 317).

Ethnography of the tacit

From the very beginning of my ethnographic fieldwork, I could see that instances of both modern therapy and traditional Orthodox cure of soul and body were variably present in my interlocutors' narratives and experiences. However, articulating the interplay of such instances through a *glocal therapeutic assemblage* has required a great deal of time, immersion, analytical efforts, critical reflection, and a continuous dialog between theory and practice (Cerwonka and Malkki, 2007). However time-consuming, ethnography is best suited to articulate taken-for-granted aspects of thought and behavior, including spontaneous verbal, emotional, and bodily reactions that standard survey methods are unable to tap into (Gupta and Ferguson, 1997). The embodied presence in the field enables ethnography of the tacit, something which is not or only spontaneously articulated in speech.

I conducted my fieldwork research between 2014 and 2017. My fieldwork included participation and non-participant observation in a church setting, including informal gatherings, clubs, church services, and choir practices. The church serves as the spiritual and social environment of a vibrant multicultural community within the parish in western Finland. Overall, I recorded ethnographic interviews with 24 practitioners, most of whom were women of Finnish, Russian, Ukrainian, and Greek origins. Most were teachers, university lecturers, accountants, researchers, and doctors, and had a university degree. I also recorded interviews with two men, but I have had numerous informal discussions with male practitioners and priesthood beyond the recorded mode. In addition, I have also read and used the periodicals issued by the OCF. My ethnographic practice has been improvisatory, interactive, and reflexive in its nature, and built on non-hierarchical and non-objectifying terms between the researcher and the researched (Cerwonka and Malkki, 2007; Ingold, 2013).

Following standard research ethics, I have anonymized all the names, the location of the church, and refer primarily to recorded interviews. Thus, women's experiences have received more attention in this chapter. Although I rely mostly on interviews, the findings presented here should be seen as part of my long-term immersion in the field. In my broader engagement with Orthodox practitioners, participant observation, informal engagement, and unexpected encounters often yielded deep insights and understandings of the researched phenomena that help to contextualize and situate the recorded interviews. Similarly, my long-term participation in choir practices and church services was vital for understating and relating to the experiences that my interlocutors narrated. For instance, over these years, the Orthodox service has unfolded for me as an event that holistically summons the acts of seeing, hearing, singing, smelling, etc. Such bodily responses combine with cognitive apprehension for the perpetual production of the sacred in a multilayered process of never-ending unveiling. In this sense, the chapter represents my experiences of an opening on the social reality of Orthodox faithful rather than an attempt at its closure (as discussed generically by Ingold, 2013). Such an opening has enabled me to analytically weave very different and diverse aspects of my interlocutors' life stories and practices into an initial ethnographic exploration, focusing on therapeutic knowledge and practices within Orthodox Christianity.

Therapeutic and *therapeia* in Divine Liturgy

My ethnographic research shows how much importance people place on participating in a church service, especially the Divine Liturgy. Liturgy stands for the recreation and celebration of the Kingdom of Heaven, as well as symbolic and actual reliving of the mystery of the Last Supper. It has been described as a 'synthesis of arts' that encompasses the art of fire or burning candles, choir singing, priestly conduct, church poetry, incense dissolved in the air, and the art of icons and frescos (Florensky, [1918] 2002). As I have discussed elsewhere, individual artistry is pertinent to unique experiences of this church art (Tiaynen-Qadir, 2017).

Receiving the Holy Communion, or Eucharist, is the culmination of the liturgy and symbolizes the cleansing and sanctification of soul and body. Thus, upon receiving the Eucharist, participants of the liturgy greet each other by saying, 'to the cure of soul and body' (*sielun ja ruumiin parannukseksi*), to which the standard reply is, 'in honor of God' (*Jumalan kunniaksi*). The texts sung and recited during liturgy, including blessings of water at certain occasions, contain numerous references to the 'health of soul and body'. These texts are mostly of ancient origins and draw on the two most frequently used liturgies developed by John Chrysostom and St. Basil the Great in late antiquity. In other words, discourses of cure and health of body and soul are age-old in the context of Eastern liturgy.

The persistence of age-old terms for cure and soul in liturgical texts does not automatically mean that practitioners perceive these words in the same way as participants of liturgy in 8th century Byzantium. Therapeutic ethos is a global phenomenon, and is increasingly bound to our modern condition (Illouz, 2008; Furedi, 2004). People globally conceive of themselves and seek to improve their lives in popular psychology terms and metaphors. Transnational therapeutic language of selfhood is circulated and reinforced by books, wellness and health style courses, TV counseling, yoga, New Age spiritualities, and a growing number of other channels, including in Finland (Woodstock, 2005; Salmenniemi, 2010, 2016; Rimke, 2000; Heelas, 2009; Lerner, 2011). Therapeutic selfhood has also affected how some of my interlocutors perceive liturgy.

For instance, some choir members pointed out that singing during liturgy helps them to keep a 'balance', that it is 'satisfying' and 'rewarding'. They emphasized a 'therapeutic' and 'calming' effect of singing during liturgy. Such formulations are in dialog with 'therapeutic' and 'cleansing' effects of Orthodox singing that have been discussed in several articles of the OCF periodicals (Sjöberg, 2013; Kallio, 2018). Moreover, it was also noted that the purpose of 'sacred songs' is not to heal or cure, but to reach for the sacred (Sjöberg, 2013).

Some interlocutors also emphasized the benefits of singing for emotional and physical well-being. Roosa has been singing in a church for over 20 years. She regularly and devotedly participates in and sings during liturgy. Roosa recollects that the first time she came to the church was by accident. She was struck by the 'beauty of singing', and immediately asked if she could join the choir. She mentioned that singing in a choir was good for her 'mental health'. At some point in her life she also attended yoga courses. In fact, she did not attend choir practices for about two years some time ago, having joined a meditation group instead. But she told me that it did not work for her in the same way, and she was eager to return to her singing in the church.

Another interlocutor, Alina, articulated quite clearly that for her 'religion is therapy'. She humorously noted that she had traveled a long path from being a 'militant atheist' to becoming a practicing Orthodox Christian. In her early twenties, along with hundreds of people, Alina was kept as a hostage for three days in the 'sadly famous' Nord-Ost siege in the Moscow Dubrovka Theater in 2002. It was a 'life-turning experience' that made her realize that dying without faith must be dreadfully disturbing and uncomfortable. Afterward, Alina turned for help to a psychologist, but also sought more ground to meet her spiritual needs. She turned to Orthodox Christianity as a tradition culturally proximate to her that she had a sense of due to her grandmother. Alina told me that she thoroughly enjoyed singing in the church choir. In a light and laughing manner, typical of her, she likened her choir singing to 'manna from heaven' and said that she especially liked the physical sensation of 'producing a sound out of her body', especially in 'company' with other people.

The very use of the term 'therapeutic' in its functional and psychologizing sense points to the effect of the modern therapeutic discourses on how liturgy and singing are perceived. However, these examples, discussed previously, also show that 'therapeutic' means quite different things for different interlocutors. While some relate it to their emotional well-being, others use this term to refer to the effect of 'sacred' singing. However, as discussed here, these psychologizing narratives are combined with the diverse range of other narration techniques that people utilize to talk of their experiences of the liturgy.

My other interlocutor Vera, a psychiatrist by occupation, stressed that liturgy could be a 'powerful support for psyche', and 'every second' among her patients 'probably needs faith' to be cured. These were her personal reflections that she shared privately in a conversation with me; naturally she was not allowed to mention church or God to her patients. Yet that was the only time when she used the language of psychology to talk of liturgy. In contrast, when she wished to share her personal experiences of liturgy, she turned to more poetic terms and even seemed to be short of words:

> Solemnity. Sometimes there is such moment in life, some kind of breakdown. Not like some kind of quarrel, but some serious stress. Somebody got sick or some problems, for instance, at a work place. And there is a feeling [*oshchushchenie*] of tearfulness, a feeling that it is bad. And then it is gone. And there is a peak of bliss. And tears stream down, I don't know... I don't know how to explain it as it is, well, difficult to do it. Well, you know, when you say that you are extremely deeply moved. There is this very feeling [*oshchushchenie*]...well, you know, it is actually overwhelming you, and there is a lump in the throat...I don't know, it is difficult to explain.

On one hand, there are some elements of the functional therapeutic explanation in this extract as liturgy figures as a way of overcoming a 'breakdown' and problems at work. On the other hand, it also illustrates how Vera resorts to description of her sensations and such uncontrolled bodily reactions as 'tears' or a 'lump in the throat' to point to the overwhelmingly moving effect of liturgy. Although the language of psychology is easily accessible to Vera due to her professional training, she does not claim liturgy to have a therapeutic effect on her, but poetically refers to 'solemnity' and 'a peak of bliss'. Vera applies the Russian word *oshchushchenie* that does not have any direct translation in English. This term is also frequently applied by other Russian-speaking interlocutors. Its use is important as this term implies a 'subjective image' of the world and encompasses the whole range of senses and sensations, tangible and emotional experiences and perceptions.

Many other women from different backgrounds utilize similar narration strategies. They describe their sensorial experiences of liturgy and unexpected bodily reactions in order to point to the importance of 'reaching beyond'. Many stress that they like the smell in the church or that choir singing 'touches the very soul' or 'moves one to tears'. They talk of the feeling of 'trembling' or 'goose bumps' on the body. Most women recounted moments when they were touched to tears during liturgy and other church services. Some men too, although more reserved verbally in their articulation of the sensorial, pointed out that sometimes liturgy is 'especially touching'. For instance, Victor mentioned to me that one has to be 'open' during liturgy, and sometimes something else 'opens' up within the self. These uncontrolled bodily reactions were talked of in a very different way from publicly encouraged articulations of bodily signs of the presence of God in Pentecostalism (de Witte, 2017). In Orthodoxy, those reactions were not to be demonstrated, but rather kept to oneself.

When people were sharing those experiences with me, they would sometimes start speaking quieter, almost whispering. One does this usually when sharing something intimate and personal. I found this carefulness in articulating the 'blessed tearfulness' – as one of my interlocutors put it – to be very much in line with the apophatic approach in Orthodoxy. According to this approach, the mystical realm of God is inexpressible in human terms and verbal expressions, and, therefore, any attempts at articulating it inevitably leads to simplifications and human-bound rationalization. Yet this reality is bodily mediated (Lossky, [1957]1976). Consequently, when people somehow reach out to this perceived reality, these experiences are not normally talked of or over-emphasized. Similarly, my interlocutors were very careful in how they talked of their experiences of the divine, and especially if and how they mentioned God. If anything, God was not perceived as a therapist, but rather as incomprehensible and indescribable in human words, as belonging to an invisible realm that surpasses human understanding and experience.

Yet, people referred to moments or glimpses of the divine presence during liturgy. Some could point to specific prayers or hymns sung during liturgy that enabled some deeper insight and experience into the beyond. It could be the ancient Trisagion prayer ('Holy God, Holy Mighty One, Holy Immortal One, have mercy on us'), which 'reaches' individuals through the medium of different languages and varying music arrangements. Some are 'deeply moved' when it is performed in Finnish as a 'Slavic melody' or as a Byzantine chant adopted for choral singing in Finnish. Others point out that it 'reaches to them' when it is sung in Ancient Greek or Church Slavonic, and as a Byzantine chant. The glocal nature of liturgy in OCF enables these various experiences for people from different backgrounds.

Similarly, the famous 'Cherubim Hymn, a song of the angels' was mentioned as one that 'moves beyond the self'. The singing choir 'mystically represents the Cherubim', and 'chant the thrice-holy hymn to the Life-giving Trinity'. For instance, Victoria told me that at some point when the 'Cherubim Hymn' was sung during one of the liturgies, the text from the Revelation (New Testament) that describes John's vision of the throne of God, 'became alive'. Likewise, Johanna and Anfisa, who sing in the choir, pointed out that sometimes there is a feeling that the hymn is actually sung through you, and the body becomes a medium or an instrument. Both mentioned that they feel blessed and happy to be able to sing to 'the glory of God'. However, the feeling of joy and happiness that they refer to seems to be quite different from psychologizing narratives of happiness:

> There is kind of self-evident in the church that you are never ready, no perfect. And it is great in any case to sing to the glory of God… All services are different, spring, winter, it all matters…sometimes very often you sing the same verses, and you want to make them sound perfect…sometimes when the choir is not so big, then the feeling of calmness comes, and alongside this feeling, there is a sense as if there is a group that sings, and as if you are actually not in the choir, but listen to what this group sings. This feeling is very rare, but it also comes with a sense of silent ecstasy (Johanna).

> These are the tears of happiness that you can be here. This is such a great blessing to be there, breathe that air, be able to sing to the glory of God. It is not possible to describe it. One has to really merely stand there and feel it. And there is always some trembling [in the body]. And when you leave the temple, and everything went well. And then you understand that it is not because of us, it is not our merits, that everything went well. But everything went fine, and there were less mistakes, and the sound was beautiful, and you feel it, and other people feel it…and then people come and thank you. But how can you explain people: "It is not me, understand me. It is not me. I am the instrument" (Anfisa).

Johanna came to the choir around 20 years ago, and seven years later had joined the Orthodox church upon realizing that 'her knowledge of Orthodoxy will never be perfect'. Anfisa joined the church three years ago, after she had migrated to Finland, and then joined the choir around one year ago. Interestingly, despite the difference in these women's life trajectories and the years of engagement with Orthodoxy, there is a great deal of convergence in how they narrate of their experiences of the divine presence during liturgy.

Their narratives of happiness, blessing, calmness, and silent ecstasy fall closely in line with Orthodox *therapeia*, in which the cure of the soul is associated with stillness of the soul, vision of God, and heavenly ecstasy (Hierotheos, 1994: 315). According to Orthodox tradition, some saints were indeed able to attain such a vision, and maintained a state of being 'cured' through their prayers and hesychia more or less permanently. Yet, for most people, such a state is attainable only momentarily, when one can 'touch the untouchable and blessed essence' (Hierotheos, 1994: 145). I find that many of my interlocutors refer to exactly this kind of therapeutic effect of liturgy, which is associated with 'joy', 'solemnity', 'serenity', 'calmness' and 'peace', and the glimpses of the divine presence. In their narratives, moving beyond the self to reconnect with the divine has been an unpredictable outcome, but at the same time a telos and cure of liturgy.

Stories of miraculous intervention and recoveries

While my interlocutors have been generally reserved in how they verbalized the realm of the Trinitarian God, they seemed to have been a bit more at ease to talk about instances of miraculous intervention and recoveries either in their own lives or the lives of relatives, friends, and acquaintances. It is important to emphasize that stories of miraculous healing have been part of the Christian tradition for centuries, and the fact that people turn to such stories is not a new phenomenon in itself. Yet in some cases they would share a story, but asked me not to refer to it in my publications. In my understanding, this carefulness partly derived from the Orthodox apophatic approach, and partly from the personal experiences of living in a predominantly secular context where such stories are readily ridiculed (see also Andell et al. in this book). Some emphasized that I should understand that in Orthodoxy such stories are not usually shared, and must remain in the domain of unspoken and personal experiences of the sacred.

Thus, the stories that I was allowed to write about are only the tip of the iceberg and many remain untold. However, these stories told by modern practitioners are important as they allude to an important aspect of the therapeutic. This is connected to the Orthodox traditional understanding of cure and illness, and challenges the secular perception of reality and the self. These stories have been part of naturally occurring conversation between my interlocutors and I, and are classified here under the following two groups only for analytical purposes.

The first group includes stories of the women that told me how their infertility was cured or their children were healed due to divine intervention. In many stories, divine intervention is mediated through the Mother of God, as Mary is mainly referred to in Orthodoxy. In Orthodoxy, the Virgin is often seen as a perfection of humankind (Schmemann, 1991). Her figure also serves as a source of identification for women: she is approached as the one who understands a mother's pain, sorrow, worries, and joy, but also has invincible powers to intercede and cure (Vuola, 2010; Tiaynen-Qadir, 2016). For instance, Marja, a mother with a Finnish background, told me that once her son got seriously ill and she had to leave him in the hospital. He was six years old at that time. She came home with a heavy heart, and prayed devotedly to the Mother of God in front of an icon that Marja's grandfather had painted for her birthday. The same day Marja received a call from the hospital that she could come and take her son home: he had recovered. She told me that she kept that story to herself, and did not share it with her friends or colleagues, who would most probably not believe her or would 'ridicule' the story. Yet, for Marja it was a miracle, and a sign of divine help and the healing powers of the Virgin.

Miira, another woman of Finnish background, told me that 12 years ago she visited the Greek island of Rhodes and came to pray in front of the famous icon of the Virgin *Panaghia Tsambika*. In Greek, the Virgin is often referred to as *Panaghia*, which can be translated as 'above all saints'. *Tsambika* derives from the local word *tsamba* that means 'a flicker of light' and has to do with the manner in which the icon was found on the peak of the mountain centuries ago. According to the tradition, this icon worked many miracles and most have to do with 'barren women who beseech the Mother of God to grant them a child'. The best-known story is about the wife of a Turkish Pasha (when Greece was part of the Ottoman Empire), who miraculously conceived a child with the icon's intervention.

Miira told me that she had to climb hundreds of stairs to get to the chapel where the icon was kept, and she 'prayed, and prayed, and prayed'. Half a year earlier, she had been told by a doctor in Finland that she would not be able to conceive a child due to health problems. However, soon after her return from Rhodes, she got pregnant and gave birth to her daughter at the age of 42. Miira told me that she was 'eternally grateful' to the Mother of God for her daughter, whom she loves dearly. Not only does Miira's story illustrate traditional Orthodox understanding of cure and healing, but it also points to the transnational nature of Orthodoxy and the transnational fame of some icons among Orthodox worldwide. In the course of my ethnographic fieldwork, I came to know that this icon is also familiar to some of my Russian interlocutors, who even arranged their family holidays in Rhodes to undertake pilgrimages to this icon.

In these stories of healing, the role of holy objects – icons, consecrated oils, holy water, myrrh-streaming relics – is vital. Significant research attests to the unique agency of 'things' in Orthodox practices (Weaver, 2011; Boylston, 2017). According to anthropologist Weaver, icons are not just symbols but agents, discursively the same as divine figures or saints they depict, and as such could act with the same authority: 'holy in themselves, they could not be contested or discredited by formal authorities either' (Weaver, 2011: 397). In Orthodox theology, icons are seen as 'windows on eternity', mediating the invisible beauty of God and God's Kingdom (Munteanu, 2013: 28). Icons point to the dignity of matter, because of its ability to participate in and to irradiate the divine beauty. Any matter, whether it is a human body or an icon, becomes sanctified when absorbing the sacred essence of the divine. Marian icons are believed to convey the essence of Mary herself. Alongside ritualistic blessings, sanctifying matter also includes remembering, reconnecting, and telling the story (Boylston, 2017). Many Marian icons are surrounded by such stories, similar to the Tsambika one. These tales add to the living tradition of Mary, and strengthen her transcendental authority in healing.

The second group of stories refer to accounts of illness as opening the doors to Orthodoxy. For instance, Victoria mentioned that her father, who was raised as an atheist in Soviet Russia, was diagnosed with leukemia. He started praying, changed his lifestyle, was eventually healed, and remained committed to his religious practices afterward. Vera told me about a similar transformation of her father, who got very ill, and for whom 'God was the only hope'. She prayed on his behalf, he got baptized and started praying himself, and in the end recovered from his illness.

A Ukrainian couple, Inna and Dimitriy went through a similar experience when Dimitriy got seriously ill. They turned to the help of a healer when conventional medicine failed them. The healer told them that they both had to turn to God, start praying and fasting, and only then Dimitriy could be cured (which eventually happened). In these three examples, illness was talked of as a symptom of the lost connection with God, which had to be somehow restored in order for the recovery to take place. Orthodoxy is presented in these stories as a cure for modernity, a set of mind and perception of reality that is based on instrumental rationality, and assigns agency, control, and power to human actors only. Interestingly, in all cases, modern medicine reportedly failed to help the suffering, but the 'traditional' turn to prayer healed the body as well.

However, there were also many stories in which there was no contradiction between conventional medical knowledge and divine intervention. One of my interlocutors mentioned that in fact her Russian doctor, a renowned surgeon who conducted her heart surgery, gave her also some spiritual guidance to prepare her for the operation. Some of my interlocutors were doctors themselves, and in their understanding divine powers could intervene in various ways, including through conventional medical practices. Many referred to and prayed to the saints Panteleimonos, Cosmas, and Damian, who were physicians themselves according to tradition. From one Greek interlocutor, I found out about a saint, Luke of Simferopol and Crimea, who was a 20th century Soviet doctor of medicine and a professor. He used to start his surgeries with a sign of the cross, irrespective of whether the patient was Christian. This again gave me a sense of how glocal living of Orthodoxy in Finland is transnationally informed both in people's understating of religion and of the therapeutic.

Toward a conclusion

I set out in this chapter to explore healing practices and knowledge within Finnish Orthodoxy, and how Finnish Orthodoxy responded to the therapeutic turn. I illustrated that OCF has responded to the therapeutic turn by emphasizing the therapeutic effect of Orthodox practices, and representing its spiritual message as suited for everybody. However, therapeutic has existed in Orthodoxy for centuries as the old-age cure of soul and body, and continues to shape Orthodox practices of cure and healing today. The therapeutic turn seemed to trigger more awareness of such therapeutic within Orthodoxy, revived as *therapeia*, based on patristic tradition.

Some of my interlocutors regularly visit the New Valaam Monastery, and have attended icon-painting or singing courses. These courses are aimed at perfecting technical artistry, and are essentially based on patristic tradition as well. Likewise, 'silent retreats' revive the age-old monastic tradition of 'hesychia'. Orthodox members after such retreats still talk of the therapeutic in the same patristic and religious terms. Yet further research is needed to distinguish responses between Orthodox and non-Orthodox participants of such courses and retreats.

My ethnographic fieldwork among Orthodox practitioners illustrates that the traditional cure of soul and body constitutes the core of the therapeutic understanding for many of my interlocutors. They utilize a variety of narration techniques – description of sensorial and bodily reactions, poetic, spiritual, and religious terms to talk of their embodied experiences of liturgy that generates stillness and glimpses of the divine. Their stories of divine intervention, which is channeled through materiality of sound, archaic-origin texts, art of icons, and holy objects, point to the importance of the beyond in the spiritual and bodily healing. Again, the glocal and the transnational nature of these experiences is evident due to the transnational Orthodox exposures and connections of my interlocutors, but also due to the glocal nature of OCF. Some interlocutors also articulate the benefits of Orthodox practices for mental health, such as singing in a choir, and frame their narratives in psychologizing terms.

To conclude, my interlocutors' experiences paint a diverse picture of the therapeutic. This picture can be seen as a glocalized therapeutic assemblage that merges these various elements with age-old Orthodox traditions of health of soul and body. These findings call for reconsideration of the totalizing effects and normalizing power of a singular therapeutic culture, and open a space for discussing various cultural therapeutics, including those that challenge *secular* psychological narratives of the self. In contrast to the psychologizing therapeutic ethos that puts self-realization and self-transformation at the center of one's life, the telos of Orthodox practices is in reaching out to the divine, within and beyond the self.

Note

1 Foremost, I am sincerely indebted to my interlocutors, who generously entrusted me as a researcher with their life stories and shared their views and experiences. This chapter is part of my postdoctoral research on the therapeutic and Orthodoxy in the project *Tracking the Therapeutic: Ethnographies of Wellbeing, Politics and Inequality* [grant number 289004] funded by the Academy of Finland and led by Professor Suvi Salmenniemi at the University of Turku. I am grateful to Suvi and other team members, Laura Kemppainen, Johanna Nurmi, Harley Bergroth, and Inna Perheentupa for their support and insightful comments on this chapter. I would like to thank all the participants of the writers' workshop, especially Felix Freigang, Julia Lerner, and Marja-Liisa Honkasalo for their thoughtful feedback which considerably improved the quality of the chapter. I also thank Dr. Ali Qadir from the University of Tampere for his detailed comments on the chapter.

References

Boylston, T. 2017. Things not for themselves: Idolatry and consecration in Orthodox Ethiopia. In *Christianity and the Limits of Materiality*, edited by M. Opas & A. Haapalainen. London, New York: Bloomsbury, 78–97.

Cerwonka, A. & L. Malkki. 2007. *Improvising Theory: Process and Temporality in Ethnographic Fieldwork.* Chicago: University of Chicago Press.

Collier, J. S. & A. Ong. 2005. Global assemblages, anthropological problems. In *Global Assemblages: Technology, Politics, and Ethics as Anthropological Problems*, edited by A. Ong & J. S. Collier. Malden: Blackwell Publishing, 3–22.

de Witte, M. 2017. Spirit media and the spekter of the fake. In *Christianity and the Limits of Materiality*, edited by M. Opas & A. Haapalainen. London: Bloomsbury Academics, 37–55.

Florensky, P. 2002. Church ritual as a synthesis of the arts. In *Beyond Vision. Essays of the Perception of Art (1922)*, edited by N. Misler, translated by W. Salmond. London: Reaktion Books, 95–111.

Furedi, F. 2004. *Therapy Culture: Cultivating Vulnerability in an Uncertain Age.* London, New York: Routledge.

Gupta, A. & J. Ferguson. 1997. *Anthropological Locations. Boundaries and Grounds of a Field Science.* Berkeley: University of California Press.

Hakkarainen, J. 2016. *Ortodoksista psykoterapiaa. Kirjoitukisa ortodoksisesta terapeuttisesta elämästä ja ortodoksisen teologian läntisestä vankeudesta.* Joensuu: Jarmo Hakkarainen, Grano.

Hanegraaff, W. 1999. New age spiritualities as secular religion: A historian's perspective. *Social Compass 46*:2, 145–160.

Hanka, H. 2008. Ortodoksinen kirkkoarkkitehtuuri Suomessa. In *Uskon tilat ja kuvat. Moderni suomalainen kirkkoarkkitehtuuri ja -taide*, edited by A. Kuorikoski. Helsinki: Suomalainen Teologinen Kirjallisuusseura, 28–301.

Heelas, P. 2009. *Spiritualities of Life: New Age Romanticism and Consumptive Capitalism.* Hoboken, NJ: Wiley.

Hierotheos, Metropolitan of Nafpaktos. 1993. *The Illness and Cure of the Soul in the Orthodox Tradition*, translated by E. Mavromichali. Levadia-Hellas: Birth of the Theotokos Monastery.

Hierotheos, Bishop of Nafpaktos. 1994. *Orthodox Psychotherapy. The science of the Fathers*, translated by E. Williams. Levadia: Birth of the Theotokos Monastery.

Husso, K. 2011. *Ikkunoita ikonien ja kirkkoesineiden historiaan: Suomen ortodoksisen kirkon esineellinen kulttuuriperintö 1920–1980-luvuilla.* Helsinki: Suomen Muinaismuistoyhdistys.

Illouz, E. 2008. *Saving the Modern Soul: Therapy, Emotions, and the Culture of Self-Help.* Berkley, CA: California Press.

Ingold, T. 2013. *Making Anthropology, Archaeology, Art and Architecture.* Oxon: Routledge.

Kallio, S. 2018. Alkukirkon yksiäänisyyden lähteillä. *Ortodoksi viesti* 2, 35.

Lasch, C. 1991. *The Culture of Narcissim: American Life in an Age of Diminishing Expectations.* New York, London: W W Norton and Company.

Lerner, J. 2011. Tele-terapiya bez psihologii, ili kak adaptiruyut self na postsovetskom teleekrane. *Laboratorium 1*, 116–137.

Lossky, V. (1957)1976. *The Mystical Theology of the Eastern Church.* Crestwood, NY: St Vladimir's Seminary Press.

Madsen, O. J. 2012. The liturgical reform of the Sunday high mass: The last attempt of Christ? The therapeutic and Christian cultures revised. *Studia Theologica 66*:2, 166–189.

Madsen, O. J. 2014. *The Therapeutic Turn: How Psychology Altered Western Culture.* Routledge.

Martikainen, T. & T. Laitila. 2014. Population movements and orthodox christianity in Finland: Dislocations, resettlements, migrations and identities. In *Orthodox Identities in Western Europe: Migration, Settlement and Innovation*, edited by M. Hämmerli & J.-F. Mayer. Surrey, England: Ashgate, 151–178.

Meyer, B. & J. Verrips. 2008. Aesthetics. In *Key Words in Religion, Media and Culture*, edited by D. Morgan. New York, London: Routledge, 20–30.

Morgan, D. 2005. *Sacred Gaze: Religious Visual Culture in Theory and Practice*. Berkeley: University of California Press.

Munteanu, D. 2013. An iconic theology of beauty: Orthodox aesthetics of salvation. *International Journal of Orthodox Theology 3*:4, 27–61.

Nehring, D., E. Alvarado, E. Hendriks & D. Kerrigan. 2016. *Transnational Popular Psychology and the Global Self-Help Industry: The Politics of Contemporary Social Change*. UK: Palgrave Macmillan.

Opas, M. & A. Haapalainen. 2017. *Christianity and the Limits of Materiality*. New York: Bloomsbury Academic.

Ortodoksiviesti. 2016. Kalenteri. *Ortodoksiviesti 05*, 41–51.

Ratinen, T. 2017. Is it a sin? The therapeutic turn and changing views on homosexuality in the Finnish Evangelical Lutheran Church 1952–1984. *Pastoral Psychology 66*:5, 641–656.

Rimke, H. M. 2000. Governing citizens through self-help literature. *Cultural Studies 14*:1, 61–78.

Robertson, R. 1995. Glocalization: Time–space and homogeneity–heterogeneity. In *Global Modernities*, edited by M. Featherstone, S. Lash & R. Robertson. London: Sage Publications, 25–44.

Roudometof, V. 2014. *Globalization and Orthodox Christianity: The Transformations of a Religious Tradition*. New-York, London: Routledge.

Salmenniemi, S. 2010. In search of a new (wo)man: Gender and sexuality in contemporary Russian self-help literature. In *Russian Media and Changing*, edited by A. Rosenholm, K. Nordenstreng & E. Trubina. London: Routledge, 134–153.

Salmenniemi, S. & A. B. Pessi. 2016. 'Herätkää pöljät!': Minuus, yhteiskunta ja muutos self-help-kirjallisuudessa. *Kulttuurintutkimus 34*:1, 3–14.

Schmemann, A. 1991. *Celebration of Faith, vol. 3: The Virgin Mary*. New York: St Vladimir's Seminary Press.

Seppälä, H. 2013. Maan tomu ylistää Luojaansa. Eräs lähtökohta ortodoksisen kirkkolaulun. *Ortodoksia 52*, 103–116.

Seppälä, S. 2010. *Kauneus. Jumalan kieli*. Helsinki: Kirjapaja.

Sjöberg, M. 2013. Pyhä laulu. *Analogi. Ortodoksinen seurakuntalehti 1*, 14–15.

Tiaynen-Qadir, T. 2016. Orthodox icons of Mary generating transnational space between Finland and Russia. *Lähde Historiallinen aikakauskirja*, 138–171.

Tiaynen-Qadir, T. 2017. Glocal religion and the feeling at home: Ethnography of artistry in Finnish orthodoxy. *Religions 8*:23, 1–14.

Tiaynen-Qadir, T. & S. Salmenniemi. 2017. Self-help as a glocalised therapeutic assemblage. *European Journal of Cultural Studies 20*:4, 381–396.

Virolainen, W. 2013. Suomenkielisen liturgian kehitys. *Ortodoksia 52*, 7–21. Accessed 11 24, 2015. https://ortodoksistenpappienliitto.files.wordpress.com/2015/02/ortodoksia_ 52_virolainen.pdf.

Vuola, E. 2010. *Jumalainen nainen. Neitsyt Mariaa etsimässä*. Helsinki: Kustannu-sosakeyhtiö Otava.

Weaver, D. C. 2011. Shifting agency: Male clergy, female believers, and the role of icons. *Material Religion* 7:3, 394–419.

Woodstock, L. 2005. Vying constructions of reality: Religion, science and 'positive thinking' in self-help literature. *Journal of Media and Religion* 4:3, 155–178.

Zigon, J. 2010. *Making the New Post-Soviet Person: Moral Experience in Contemporary Moscow*. Boston: Brill Academic Publishers.

Zigon, J. 2011. *'HIV Is God's Blessing': Rehabilitating Morality in Neoliberal Russia*. Berkeley: University of California Press.

5 Saving the Post-Soviet soul

Religion as therapy in the narratives of Russian-speaking migrant women

Julia Lerner

Kathrin Lofton, scholar of contemporary forms of religion, points to the long-standing interconnection between the religious and therapeutic logics:

> Psychology and theology do not offer the same gospels. But it may be useful to think about the gospel function within therapeutic discourse – especially as the therapeutic idiom begins to pervade even the most conservative religious cultures. Religion has long existed within, and been diagnosed by, therapeutic culture, just as therapeutic culture has existed within, and been diagnosed by, religions. Once we understand the interconnection of these two categories we can hope to better interpret their ongoing effects and appropriately critique their transformative limits.
>
> (Lofton, 2015: 36)

Embarking from far-reaching historical interrelations between religion and therapy, this chapter aims to examine the contemporary interplay between the two spheres using the particular case of ex-Soviet immigrants.[1] As I will show, these neo-religious subjects simultaneously acquire therapeutic and religious languages through which they perceive themselves and give meaning to their lives. In doing so, they illustrate the constitution of a new type of subjectivity which is at once therapeutic and religious.

Today, the historical correlation between therapy and religion appears in a new form, namely, a therapeutic-religious assemblage emerging alongside the seemingly global triumph of therapeutic culture (Tucker, 2002). The notion of 'assemblage' allows us to depict a moment of a contextual and flexible constellation that accompanies the most significant historical processes headed by neo-liberal ethos, religious revival and super-individualization. Recalling Weber's classical 'elective affinities' (Weber, 1958) that created a contextual historical assemblage of Calvinism and capitalism, the religious and therapeutic cultures, many of whose elements are mutually antithetical, also share important similarities. Paradoxically, they even serve to strengthen each other. The incorporation of therapeutic language into the religious mindset and the religious way of life creates the possibility of constituting a type of subjectivity that is, at once, well-functioning self-managing neoliberal and deeply religiously committed.

This newly emerging assemblage is particularly visible among neophytes of the religious ethos and the capitalist spirit. In the case of the ex-Soviet subjects I study, the therapeutic-religious blend is refracted through the characteristics of the post-Soviet cultural condition as well as through the immigrant experience. Hence, in my examination of the manifestations of their therapeutic religiosity, I consider accounts of post-Soviet religiosity and subjectivity as well as the trans-formation of religion in migration. Both the transformative post-Soviet experi-ence and the experience of migration prompt a reconsideration of the self and encourage the acquisition of new cultural languages. I suggest that the search for 'saving the modern soul' (Illouz, 2008) appears in the narratives of these migrants as 'saving the post-Soviet person'.

Focusing on three rich biographical cases of Russian-speaking immigrant women, I will probe their narratives of personal well-being and happiness gained through the religious way of life and articulated in therapeutic language. In my interpretative encounter with these narratives, I was interested in not only the personal reasons for their religious transformation, but, first and foremost, the cultural resources and languages that made such a transformation possible and that were adopted for articulating the personal meaning of this transformation. As an outcome of the narrative analysis, I suggest a further discussion of the broader meanings of the subjectivity shaped by therapeutic religiosity: How does this subjectivity relate to the therapeutic and neoliberal model of the subject that dominates contemporary culture and research? How is this self-centred therapeu-tic subject assembled with a religious identity and way of life? And how does the assembled therapeutic religious subjectivity affect the distinction between reli-gious and secular mindsets?

Explaining immigrant religiosity

This analysis emerges from a longitudinal, ethnographic and narrative study that followed the phenomenology of various routes of Russian-speaking religiosity situated in the wider spectrum of religious groups in Israeli society.[2] The study was conducted in nine communities and study groups, including the Hasidic and Chabad communities in Jerusalem and Beer Sheva, through modern Kabbalah studies to Jewish Christians and Seventh-Day Adventists in Beer Sheva and Russian-Orthodox groups in Haifa. In addition to direct observations in the com-munities and biographical interviews, an interpretative discourse analysis of the selected media texts closely connected to the religious identities under study was conducted.[3] Aiming to clarify the particular local Israeli features of new Russian-immigrant religiosity as well as its global post-Soviet characteristics, the study was enriched by a comparative perspective through research exchanges[4] and interviewing post-Soviet religious immigrants outside of Israel.

From the very outset of this study, I was puzzled by the question of why mostly irreligious post-Soviet immigrants become religious as part of their relocation experience, and what kind of religiosity they develop. Scholarship on the increas-ing religiosity that accompanies migration has tended to understand religion as a tool of repair and stabilization. Following this logic, research on immigrant religiosity in the United States and Europe considers religion as a device of integration, due to the many resources (cultural, social, psychological and economic) that religious institutional frameworks offer to immigrants (Cadge & Ecklund, 2007). Thus, immigrants employ religion as a source of identity, as religion provides symbols, rituals and practices that immigrants can use to affirm or reinvent who they are vis-à-vis the host and the home countries (Yang & Ebaugh, 2001). Moreover, established immigrant communities function as an extended family for their members, symbolically replacing distant relatives (Hagan & Ebaugh, 2003; Warner & Wittner, 1998). This approach stresses the facilitating power of religion in transitional states in general, and considers religion in immigration as a strong device of belonging and well-being (Chen, 2008; Levitt, 2007; Mooney, 2009). Generally speaking, it has described religion as a 'therapeutic' device.

The scholarship on Russian immigrant religiosity[5] in Israel follows similar lines. Their religious transformation is often explained as 'Israelization' through religion and seen as a way for Russian speakers in Israel to cope with their doubly questioned Jewishness (Raijman & Pinsky, 2011; Remennick & Prashizky, 2012). Others suggest viewing this multi-variant Russian-immigrant religiosity through the prism of the post-Soviet crisis and the quest for new ideological and spiritual meaning, in the context of the transnational phenomenon of the post-Soviet religious revival (Elias & Lerner, 2016). Presenting the unsettling conditions of civic-political nature as reparable through religion, researchers presuppose the universal psychological character of a religious mindset. The assumption here is that religion, as a way of experiencing the world, stabilizes an unstable condition. As such, the religiosity will intensify in periods of crisis, anomie and transition (generational, family, national, psychological and state). Supplying strength in weakness, it will appear as an answer for traumatic states, whether individual or collective.

In my attempt to account for the religious transformation of Russian speakers in Israel, I have taken a critical stance towards the notion of religiosity as a resource of repair in migration, as I perceived a tendency to over-psychologize both phenomena – religiosity and migration. However, the more I observed the new Russian-speaking religious field in Israel, the more I myself experienced the clear presence of a therapeutic dimension in this immigrant religiosity. I was intrigued by the fact that, in many of my informants' narratives, their religious experience features a therapeutic aspect reflected in the way they articulate themselves. In their narratives they appear as satisfied, autonomous individuals, making their own choices and carrying within an inner harmony. One hears stories of new religiosity combined with success in managing a normative life, including the tasks of profession and family demands, as well as the organization of emotions and time. In other words, their new religious subjectivity resembles the meanings of a neoliberal, therapeutic individualistic well-being. This intriguing result of my inquiry into accounts of neophyte religiosity confronts us with a therapeutic neoliberal subject. In what follows, I suggest an interpretation of this assemblage of religious and therapeutic languages that emerges in the narratives of immigrant women.

Narratives of well-being through religion

In what follows, I present the interpretation of biographical stories of three religious, Russian-speaking immigrant women. The cases examined here represent voices from the wide and multi-vocal empirical corpus of biographical and thematic narratives that comprise the research data (more than one hundred open-ended and focused interviews). In these three cases, I applied narrative ethnography (Holstein & Gubrium, 2011) – an approach that combines interviewing subjects together with a deep ethnographic knowledge of their everyday life absorbed through personal relationship with them. These cases are representative of the narratives of therapeutic religiosity, and I have chosen to use them as illustrations. First, these women share some structural sociocultural similarities, as they all belong to the first post-Soviet generation, as well as to a wide but distinct sociocultural-educational milieu. Second, the three share a professional orientation, namely, one connected to the social sector and institutions of care. And finally, they have situated themselves within dramatically different religious creeds – Orthodox Judaism, Messianic Christianity and Sunni Islam, adopting related religious cosmologies, lifestyles and everyday practices. Two of these women share a Jewish origin and lived in Israel at the time of the interview, and one lives in Finland and is linked to the Israeli context by the Palestinian origin of her husband. The similarities and differences in their biographies and narratives make the joint analysis highly intriguing. Thus, striving to consider not only the typical features of these narratives but also their exceptional characteristics, I shall present them one by one through focused biographical analysis.

Esther and Diana grew up in central Russian cities – Moscow and St. Petersburg, respectively. Elena was raised in a small town in Estonia with a Russian-speaking majority. They were all brought up among Soviet intelligentsia – academics, teachers and engineers. They all describe their families, as do most Russian immigrants of this generation, as a-religious or anti-religious. Esther and Diana discovered their Jewishness during their teenage years, and the discovery was almost devoid of meaning for them. Elena, for her part, describes an encounter with Russian Orthodox church in post-Soviet Estonia as alienated: 'I grew up in atmosphere of godlessness *(bezbozie)*', she says. Esther and Diana came to Israel with a big wave of immigration, while Elena immigrated to Germany as part of her search to study abroad. The three of them are well educated; each earned a master's degree. Esther and Diana work in the third sector in the area of social support. Elena also dreams about finding work as a cultural broker in the area of immigrant integration in Europe, assisting people to find and fulfil their potential in their new circumstances.

Today, all three women, Esther, Diana and Elena, are deeply religious – on both the levels of doctrinal thought and everyday practice. Esther, a married mother of six, is a member of an ultra-orthodox Chabad community. Diana, who is single, is an active member of a messianic Christian community in Israel. As a type of modern nun, she is celibate for religious reasons and shares a home with two other women from her community. Elena, for her part, is married to a

Palestinian refugee from Gaza; she is Muslim, orthodox and 'veiled' (*pokritaia* as she says in Russian), the mother of three boys. All three women have acquired and developed their religiosity in the course of their migration, as part of the cultural transition and reaching adulthood.

As I listened to the stories of these women, I was struck by the statement, made by one after the other, that they were 'happy'. Their narratives were anchored in terms of achieving well-being, harmony, psychological calmness and even happiness. In what follows, I seek to unpack this happiness in relation to their religiosity, on the one hand, and to the therapeutic ethos and the imperative for happiness, on the other.

In the course of their biographical stories about the discovery of their true religion, all the women interweave the idea of personal choice and the narrative of the search for the inner self, but also serendipitous reasoning. Something important that happened to them by mistake or absolutely accidentally becomes *hashgaha pratit* (Hebrew for personal providence), signalling the presence of God in their private lives. All of the stories feature a traumatic mystical experience marking this very presence.

Consider the following story, in which Esther recounts the death of a schoolmate:

> I was asking myself questions about death and why we live at all. I took it very, very hard; I could not function, and my parents were worried about me.

Or Diana, who recalls a severe anxiety attack:

> I had a very difficult experience in my teenage condition, I did all kinds of silly things.... I did not look for God, just felt very bad. This one time I could not sleep and went crazy. And thought to myself: I will take this magic book 'Biblia'...at that time these books were only beginning to appear in people's houses. So, I started to read it with the attitude that there is no God and that all this is total nonsense, but I finished convinced that God exists and that I am doing things that do not please Him. And I had a strong feeling that I am going to die here and now.

Elena remembers that 'things' she could not explain happened to her all the time. For example, at age fifteen, just after her parent's divorce, she was biking with her brother in the forest and struggling to ride up a steep hill when she felt an invisible hand pushing her from behind:

> This was the moment I discovered that there is something [there].

The paradigm of religion as a response to a personal psychological problem or difficult socioeconomic condition appeared in most of the biographical narratives of the Russian-speaking immigrants who became religious just before or after the migration. This was particularly evident in the narratives of single mothers, lonely elders, those who lost their profession in migration, and people who were challenged by serious illnesses or who went through painful divorces. So, in this sense, Russian immigrants articulated their religious transformation by reproducing the classical narrative of conversion or return to religion, or that of a religious conversion that involved overcoming trauma (Rambo, 1993).

Concomitantly, the religious revival of these women is characterized by its specific post-Soviet appearance. The transformation of their late-Soviet mindset into a religious one can be viewed as resistance to the Soviet indoctrination of atheism or as a smooth adaptation to, or even fulfilment of, the exported Soviet ideological and cultural repertoire. First, the Soviet cultural background made Russian immigrants highly ambivalent towards religiosity. Indeed, historically, while Soviet ideology did strive to create a 'New Man' inspired by materialist and scientific worldviews, on a more symbolic cultural level, the dogmas and beliefs of Marxist–Leninist ideology operated rather like theological and eschatological religious systems (Frouse, 2008; Thrower, 1992; Zilberman, 1977). Similarly, the Soviet code and rituals worked in the everyday life of the Soviet people as almost religious attributes (Yurchak, 2005). Moreover, not all domains of the Soviet way of life were directly and exclusively determined by atheism and anti-religious views (Luehrmann, 2011). This permitted a peculiar translation of Soviet ideas into the prevailing ideas of spirituality (*dukhovnost'* in Russian) and encouraged a permanent quest for 'the meaning of life' rather than for material prosperity and 'work upon oneself' (*rabota nad soboi* in Russian). In this way, the 'religious unconscious' was preserved within the Soviet discourse and experience (Epstein, 1994). Finally, the religious arenas existing at the margins of Soviet ideology and society acquired political and cultural meaning as a counterforce to Soviet collectivistic values. Religion came to be associated with the private sphere and was perceived as embodying resistance to the regime and its indoctrination (Kornblatt, 2004).

Later, the ideological-political but also everyday cultural collapse of the Soviet frame brought about dissolution of limits on religion, and also a moral and ideological vacuum, resulted in a massive post-Soviet religious awakening, described by scholars from the late 1980s as a 'supermarket of religions' (Pelkmans, 2009; Wanner, 2012). Faith, disconnected from any particular religious doctrine and lacking a communal framework, can be seen as a response to official Soviet atheism, promoting what the literature calls post-Soviet inclusive or 'minimal' religion (Epstein, 1999; Sutton, 2006). While in contemporary Russia the mainstream religiosity takes a statist institutional form, this post-Soviet inclusive and universalistic form is manifest today in the religious beliefs and practices found in the broader space of the post-Soviet diaspora, including those in Israel.

Like many other Russian-speaking religious immigrants, Esther, Diana and Elena describe an experience of the post-Soviet 'religious supermarket'; a chaotic assortment of open religious and spiritual trajectories – all of them eclectic and foreign. Diana first came in her search to a synagogue in St. Petersburg, after which she arrived at a Russian-Orthodox church. Then, a friend took her to one of the newly established evangelical communities in the city. It was there that she later met a messianic figure who became her religious guide. Esther went in a different order – a schoolmate took her to a Russian-Orthodox priest, and only after that did she arrive at the circle of Judaism, join a Jewish school and later find her true place in the Chabad movement. Elena recalls how she tried to become part of Russian-Orthodox life in Estonia but 'something' did not accept her there, as she describes. She tells how, in her teenage years, their grandmother took her and her brother to baptize them in the Russian church when they visited her in Latvia. Elena took with her a cross on a silver chain but, just as the priest was supposed to place the cross on her neck, the chain broke and the cross fell to the floor. Alienated, she sought other options. She and her mother became interested in esoteric literature and astrology, but the search continued until she found Islam.

Within the post-Soviet religious trajectories, these three women explored the repertoires of different religious doctrines and shaped their lives in accordance with the demands of ultra-Orthodox Judaism, Messianic Christianity and Islam. In spite of the deep differences between the women, the narrative of their inner harmony is strikingly similar. All tell a therapeutic story. First and foremost, one hears of a journey to discover their true self, of overcoming a personal difficulty, of gaining control of their lives, time and emotions. The narrative of identifying problems (or finding a pathology), probing the unconscious, making connections with past events or even one's childhood, and summoning the self onto a path of healing and the elimination of suffering is the basic narrative of the therapeutic culture (Cushman, 1995; Illouz, 2007; Furedi, 2004). The organizing theme of personal choice, the ability to manage one's successes and take responsibility for one's failures signals the presence of therapeutic neoliberal subjectivity (Rose, 1990, 1996).

That Diana, Esther and Elena speak in terms of 'autonomous responsible subjects' concomitantly with becoming religious is, by itself, a result of a transformation that is both post-Soviet and religious. For them, both sets of assumptions – that of a religious mindset as well as the assumptions of modern psychology – are not obvious at all, nor is the more contemporary therapeutic neoliberal pursuit of happiness.

Despite the enthusiastic early phase that psychoanalysis enjoyed in Russia at the beginning of the 20th century (Etkind, 1993), psychoanalysis and post-Freudian psychology never truly shaped Russian and Soviet culture and social relations. The socialist regime, by contrast, critically shaped the Russian emotional style, and obliged the Soviet person not only to think but also to feel in a specific, socialist way (Steinberg & Sobol, 2011). If, in the Russian and Soviet context, the therapeutic narrative – including its language and model of subjectivity – was absent, today, a version of the therapeutic culture that assembles 'emotional socialism' and the global therapeutic language has already become evident in post-Soviet Russian articulations of selfhood, emotions and personal relations (Lerner, 2015; Lerner & Zbenovich, 2013; Leykin, 2015; Matza, 2018; Salmenniemi, 2017). In the case of the narratives of the immigrant women, the post-Soviet therapeutic language is also assembled with post-atheist religious beliefs.

Therapeutic cultural logic appears to clash in several important ways with generalized religious ethos: the high value the former ascribes to individual needs and their satisfaction, its basic belief in self-regulating individual autonomy, its distancing from moral judgement while turning guilt and suffering into weaknesses or even pathologies. However, it appears that, in the contemporary assemblage, the discourse of religiosity is undergoing a 'personal development' turn (Heelas, 2009; Tucker, 2002) and the contradictions between modern psychology and religious consciousness are solved on the level of doctrines, theology and in the everyday cosmologies of religious subjects. The assemblage of therapeutic religiosity presents religion as one route towards development and self-management. In what follows, we will see how the religious and the therapeutic logic are assembled in the three cases under study as means to manage the soul and its practice.

Esther: managing spiritual time

Let's begin with Esther's narrative of well-being through management of time. Esther is a busy woman. She has six children, a full-time job and is enrolled in a doctoral programme. She strictly practices an ultra-orthodox version of Judaism in her everyday life while she keeps her family life within the frame of the Chabad community. This is how she describes her current life:

> I'm feeling very good... and also proud [of myself]. Every moment we can decide what we do. The choices I made in my life – I'm proud of them all and happy about the process I went through. Of course, everybody makes mistakes, but I think these mistakes only came to teach me all kinds of lessons in life. First of all, I'm a mother of six; I'm very, very glad that I'm a part of such a big family. I am married to a man I love very much, together with a big and happy family. This place of family is very important. Beyond this, I continue to do my research that I love; I believe that it will advance properly... The fact that I'm doing one thing, and another thing and another... suddenly, this puzzle of me is created, and the tower that I want to build and advance (*lekadem*). I hope very much that I will come to that place I want to be in... in peace with myself (*shlema*), connected to myself, giving an education to my children, and my own personal example – I want them very much to see my example in their eyes.

Esther is proud and happy. Narrating on her self – building it, cultivating and developing it, fulfilling it and eventually being happy with it – is central to Esther's religious language and experience. In her 'life world', the value of self-development is linked to both her religious and professional identities. She uses life-coaching terms such as 'taking choices', 'advancing yourself' and 'being true to yourself' and 'fulfilled' simultaneously with Hebrew spiritual concepts, signalling religious metaphysics. In this way, the religious language is psychologized and the therapeutic terms gain religious content.

First, the focusing on the self as a value and its proper management can be found in discourses and practices of many religious movements. The similar discourse of self-management and self-development also dominates some professional sectors and institutions of care that serve as the main carriers of the therapeutic, neoliberal, psycho-managerial logic. Esther is part of this professional milieu; she works as a public relations director in an NGO that assists people in overcoming poverty. I ask Esther to describe the ideology of the organization, which she communicates as part of her job. She tells me that the ultimate principles that stand at the heart of the objectives of this NGO proclaim work of reparation, reducing the evil by investing conscious personal efforts. People are encouraged to push themselves harder, to take themselves out of the misery, to take responsibility for their budget and habits, and to control their life. People learn that Esther identifies herself with this approach. Moreover, Esther herself fulfils this principle in her everyday life while she combines it with religious meanings. She tells me that in no other place has she found what she finds in religion:

> Religion tells me how I should fill my time. There is something flat in all rest of reality. So today I am trying to fill in this place for myself. Religion gives content to it, depth.

When I ask her about this 'depth', she answers:

> Today the big issue in my life is time. I have just very little time, so how should I fill it and manage it? I have a way to evaluate what I do with my time. If I now invested half an hour in my child, I did the maximum in my life to advance myself. Or if I have invested half an hour in studying [...]. Today, I think that my life is very limited in time and in my ability to achieve my objectives, so I should know the correct goals and how to manage the time. Before I go to sleep, I write down the tasks of the next day. I write numbers: one two, three. And within the first I have A, B, C. I know how to manage myself. I know that if 3C will not work, it's ok. But if I do not plan, it will not happen at all. But how do I know what is important to do? [If I] just go to a coffee shop...I will feel emptiness. I had periods like this, it happened; I felt that I was standing in one place, not advancing what is important to me. And advancing in a spiritual dimension and in my work is most important to me. Now, for me, [whether] to explain to my child about what kinds of trees he sees in the forest or what kinds of animals are in the zoo or, alternatively, his ancestors; of course, I would choose to tell him about Avraham [and the origin of the Jews].

I suggest reading Esther's story as a therapeutic narrative of self-management, self-empowerment and self-development through the management of time. She employs the logic and the style of life coaching while adapting it to her spiritual religious goals and needs. She learns to manage time well in order to have time to give her children the basics of their religious knowledge. Hence, in her narrative, the recognizable neoliberal therapeutic discourse is assembled with meanings that derive from the Jewish religious cosmology.

Diana: managing vocation

Diana's story, too, is a narrative of self-fulfilment, with a focus on the search for and investment in her true mission. In Diana's scenario, this investment yields happiness.

Diana tells me her biographical journey, recalling how she coped with a difficult teenage period, and a family crisis that resulted in drug addiction. At that time, she discovered God and her Jewishness, and made peace between the two:

> I just felt that God was angry with me and I had to make peace with him.

This harmony Diana found much later, in her mission of serving God in Israel while working for the messianic Jewish-Christian community there. But earlier, as a lost young woman, as she describes herself, she sought salvation everywhere. After one stormy mysterious night with a bible in her hands, Diana first 'ran to a synagogue':

> The Chabad rabbi there started to explain to me something about God as a 'remarkable notion'. And I was furious. I already felt that I did not know a lot about God, but I knew that He is not a notion. I wanted to die for him.

At that time, the next natural place to turn was a Russian-Orthodox monastery, and, indeed, that is where she ran: 'I came and told them – please accept me, I want to be a nun!' Later, Diana discovered a young Evangelical community. At some point, her God became her career, and she worked as a missionary in St. Petersburg. This is when Diana began to tell herself and others: 'My parents are Jewish; I am not'. But a speech given by a messianic Jew from Canada living in Israel that came to Diana's community changed all that. Diana discovered her true mission of being a Christian Jew, moved to Israel and devoted her professional and personal life to the service of God:

> In my character, I'm a total extremist. For me, it is all or nothing; if you are into something – so, only totally and until the end. That's why I think that everything in my life is part of my faith and colored by it.

Diana established an organization that assists immigrant families in need. To the Israeli state authorities, it is an NGO supporting immigrant single mothers, and for her Christian world it is her 'ministry'. She travels throughout the world, raising money among messianic communities for her ministry, something at which she is highly successful. Diana is in charge of all the activities of the organization, from distributing food to organizing educational activities for children, cultural events and camps for the young and accompanying her care recipients to state authorities and the courts.

She explained her decision to live without intimate relationships and with no children in theological terms. But she also says:

> Actually, I cannot see myself doing what I'm doing with a partner and kids: it's impossible, my mission and work are total for me. I can live only according to God, and not to my husband. I am autonomous and independent, and there is a sort of *Blagodat'* (Grace of God or Happiness).

Diana adopts the value of therapeutic autonomy and self-fulfilment in a remarkable way as she subordinates it to the Holy Spirit and religious mission. In her narrative, the self and the work are inseparable. It is the total investment in them both that results in her well-being.

When I ask about the attitude of her irreligious family to her way of life, she answers:

> My father understands me, and he always protects me in front of others. My grandmother always reproaches me because of living alone with no sex and with no option for children. But my father says to her – leave her alone; don't you see that Diana is happy? In fact, when I met my extended family around the table and someone asked: who among us would continue to do what he does if there is no need for money? I was almost the only one to say that I'm absolutely happy with who I am and what I'm doing.

Diana is indeed committed to the task she has built for herself. Like the logic of the organization for helping the poor where Esther works, Diana's work with immigrant single mothers is 'to help them to help themselves'. Her task is to bring them to the point where they become independent subjects and assume personal responsibility for their lives.

'Personal responsibility' is a concept central to the therapeutic discourse, especially in its neoliberal variant of self-managerial discourse. Contemporary critique ties the triumph of the therapeutic logic to the neoliberal economic and cultural regime that promotes the autonomous self-regulating subject taking 'personal responsibility' for his functioning. The personal responsibility for one's choices, for personal failures but also a commitment to achieve well-being, is part of what is discussed in the critical literature as the contemporary 'happiness regime' (Ahmed, 2010; Binkley, 2014). Linked to the economic system and moral normative perceptions anchored in the lifestyle of the professional middle class, the discourse of happiness is developed in particular in certain academic areas (such as positive psychology) and therapeutic professions, and also informs the agenda of organizational counselling and all sorts of life coaching, which translated it into the operational level of recommendations (see Yankellevich in this book). The logic of personal responsibility in the quest for happiness penetrates more spheres of life, becoming visible not only in private domains (parenthood, marriage or food) but also in the public sphere (educational institutions, collective memory and politics). In the therapeutic discourse, taking responsibility corresponds to neoliberal logic; in Esther's and Diana's narratives, it is assembled with religious logic and appears as a spiritual practice. In Elena's story, which follows, the responsibility also becomes embodied.

Elena: managing femininity

Elena's story of saving the soul is also a narrative of management. She acquired religiosity as a tool to manage her femininity and sexuality. In portraying her immigration, the search for her 'self' and for a life-partner, and of coming consciously to the observance of Islam, she returns time and again to her family story, and especially to her grandmother and her father – who committed 'many sins' in their turbulent sexual and romantic lives. As a growing girl, Elena lacked confidence: 'Nobody looked at me in our town'. It was later in Germany, working as an au pair, that she discovered herself as an attractive young woman. Her experience of immigration was all about discovering the world of interpersonal relationships and relations with men. After a year in Germany she went back to Estonia, but was seeking a way to return to Germany in order to study and settle down. Shortly thereafter, Elena made this move, but freedom in Germany brought new difficulties. She was falling in love, she was fascinated by the relationships she had or fantasized about having, but she also was 'keeping herself', as she says, refraining from sexual relationships. In this period, as a young woman alone facing a new environment, language and culture, and seeking companionship, she found herself in dangerous situations with men. This frightened her, and she became more cautious. The freedom that had attracted her now became a threat:

> I understood then how I looked from their point of view. I was dancing at the bar, I'm easy to take, I will follow everyone… My naiveté left me. I see how this lightness and easiness is superficial and deceptive. It was a new period of understanding of myself.

Sometime after that, Elena met her future husband, a young scientist of Palestinian origin. He introduced her to Islam but, as she says, made no attempt to force her to convert or to become observant. She took Islam upon herself slowly, discovering how close its theology was to her mind but also realizing 'how much good it does for her' and her self-feeling. She describes a decision 'to cover' herself (wear a veil on her head) as a meaningful step in her journey:

> I've accepted Islam as my religion. And it was clear for me that all that is included in the frames of Islam, I need just to accept, regardless of whether I like it or not. And indeed, after I did it I understood how right it is, that it works. Men stopped talking to me. They stopped looking at me as a woman. Before that, even when I was married, you know how it is… they could say something or sit next to me and start talking […] Islam is a journey of my

own choice [and now] it gave me... I would not say happiness, but I came to some calmness, for my inner balance. My search has ended. There is a movement, of course, to learn more about my religion. But I do not take wrong decisions anymore [...] I feel pure. I do not attract the gazes of men. I do not interest them anymore.

Elena's calm and rational narrative is organized by the frames of a self-seeking journey and acquiring her sense of being through self-control. It is presented in terms of 'the difficulty', then 'taking the choice' and performing 'the personal responsibility'. In her story, the domain of difficulty is closely linked to femininity and should be understood in relation to gender aspects of the therapeutic culture. The therapeutic narrative has been a crucial tool for female empowerment in the feminist movement. Through this narrative, the movement has created a space and language in which women could expose their experiences, come to terms with their positioning and learn to gain control of their lives (Plant, 2015; see also Perheentupa in this book). In Elena's narrative, this recognizable narrative of women's self-awareness is incorporated in the religious journey and packaged together with the practice of the corporal restrictions prescribed to a Muslim woman. Today, for Elena, being religious and being true to herself means being a woman in control of her body.

From religion as therapy to neoliberal therapeutic religiosity

The narrative accounts show that Esther, Diana and Elena discovered religion alongside learning the therapeutic way of thinking as part of their migration to Israel and Europe. They adopted the therapeutic logic particularly in the frames of their professional occupation in the 'third sector', social-care oriented NGOs, which implement the therapeutic logic in their activities and translate it into their practices. Moreover, the women were exposed to religion when it already spoke the language of psychology. The assembled religious-therapeutic mindset provided them with the resource of self-fulfilment in spiritual terms, but also as functioning normative individuals, women and mothers, and moral persons. Their religiosity appears as a way for up-to-date life-management: management of feelings, time, sexuality, work and family. Thus, the adoption of the assembled religious discourse turned Esther, Diana and Elena into 'successful people'. For them, religion sparked the idea of personal choice, a crucial value in the therapeutic individualist logic. It allowed them to push themselves to go beyond themselves, to change their lives while staying within the strict boundaries of their religious prescriptions. It created an experience of authenticity, freedom and autonomy. In their eyes, religiosity renders them successful, normative 'healthy' and 'proper' subjects. Therefore, in this reading of the post-Soviet religiosity in migration, I argue that the religious and therapeutic discourses merge to produce a neoliberal subject in the narratives of these women.

The reconfiguration of the therapeutic dimension of religious experience into a narrative of flexible, autonomous, self-managing subjectivity requires further discussion. To start with, the perception of religion as a form of therapy has a long history. Assumptions that shape the understanding of religion as alleviating pain, as providing a remedy, a coping resource, a boost at times of weakness and a recharge at moments of emptiness may be the oldest and most entrenched social thoughts about religion. They are present in theological discourse, embodied in religious healing practices, but are also evident in the scientific and ideological discourse that is critical of religiosity. In the contemporary scholarly domain, this perception dominates psychology, which is preoccupied with measuring the influence of religion on well-being (e.g. Zel & Baumeister, 2013). They consider religion as a universal 'emotional therapy' (Asma, 2018). A great deal of psychological research has linked religious affiliation and belief with physical and psychological well-being and demonstrated how religiosity can serve as a resource for people in precarious life conditions (Watts, 2017). The particular area where the therapeutic nature of religiosity is assumed is the study of 'conversion', especially a personal dimension of conversion as a repair of traumatic condition (Rambo, 1993). The assumption that increasing religiosity is related to traumatic experiences, crisis or unstable social conditions also might explain why the perception of 'religion as therapy' serves as the dominant explanation for immigrant religiosity and the religious transformation of immigrants. Indeed, migration is considered a state that disrupts personal and collective stability. Thus, one can readily see that the aforementioned notion of religiosity in migration as a stabilizing factor and a resource is another manifestation of the 'religion as therapy' approach.

Today, however, we are witnessing a new turn in relations between religion and the idea of therapy, as well as between religion and psychology in general. Religion and the new religiosity are one of the most obvious and complex assemblages within the therapeutic turn, one that calls for close examination. Discussing the presence of a new relation between psychology and religion, Frank Furedi (2004) argues that therapeutic culture seems to thrive at times when religion is surpassed in authority and popularity by psychological culture. Recognizing the empowerment of the individual self in 'therapeutic religion', James Tucker places this type of religiosity outside the traditional religious institutions and limits its significance (Tucker, 2017). Scholars of religion and spirituality, have noted that mainstream contemporary religion has also adopted the elements of the global therapeutic discourse and uses it to strengthen itself. Kathryn Lofton, who has interpreted the Gospels in the light of therapy, suggests that the two projects have much in common: both contemporary religion and therapeutic gospel are built on a double solicitation – 'by asking to change your life [...] while suggesting that "your life needs changing"' (Lofton, 2015: 35). Tanya Luhrmann, in her work on the new intimate relations with God in American Evangelism, discusses the perception of 'God as therapist' (Luhrmann, 2012). As an example of a revived therapeutic dimension of mainstream theology, Tatiana Tiaynen-Qadir in this book brings a case of *therapeia* within the sources of Orthodox Christianity. Thus, one way or another, the psychological discourse has become an inseparable part of an emergent therapeutic religiosity. Moreover, it appears that, today, the scholarly understanding of religiosity as a calming agent actually overlaps with the therapeutic language of the new religiosity itself. Religious subjects and their researchers alike assume the therapeutic logic in the religious logic.

All of the above drives my attempt to develop a critical understanding of religiosity as therapy. I argue that we cannot ignore the therapeutic dimension of the religious experience – but that we ought to change the way we interpret it. Instead of seeking the therapeutic reasons for religious transformation, we should analyze the language of its reasoning to follow the ways in which religiosity is articulated and to reveal its therapeutic rhetoric. Without assuming that religion is adopted as an act of therapy or a resource for repairing and belonging, we can try to understand the ways in which people in general and immigrants in particular acquire therapeutic religion that speaks the language of calmness, belonging and well-being. Thus, the language of contemporary religion, or at least this kind of religion, constitutes a normative proper subject, one who is successful and happy. This outcome is worked out in the new relations between religious ethics, psychological discourse and neoliberal morality.

It would be an overstatement to claim that, today, each and every newly acquired religiosity speaks the therapeutic language. An intersectional combination of social positioning, generation, professional occupation, as well as of gender disposition,[6] exposes individuals and groups to the language of well-being and to a religious way of life at one and the same time. The intersection of religious agents and consulting institutions, such as nonprofit organizations of social and communal support, forges a new assemblage of therapeutic discourses and institutional practices. In this condition, the difference between the religious and areligious subject indeed becomes blurred, as both types of individual seek well-being and self-development. As in Weber's model of elective affinities, introduced to describe relations between capitalism and Protestantism, the religious and therapeutic cultures, in many respects mutually antithetical, also share some important similarities and paradoxically strengthen each other. In this way, it seems that religion could strengthen (or even create) a neoliberal subject no less than does life coaching or a course of self-development.

However, one might wonder about the nature of the similarity and blurredness that this assemblage produces. Specifically, does it organize all the spheres of private and public life of the religious therapeutic subjects? Where does it limit or fail to keep the mélange? The three women whose narratives I have discussed here conduct their lives within clearly demarcated communities and according to clearly delineated rules. Moreover, as actively religious women working with third sector institutions, their everyday lives are committed to the needs of their own community, and to the public good in general. In working on her individual self, each woman strives to achieve not only personal well-being but also to satisfy the imagined transcendental authority and its rule. Hence, the similarity of religious and therapeutic self-discourse does not abrogate the total nature of the religious way of life. Nor does it efface the distinct metaphysical authority that religious subjects follow. In this sense, the therapeutic religious assemblage illustrates the potential for the extension of the psychological logic to the new communal, public and collective realms. If the critique tends to assume that the therapeutic logic empties the self of its communal and political content and diminishes collective and communal attachments, the examined therapeutic religious assemblage illustrates the potential of the therapeutic culture to cooperate with and augment the authoritative transcendental and communal discourses.

Notes

1 The research that provides the basis for this chapter was supported by The Israel Science Foundation (grant number 449\10 and 16\496).
2 Surveys conducted in the past decade have shown that nearly one-third of Russian-speaking Israelis define themselves as 'religious', and only about the same number define themselves as 'non-believers', making the percentage of Russian immigrants affiliated with some sort of faith even larger (Remennick & Prashizky, 2012). Similarly, there is strong ethnographic evidence (including my own study) of Russian-speaking immigrants' active participation in local religious communities, both Jewish and Christian.
3 Data gathering in the Christian communities was based on observations of about 60 events in messianic communities (meeting groups and churches), in a Russian-Orthodox study group, and in the Seventh Day Adventist Church, as well as on more than 50 interviews with the members of these communities. Our data collection on Russian-Jewish religiosity focused on Orthodox Judaism (Chabad and National-Religious communities), the Kabbala La-am Movement and the Russian-language media.
4 For example, the international workshop titled 'New Religiosity in Migration', Ben-Gurion University of the Negev, May 2014.
5 Being granted citizenship according to the Israeli law of Jewish return to the Jewish historical homeland, more than 30 percent of Russian-speaking immigrants belong to 'ethnically mixed' families, and many of them cannot be considered Jewish according to the *Halakha* (Jewish religious law, which defines Jewishness largely on the basis of matrilineal descent). The 'Jewish problem' of Russians in Israel also stems from their cultural distance from Jewish religious knowledge and habitus. During the Soviet era, Jews defined their Jewishness in ethnic and not religious terms.
6 The gender aspect of the therapeutic religious assemblage should be mentioned particularly, because women constitute the main subject of both the new religiosity and the therapeutic culture. Moreover, they are patently present in third-sector professions.

References

Ahmed, S. 2010. *The Promise of Happiness*. Durham, NC: Duke University Press.

Asma, S.T. 2018. *Why We Need Religion: An Agnostic Celebration of Spiritual Emotions*. Oxford: Oxford University Press.

Binkley, S. 2014. *Happiness as Enterprise: An Essay on Neoliberal Life*. Albany: Suny Press.

Cadge, W. and Ecklund, E.H. 2007. Immigration and religion. *Annual Review of Sociology* 33, 359–379.

Chen, C. 2008. *Getting Saved in America: Taiwanese Immigration and Religious Experience*. Princeton University Press.

Cushman, P. 1995. *Constructing the Self, Constructing America: A Cultural History of Psychotherapy*. Cambridge, MA: Perseus.

Elias, N. and Lerner, J. 2016. Post-Soviet immigrant religiosity: beyond the Israeli national religion. In *The New Jewish Diaspora: Russian-Speaking Immigrants in the United States, Israel, and Germany*, edited by Z. Gitelman. New Brunswick, NJ: Rutgers University Press, 213–228.

Epstein, M. 1994. *Вера и образ. Религиозное бессознательное в русской культуре 20-го века (Faith and Image: Religious Unconscious in the Russian Culture of the 20th Century)*. Tenafly, NJ: Hermitage Publishers.

Epstein, M. 1999. Minimal religion and Post-atheism. In *Russian Postmodernism: New Perspective on Post-Soviet Culture*, edited by M. Epstein, A. Genis, and S. Vladiv-Glover. New York: Berghahn Books, 345–393.

Etkind, A. 1993. *Eros nevozmozhnogo: Istoriia psikhoanaliza v Rossii (Eros of the Impossible: A History of Psychoanalysis in Russia)*. St. Petersburg: Meduza.

Frouse, P. 2008. *The Plot to Kill God: Findings from the Soviet Experiment in Secularization*. Berkeley, CA: University of California Press.

Furedi, F. 2004. *Therapy Culture: Cultivating Vulnerability in an Uncertain Age*. London: Routledge.

Hagan, J. and Ebaugh, H.R. 2003. Calling upon the sacred: Migrants' use of religion in the migration process. *International Migration Review 37*:4, 1145–1162.

Heelas, P. 2009. *Spiritualities of Life: New Age Romanticism and Consumptive Capitalism*. Hoboken, NJ: Wiley.

Holstein, J.A. and Gubrium, J.F. 2011. *Varieties of Narrative Analysis*. Thousand Oaks, CA: Sage.

Illouz, E. 2007. *Cold Intimacies: The Making of Emotional Capitalism*. Cambridge: Polity Press.

Illouz, E. 2008. *Saving the Modern Soul: Therapy, Emotions, and the Culture of Self-Help*. Berkeley, CA: University of California Press.

Kornblatt, J.D. 2004. *Doubly Chosen: Jewish Identity, the Soviet Intelligentsia and the Russian Orthodox Church*. Madison: University of Wisconsin Press.

Lerner, J. 2015. The changing meanings of Russian love: Emotional socialism and therapeutic culture on the post-soviet screen. *Sexuality and Culture 19*:2, 349–368.

Lerner, J. and Zbenovich, C. 2013. Adapting the therapeutic discourse to post-soviet media culture: The case of Modnyi Prigovor. *Slavic Review 72*:4, 828–849.

Levitt, P. 2007. *God Needs No Passport: Immigrants and the Changing American Religious Landscape*. New York: New Press.

Leykin, I. 2015. Rodologia: Genealogy as therapy in Post-Soviet Russia. *Ethos 43*:2, 135–164.

Lofton, K. 2015. Gospel. In *Rethinking Therapeutic Culture*, edited by T. Aubry and T. Travis. Chicago: University of Chicago Press, 34–45.

Luehrmann, S. 2011. *Secularism Soviet Style: Teaching Atheism and Religion in a Volga Republic*. Bloomington: Indiana University Press.

Luhrmann, T.M. 2012. *When God Talks Back*. New York: Vantage Books.

Matza, T. 2018. *Shock Therapy: Psychology, Precarity, and Well-Being in Postsocialist Russia*. Durham, NC: Duke University Press.

Mooney, M. 2009. *Faith Makes Us Live: Surviving and Thriving in the Haitian Diaspora*. Berkeley, CA: University of California Press.

Pelkmans, M. 2009. *Conversion after Socialism: Disruptions, Modernisms and Technologies of Faith in the Former Soviet Union*. Oxford, UK: Berghahn Books.

Plant, R.J. 2015. Motherhood. In *Rethinking Therapeutic Culture*, edited by T. Aubry and T. Travis. Chicago: University of Chicago Press, 72–84.

Raijman, R. and Pinsky, J. 2011. Non-Jewish and Christians: Perceived discrimination and social distance among FSU migrants in Israel. *Israel Affairs 17*:1, 26–142.

Rambo, L.R. 1993. *Understanding Religious Conversion*. New Haven and London: Yale University Press.

Remennick, L. and Prashizky, A. 2012. Russian Israelis and religion: What has changed after twenty years in Israel? *Israel Studies Review 27*:1, 55–77.

Rose, N. 1990. *Governing the Soul: The Shaping of the Private Self*. London: Routledge.

Rose, N. 1996. *Inventing Ourselves: Psychology, Power, and Personhood*. Cambridge, UK: Cambridge University Press.

Salmenniemi, S. 2017. 'We can't live without beliefs': Self and society in therapeutic engagements. *The Sociological Review 65*:4, 611–627.

Steinberg, M.D. and Sobol, V. 2011. *Interpreting Emotions in Russia and Eastern Europe*. DeKalb: Northern Illinois University Press.

Sutton, J. 2006. 'Minimal religion' and Mikhail Epstein's interpretation of religion in late Soviet and post-Soviet Russia. *Studies in East European Thought 58*, 107–135.

Thrower, J. 1992. *Marxism-Leninism as the Civil Religion of Soviet Society: God's Commissar*. Lewiston, NY: Edwin Mellen Press.

Tucker, J. 2002. New age religion and the cult of the self. *Society 39*:2, 46–51.

Tucker, J. 2017. New healers and the therapeutic culture. In *Therapeutic Culture: Triumph and Defeat*, edited by J.B. Imber. New York: Routledge, 153–172.

Wanner, C. 2012. *State Secularism and Lived Religion in Soviet Russia and Ukraine*. New York: Oxford University Press.

Warner, R.S. and Wittner, J.G. (eds.) 1998. *Gatherings in Diaspora: Religious Communities and the New Immigration*. Philadelphia: Temple University Press.

Watts, F. 2017. *Psychology, Religion and Spirituality*. Cambridge: Cambridge University Press.

Weber, M. 1958 [original 1905]. *The Protestant Ethic and the Spirit of Capitalism*. New York: Charles Scribner's Sons.

Yang, F. and Ebaugh, H.R. 2001. Transformations in new immigrant religions and their global implication. *American Sociological Review 66*:2, 269–288.

Yurchak, A. 2005. *Everything Was Forever until It Was No More: The Last Soviet Generation*. Princeton: Princeton University Press.

Zel, A. and Baumeister, R. 2013. How religion can support self-control and moral behavior. In *Handbook of the Psychology of Religion and Spirituality*, edited by R.F. Paloutzian and C.L. Park. New York and London: The Guilford Press, 498–516.

Zilberman, B.D. 1977. Orthodox ethics and the matter of communism. *Studies in Soviet Thought 17*, 341–419.

6 Coaching for the nation

A new 'moral and ethical assemblage' for Israel's last republican generation

Ariel Yankellevich

Since the early 2000s, coaching has enjoyed great popularity in Israel, both in the workplace and in the sphere of personal life.[1] A myriad of for-profit institutes and higher-learning institutions offer coaching training programs and thousands of Israelis have become certified coaches.[2] Moreover, coaching has made its way into mainstream media culture, as indicated by the proliferation of reality TV-shows, radio talk-shows and self-help books dedicated to the topic. The ascendancy of coaching in Israel is not an isolated phenomenon, but can be seen in the context of the rapid expansion of a personal development industry including workshops, seminars, popular success literature and a wide variety of consulting and therapeutic services. Starting in the eighties as a somewhat fringe phenomenon (Beit-Hallahmi, 1992), this industry has flourished in Israel in the last twenty years as a counterpart to the increasing individualization and neoliberalization of Israeli society. As Israeli sociologists have noted, following the decline of the Labor Zionist collectivistic ethos in the late seventies, (mostly) middle-class secular Israelis began looking for meaning and self-fulfilment in the private sphere (Almog, 2001; Ram, 2000, 2008; Shafir & Peled, 2002).

The growing popularity of coaching among Israel's middle-class may thus be interpreted as reflecting this individualization trend (see Pagis, 2016). As a new therapeutic practice that blends psychological and managerial discourses, coaching aims at the production of autonomous, self-responsible, 'enterprising selves' (Du Gay, 1996; Rose, 1996) attuned to the challenges of work and life under neoliberalism. At the same time, it regards all forms of dependence and collective commitments as problematic remnants of an outdated economic and social configuration (Binkley, 2011b). As Mäkinen explains, 'the conception of selfhood that is constructed in coaching is a variation of a theme that is by now familiar from countless other contexts, namely the ideal subject of neoliberal individualism' (2014: 826). But as I will argue in this chapter, in order to better understand the appeal of coaching in contemporary Israeli society, we need to move beyond a monolithic and linear interpretation of neoliberal rationalities of government and look into the ways that these rationalities are 'reorganizing subjectivities tied to earlier social ways of governing [...] rather than simply challenging or replacing them' (Brady, 2014: 30). Such an approach places analytical emphasis on processes of assembly rather than on resultant formations and therefore highlights the contingency and provisionality of neoliberal governmentalities. As Higgins and Larner (2017: 5) argue, 'these emergent assemblages may cohere in ways that constitute spaces, sites and subjects as "neoliberal", but they may also at the same time involve multiple, contradictory and overlapping projects and practices that exceed any straightforward reading as neoliberalism'. Hence, instead of assuming coaching's individualizing and depoliticizing effects, we should ask how its core ideas and practices enter into assemblages that also include existing local discourses and traditions of the self and its involvement in public life.

This chapter is based on a case study of Israeli coaches from what I term 'the last republican generation.' Members of this ethno-class generational unit were born in the fifties and early sixties and had their formative experiences in the era before the neoliberal economic turn in Israel (generally dated to the mid-eighties). As members of the veteran,[3] mostly Ashkenazi (Jews of European origin) social elite,[4] they were socialized into the Labor Zionist collectivistic and nationalistic ethos, which tied individual self-realization with the fulfilment of collective goals (such as national security, immigrant absorption, frontier settlement and the building of national institutions) and loyalty to the state. This ethos was crystallized in a republican discourse of civic virtue that placed this group as a 'service elite' and rewarded it accordingly (Shafir & Peled, 2002). On the other hand, this was the first generation of the veteran middle-class that adopted a culture of hedonistic individualism and sought to realize its personal and professional abilities in the spheres of work and leisure (Almog, 2001; Ram, 2008). The recent turn of many of its members to the burgeoning field of coaching,[5] often after long careers as salaried employees in large bureaucratic organizations, seems to conform to this generational pattern of withdrawal into the private realm and increasing preoccupation with the self. But as I will show in this chapter, the adoption of the neoliberal therapeutic discourse of coaching by this dominant social group cannot be reduced to a single and coherent cultural logic of individualization, as it defies the opposition between individual self-development and social and political engagement. Rather, coaching takes part in a new 'moral and ethical assemblage' (Zigon, 2010; 2011) that combines neoliberal rationalities with the Labor Zionist republican ethos.

The data for this chapter comes from 42 in-depth interviews with members of the last republican generation who chose coaching as a second (or third) career. The interviews were conducted between 2016 and 2017 in different locations in Central and Southern Israel and lasted two hours on average. All interviews started with the open question 'tell me about yourself; you can start wherever you want,' and subsequently turned to the participants' career paths and their involvement in coaching. Research participants were initially recruited from personal websites, via an e-mail sent to affiliates of the Israeli Coaching Bureau (one of the two main coaching professional associations in Israel) and through personal acquaintances. I then used a snowball sampling technique, asking interviewees to provide the names of friends and acquaintances who are also involved in the field of coaching. Roughly two-thirds of participants were women, which seems to reflect their predominance in the profession. Most interviewees had training in various self-development techniques besides coaching, such as Neuro-Linguistic Programming (NLP), alternative medicine, mediation, management consulting and more. Moreover, their coaching practices varied considerably, ranging from business and career coaching to more life-focused forms of coaching, such as relationship coaching, coaching for adults and children with attention deficit hyperactivity disorder (ADHD), ontological coaching (a 'spiritual' brand of coaching roughly inspired by the Landmark Forum), retirement coaching and more. Notwithstanding this variation, virtually all interviewees adhered to some basic principles and techniques that are characteristic of coaching, such as goal-setting and strategic planning, identification and reinforcement of personal abilities and strengths, a focus on short-term processes and results and an orientation to the future.

The chapter begins with an introduction to contemporary debates on neoliberal subjectivity and the role of therapeutic culture. The following sections examine different modes of articulation between neoliberal therapeutic discourses and the Labor Zionist collectivistic ethos through the interviewees' stories of involvement in coaching. The concluding section will wrap up the chapter by suggesting a look at these articulations through the lens of assemblage theory.

Neoliberal subjectivity and the critique of therapeutic culture

In the last twenty-five years, a growing body of literature in the social sciences has been preoccupied with the construction of subjectivity under neoliberalism. Inspired by the Foucauldian tradition, these studies analyze neoliberalism as a form of governmental reason that aims to 'conduct the conduct' of free subjects (Foucault, 1991). Neoliberal governmentality works through the cultivation of autonomous, entrepreneurial dispositions within subjects and the marketization of social relations (Binkley, 2014; Rose, 1996). As Foucault argued in *The Birth of Biopolitics*, neoliberalism generalizes the enterprise form within the social body and makes it a model of social relations and of existence itself (2008: 241–2). This entrepreneurialization of society has profound social consequences:

> the organization of society around a multiplicity of individual enterprises profoundly depoliticizes social and political relations by fragmenting collective values of care, duty and obligation, and displacing them back on to the managed autonomy of the individual.
>
> (McNay, 2009: 65)

This process of social desolidarization (Hartmann & Honneth, 2006) results from the coronation of economic interest and free choice as irreducible principles of human action. The neoliberal subject, or *homo economicus*, is driven solely by his own egoistic self-interest, which is aimed at the maximization of his own happiness and well-being. Moreover, the construction of this neoliberal subject includes practices of desubjectification aimed at eradicating former collectivistic and dependent dispositions rooted in earlier forms of social governance (Binkley, 2009, 2011a, 2011b). In this sense, the neoliberal governance of the self atomizes our understanding of social relations and erodes conceptions of the public domain (McNay, 2009: 64). Neoliberal subjects tend to recast social and political problems as personal ones and seek for individualized solutions (Scharff, 2016).

In this respect, the neo-Foucauldian critique of the neoliberal governance of the self shares certain key assumptions with what Aubry and Travis (2015) have recently termed 'the canonical critique of therapeutic culture'. This strand of critique, best expressed by commentators such as Phillip Rieff, Christopher Lasch, Richard Sennett and Robert Bellah (and more recently by Frank Furedi, Philip Cushman and James Nolan Jr.), posits that late modernity is characterized by the rise of a therapeutic ethos that encourages an individualistic conception of the self and depoliticizes and privatizes social life. The 'fall narrative' offered by these critics blames therapeutic culture for the decline of public life and the lack of commitment to social institutions. As Eva Illouz (2008: 2) summarizes this critique:

> in calling on us to withdraw into ourselves, the therapeutic persuasion has made us abandon the great realms of citizenship and politics and cannot provide us with an intelligible way of linking the private self to the public sphere because it has emptied the self of its communal and political content, replacing this content with a narcissistic self-concern.

More recent accounts of therapeutic culture, though more nuanced and less condemnatory, still draw a dichotomy between individualized self-development and political and social engagement (Gill & Orgad, 2015; Matza, 2009; McGee, 2005; Nehring et al., 2016; Salmenniemi, 2012). While they often acknowledge the multifaceted nature of therapeutic culture and explore its entanglement with local discourses, many of these studies ultimately see therapy as an individualizing and depoliticizing force. In this chapter, I would like to challenge the dichotomous view that opposes 'the therapeutic ethos to a model of civic virtue or political engagement' (Illouz, 2008: 223) by suggesting that the adoption of neoliberal therapeutic discourses and practices does not necessarily entail a withdrawal into the private realm nor the abandonment of a vision of the common good. On the contrary, it may give way to new forms of political and social engagement.

The last republican generation: between coaching and *hagshama*

The ethno-class generational unit I termed 'the last republican generation' has been described by critical Israeli sociologists as the bearer of a liberal, individualistic turn in Israeli society. From its early days as a colonial frontier society, the Zionist settlement in Palestine was constituted as a community of republican virtue built around an ethos of 'pioneering' (*chalutziut*) that placed self-sacrifice and unselfish work for the nation's common good as ultimate values. This ethos was a central pillar of the Labor Zionist collectivistic and nationalistic ideology that was hegemonic in Israel until the late seventies. Despite its socialist rhetoric, this ideology served as the legitimation basis for a hierarchical incorporation regime that arranged and rewarded different groups of citizens according to their conceived contribution to the common good of the nation as defined by the Zionist vision. The veteran Ashkenazi elite was placed at the top of this regime, as it allegedly embodied the republican virtue of pioneering (Shafir & Peled, 2002).

Beginning in the mid-seventies, as a result of a combination of several local and global political, economic and sociocultural processes,[6] the Labor Zionist republican ethos entered an ongoing crisis and started its decline. For the veteran Ashkenazi elite, which was heavily invested in this ethos, this fall from grace spurred an identity crisis and many of its members began searching for meaning and purpose through less collectivistic ideologies and projects (Almog, 2001; Beit-Hallahmi, 1992; Katriel, 2004; Kimmerling, 2005; Ram, 2008; Roniger & Feige, 1992; Shafir & Peled, 2002). The halt to the peace process and the election of right wing Netanyahu as prime minister in the mid-nineties reinforced in this social group 'a sense of alienation not only from collectivism but also from the collectivity itself' (Ram, 2000: 227).

It is in this context that we should analyze the turn to coaching by members of this generational unit. At first glance, many of the interviewees' stories of engagement with coaching seem to fit the macro-sociological picture presented by Ram and others. Take for example the case of Kobi, a coach in his sixties that works mainly with families and children. A retired military person, Kobi makes a living as a freelance high-tech contractor besides his coaching activity. In this sense, he is a rightful representative of 'the middle-class successors of the older state and military elite [who] are withdrawing from the older career-path and turning to the more attractive and rewarding trajectories offered by civil society and the burgeoning market' (ibid.). During our interview, Kobi told me about his plans to leave the business world in order to dedicate himself fully to coaching: 'I am in a phase out from the business world. I want the soul, I want to contribute and I want to make things better.' Later in our conversation he expanded on the reasons for taking up coaching as a profession:

> I did a lot of things in my life and I got fed up. And then I said that I need something for the soul, something that will do me good. Today I can define it; back then I didn't know how to define it. The choice of [working with] families and children came while I was undergoing coaching myself. During my studies I understood that the area where I will have the most influence, the area that suits me the best, is the work with children.

Kobi's account reveals two interrelated motivations for becoming a coach. On the one hand, he turned to coaching because he wanted 'something for the soul' after many years in the military and hi-tech sectors. This motivation appears in many sociological and journalistic descriptions of the wide appeal of self-development technologies, especially among the professional-managerial class. These technologies provide overworked professionals in the post-Fordist economy an escape from the cold and hyper-rational world of work and let them do something more humane and self-rewarding (George, 2013; Mäkinen, 2012; Salmenniemi et al. in this book). On the other hand, Kobi turned to coaching because he wanted to contribute to society and have more social influence. Doing something for his soul in his case does not entail turning inwards, but outwards. In his view, his personal growth and success are deeply tied to his contribution to society. Hence, Kobi also volunteers as a coach among underserved populations, leads community-building programs and has plans for establishing an integrative clinic for families and children. As he said: 'I decided very quickly that in this stage of my life it is time to give back to society.'

This same motivation to contribute to society underpins many interviewees' coaching activities. Liora, a kibbutz member in her early sixties, talked about searching for new fields of action as a coach:

> We [she and her associate] looked for something to do and we got to all kinds of organizations of the type we knew: hi-tech, telecommunications, things like that, but after a year we both said that we feel that where Israel needs us most is in the field of education. We want to bring the option of coaching to education. So we started little by little, at first in his hometown, he went to the high school principal and he offered a free intervention.

In this excerpt we see how collectivistic dispositions rooted in the Labor Zionist republican ethos inform Liora's new identity as a coach. Her choice of a field of action is not dictated by individualist concerns (like making money or gaining prestige by working in leading industries), but by a sense of responsibility for the fate of the nation. In this sense, Liora still sees herself as a member of a service elite committed to the achievement of the nation's common good. Coaching is only a new and powerful tool that helps her fulfil this self-appointed social mission. Moreover, much like Kobi, she does not draw a distinction between her social engagement and her individual self-development. In her view, both are deeply related and resonate with each other. She describes herself as an 'enabler', a person that through her own self-growth can make the world a better place. As she explained:

> I really believe that things must start from the person; not from an egoistic standpoint, but from the standpoint that I am the source of my own world. If the things I need are not provided, I can't give. I can give from what I have; I can't give from what I don't have. Hence my duty is to increase what I have.

Liora and Kobi's stories exemplify the entanglement of a therapeutic neoliberal discourse of individual self-development with the Labor Zionist ideal of *hagshama*. Translated as 'realization' or 'consummation', the practice of *hagshama* refers to 'the personal implementation of pioneering values' (Almog, 2000: 296). As Shafir and Peled explain, in the pre-state years, *hagshama atzmit* (literally 'self-realization', not to be confounded with *mimush atzmi*, which is the contemporary Hebrew term for individual self-realization or self-fulfilment) expressed the strongest commitment to national goals as defined by the Labor Zionist movement:

> *Hagshama atzmit* was not an individual's act but the self-realization of the virtuous citizen, namely, the carrying out of the movement's pioneering goal by the individual member as his/her duty *qua* citizen. *Hagshama atzmit* meant personal participation in the collective endeavor of transforming Palestine into a Jewish homeland.
>
> (Shafir & Peled, 2002: 43)

In this way, the Labor Zionist republican ethos tied individual self-realization with the fulfilment of collective goals and service to the nation. While the actual practice of *hagshma* was confined to a small Ashkenazi pioneering elite (and was rewarded accordingly, both materially and symbolically), it became an ideal to which the younger *Sabra* (native-born Jewish Israelis) generations were socialized and measured up to (Almog, 2000; Shafir & Peled, 2002). In recent decades, following the weakening of the republican citizenship discourse, the *hagshama* ideal and its accompanying pioneering ethos have lost much of their appeal for younger generations of Israelis, especially among the secular middle-class.[7] But as my interviewees' stories show, this collectivistic ideal (and the social responsibility that comes with it) is still a part of their generation's moral landscape and unreflective, habitual dispositions. Therefore, I would like to argue that their use of coaching in the service of collective goals is not just an expression of an ethics of doing good that characterizes the therapeutic professions (Rose, 1996), but is part of a wider identity project aimed at negotiating their complex position as a waning but still powerful elite in search of new sources of social legitimation. In this project, individual self-development and social engagement are assembled together.

In the remainder of this chapter, I will describe two central ways of articulating the neoliberal therapeutic language of coaching with the Labor Zionist practice of *hagshama*. First, as Liora's story shows, therapeutic self-change has become a condition to engage in work for the sake of others. As many interviewees testified, they only felt that they could bring about social change after they underwent change themselves. Second, the forms of social engagement endorsed by the interviewees, while still addressing the common fate of Israeli society as a whole, focus on the ripple effect of individual change instead of political or collective solutions. In this way, they reproduce a vision of the nation's common good that is in line with neoliberalism.

Transforming oneself in order to contribute to society

In most of the interviewees' stories, social engagement is described as a relatively new facet of their lives. While many of them were public or semi-public employees in their first careers (teachers, social workers, military persons), they rarely see their former work in the public sector as a significant form of social engagement or contribution to the welfare of society. Moreover, virtually none of them mentioned contributing to the common good of the nation (or just '*zionut*', as this kind of altruistic motivation is usually called in Israel) as a central motivation for their early career choices. This seeming contradiction is explained by the institutionalization of the pioneering ethos in the transition to statehood, which turned collectivism from a voluntary, grassroots ideology to a chief principle of government (Rozin, 2011; Shafir & Peled, 2002). For many interviewees then, entering public service was an opportunity to pursue their individual professional aspirations in what was still a state-centered economy (Maman & Rosenhek, 2012; Shafir & Peled, 2002; Shalev, 2000). It was also a common occupational path for middle-class Ashkenazi young professionals entering the workforce in the late seventies and early eighties.

Take for example the case of Nirit, a coach in her early sixties. A social worker by training, she worked for more than twenty years as a public welfare official in her hometown social services office. During her tenure there, she became acquainted with the pensioner population and its specific problems. As her interest in this age sector grew, she started to think about new ways to help them beyond the existing institutional frameworks, but she did not dare to leave her secure job and to embark on an independent project. It was only through her personal experience of coaching that she took courage and made the first steps in that direction:

> Only when I started studying coaching and it shook all the furniture inside my head and ordered them in another way… and suddenly I realized that everything is possible, everything I want. […] We learned to set goals and have dreams and develop visions. I knew that I wanted to establish a pensioners' centre, because there is not such a thing in Israel, and in this centre I want to let pensioners and their families come and get advice and get a push for starting the journey, what do we do when we retire. And I dreamed about it in such a way that it excited and enthused me so much, so I decided to take a sabbatical year.

In Nirit's story we find again the same entanglement between individual self-development and collective commitment. As we learn from the above quote, Nirit's involvement in coaching did not lead to withdrawal into the private sphere, but reinforced and opened new possibilities for social engagement, as she used her newly acquired ability to 'set goals and have dreams and develop visions' in order to contribute to society. Moreover, her newfound realization that 'everything is possible' sparked a renowned interest in direct political participation and in recent years she has been involved in the Israeli pensioners' party and even ran for office.

Nirit's story of renewed social and political engagement following her training as a coach is far from unique. Other coaches also related how the self-transformation they experienced through coaching made them more emotionally available and skilled for pursuing interests beyond their own selves. As Tami, a coach involved in local politics told, 'when you feel complete, peaceful, accomplished, successful, you have something to give others. [...] I think that if it were not for my work as a coach I wouldn't get too far [in politics].' In a telling reversal of the sociological critique of therapy, many interviewees talked about how in their previous lives *before* the discovery of coaching they were extremely self-absorbed and preoccupied with their own private issues. Their excessive focus on the self and its problems did not leave room for thinking about social and political issues, let alone do something for the nation's common good (even if in their daily jobs as public servants they were actually engaged in such endeavour). It was only *after* they studied coaching that they started to look beyond themselves and became preoccupied with the fate of Israeli society. By instilling in them new empowering beliefs, qualities and abilities, coaching allowed them 'to put the head out' of their 'little' private fears and troubles and get involved in public life (see also Salmenniemi et al. and Perheentupa in this book). As Yael, a coach and lecturer on feminist issues, told, being a coach taught her 'to keep silent, to listen, to be there for someone', to be less stressed-out and fearful, and this in turn was reflected in her activism for the sake of disadvantaged women.

In this sense, it seems that for the last republican generation, the turn to coaching does not signal a further turn away from the collective, but rather reconnects it (both practically and emotionally) to its historic role as a service elite who sees itself as responsible for the fate of the nation. But as we will immediately see, the form of contribution to the nation's common good that its members now endorse is far from the old Labor Zionist collectivistic repertoire. Instead, as Nirit's dream of a pensioner's centre shows, their social initiatives espouse and reproduce the neoliberal language of entrepreneurship and individual choice.

Collectivistic entrepreneurship: fostering individual change in the service of the nation

As shown earlier, contribution to the common good of the nation is a central motive in the interviewees' stories of involvement in coaching. Some of them even described their coaching activity as a mission (*shlichut*),[8] a personal calling to act in the benefit of society. But as I already hinted, the kind of contribution they have in mind differs from earlier collectivistic endeavours in significant ways. First, in contrast to the days of Labor Zionist political and sociocultural hegemony, in today's neoliberal Israel it is they (as private but concerned citizens), not the state, who get to choose what the national goals are. Since the mid-eighties, the Israeli state has largely withdrawn from its role in welfare provision and its vacant place has been occupied by a whole field of NGOs, in a process that has been referred to as 'the NGOization of civil society' (Herzog, 2008). Initiatives like Nirit's pensioners' centre, Kobi's integrative clinic for families and children and Liora's project of coaching at school, among others, adopt this logic of action and concentrate on niches of activity that were formerly under full state responsibility and have been increasingly privatized in recent years. Hence, whether in the Labor Zionist past members of the veteran Ashkenazi elite were 'called to the flag' in order to perform national missions defined by the state, now they follow flags of their own liking. But still, these flags are nonetheless national and collective, not individual.

Second, for most interviewees contributing to the nation's common good is less a matter of participating in collective endeavours or engaging in outright political activity (though as we saw in the cases of Nirit, Tami and Yael, there is also room for that) than of fostering individual change and self-development. Hence, although they often voiced ardent political criticism of Prime Minister Netanyahu's right wing government and policies during the interviews, they seldom spoke about the need for profound structural change, especially in economic matters. This is less due to feelings of political powerlessness than to their structural position as the 'winners' from the liberalization of the Israeli economy (Ram, 2008; Shalev, 2000). Thus, while they sometimes decried the 'excesses' of the capitalist turn in Israel and the retrenchment of the welfare state, for the most part they did not want to go back to the old Labor Zionist 'socialist' model. Instead of political, structural change then, they conceived societal change as stemming from the ripple effect of individual transformation. As Dov, a coach in his early sixties, argued:

> I think that when someone undergoes coaching and comes to it to make a change from a positive place, the change in the end influences his family group, also his extended family, also his group of friends, also his community.

According to this approach, if each of us understands that 'things must start from the person' (to quote Liora) and takes responsibility for himself, the nation as a whole will benefit. Like with Adam Smith's invisible hand, the sum of each individual's autonomous efforts will result in a maximization of the common good (see Klin-Oron, 2014 for a similar argument from the field of spiritual channeling in Israel). Dov provides a vivid example of this neoliberal approach when he describes his project of establishing a 'school for entrepreneurs' that will provide business coaching to small business owners and developers. He came to the idea after he learned that a majority of small businesses in Israel close down after one or two years of activity. While he acknowledges that large economic forces beyond any business owner's control impact on his chances to succeed, he ultimately blames their failure on a lack of entrepreneurial skills. As he says, 'if forty-four thousand businesses closed [last year], this means that at least forty-four thousand people made a mistake at some point.' By teaching them how to navigate a constantly changing economy and think in a strategic, entrepreneurial fashion, he hopes not just to help each individual business owner but to make a significant impact on the national economy. As he explained:

> One of our thoughts regarding the school for entrepreneurs that we want to establish is that the more successful businesses there are, it contributes to GNP [Gross National Product] in the end. That is, it helps also at the national level.

While most interviewees did not frame their national contribution as coaches in such an explicit and articulate way, the enlistment of coaching's neoliberal individualized therapeutic approach to the solution of what they saw as national problems was far from unique. Interviewees often described coaching as a new gospel that can provide innovative answers to Israeli society's most acute problems, such as educational underachievement, social inequality, poverty relief and social and political polarization. Even Israel's arguably most intractable national problem, the Israeli-Palestinian conflict, was deemed a legitimate target for coaching intervention. As Haim, a very active coach in his mid-sixties, explained:

> I started with the vision that this work will cross borders and I will be able to make some kind of impact in countries beyond our political side. [...] Coaching creates bridges of communication between people, both within themselves and with others. That is, we can learn to send to each other travelers instead of missiles [both words sound similar in Hebrew], tourists instead of terrorists. Being able to learn how to agree while we have disagreements in many areas and to respect the fact that we disagree, that he thinks X and I think Y, and I will respect him that he thinks X and he will respect me that we think Y and we don't have to kill each other. And through this coaching approach, this coaching language, I really believe that it's possible.

In this excerpt, Haim provides an interpretation of the Israeli-Palestinian conflict based on the therapeutic ethos of communication (Illouz, 2008). In his view, the key to avoiding violence is to create 'bridges of communication' between both sides of the conflict by fostering open dialogue and acknowledging and respecting their mutual differences. In this way, he simplifies a national problem with complex structural causes and scales it down to the individual level, much like Dov did in the small businesses case. By reducing it to a problem of (mis)communication, Haim depoliticizes the conflict and makes it amenable to therapeutic intervention.[9]

But as I have argued throughout this chapter, the adoption of coaching's highly apolitical and individualized language by members of the last republican generation like Haim does not mean that they have withdrawn into their private affairs and lost their stakes in national issues. If we pay close attention to Haim's words, we can discern the use of the collective 'we' when referring to the Israeli side of the conflict. This use of the collective 'we' betrays a sense of belonging to a bigger collective, an almost natural identification with the nation. In forging a vision to use coaching to solve the Israeli-Palestinian conflict, Haim is not acting as a private individual but as a representative of the nation, a self-appointed ambassador of peace. In this sense, I would like to argue that his turn to coaching does not signal a rupture in his commitment to the nation nor a sense of alienation from the collective (Ram, 2000), but rather provides him with a new and more effective tool to fulfil his *schlichut* as a member of Israel's service elite. Therefore, much like in the other cases I presented in this chapter, the neoliberal logic of coaching does not stand alone, but is enlisted to and interwoven with this generation's republican mission to contribute to the nation's common good.

A new moral and ethical assemblage?

In a programmatic text on the emergence of global assemblages, Ong and Collier (2008: 13) argue that 'neoliberalism's actual shape and significance for the forms of individual and collective life can only be understood as it enters into assemblages with other elements'. They define an assemblage as 'the product of multiple determinations that are not reducible to a single logic' (ibid.: 12). In this chapter, I have tried to show how such an assemblage is being constructed in the new field of Israeli coaching. I have argued that we should not interpret the emergence of this field as expressing a single individualization logic in Israeli society, but rather look at how coaching's neoliberal therapeutic rationality enters into dialogue with local discourses and traditions of the self as it is adopted by different social groups.

Focusing on the case of coaches from Israel's 'last republican generation', I have pointed at how life-coaching provides them with a new language for 'linking the private self to the public sphere' (Illouz, 2008: 2). This language seems to have replaced the Labor Zionist collectivistic ethos that has lost much of its former relevance in contemporary neoliberal Israel. But as I have tried to show, this does not mean that this ethos and its associated republican dispositions to act for the common good of the nation have disappeared from this generation's moral landscape. Instead, they partake in a new 'moral and ethical assemblage' (Zigon, 2010, 2011), which also includes neoliberal discourses of entrepreneurship, individual autonomy and self-development. As Zigon (2011: 44) argues, 'within moral and ethical assemblages diverse and seemingly contradictory discursive traditions can uniquely combine and support one another in ways perhaps unrecognized by those participating in the assemblage'. Hence, 'they offer a greater range of possibilities for morally being in the world and ethically working on oneself than any one of these traditions on its own' (ibid.: 47). For members of the last republican generation then, such an assemblage provides a context for remaking their complex identities in neoliberal Israel.

Finally, this chapter joins a growing body of research showing the implication of self-improvement discourses and practices in the (re)construction of national communities and identities in the wake of neoliberal reform, especially (but not exclusively) in the post-socialist context. In this process, old-time local notions of citizenship, patriotism and the common good are reworked in creative and often unpredictable ways, as they articulate with neoliberal political rationalities (Hemment, 2012; Hoffman, 2006; Matza, 2009). Thus, without overlooking therapy's role as a globalizing and homogenizing force (Illouz, 2008; Nehring et al., 2016), future research should also consider how it is deployed in efforts to reassemble the nation.

Notes

1 This research was supported by The Israeli Science Foundation (grant No. 16\496).
2 Like in most parts of the world, coaching is not a state-certified profession in Israel, so there are no official statistics on the number of trainees and practitioners. Available data from local coaching associations suggests that over 10,000 Israelis sought coaching

training, allegedly making Israel the country with the highest number of trained coaches per capita in the world (see Kaneh-Shalit, 2017). However, it is important to note that most certified coaches do not end up working in the field, so that the number of actually practicing coaches is much lower.

3 In an immigrant society such as Israel, the term 'veteran' is used to distinguish between older and newer Jewish immigrants. Veterans were those that immigrated to Israel prior to the state declaration in 1948, mostly from Eastern Europe, and conformed the local social elite (see Peled & Shapir, 2005; Kimmerling, 2001).

4 Following Israeli researchers of ethnicity, I treat the Ashkenazi ethnic label as a performative rather than as ascriptive identity (see Sasson-Levy, 2013). Thus, my sample includes a few 'pure' Mizrahim (Jews from North Africa and Middle Eastern countries) and individuals of mixed ethnicity that resemble and act as Ashkenazim in most respects.

5 Again, there are no official statistics on the age-distribution of certified coaches in Israel. Nonetheless, the central role of members of this generational unit in the coaching field is hard to miss. For example, most of the founders and original members of the two major coaching associations in Israel come from this social group (for similar findings in the U.S., see George, 2013: 191).

6 These include, among others, the trauma of the 1973 War, the political turnover of 1977, which ended Labor's forty years of continued government, the liberalization of the economy and the increasing penetration of Western consumer culture.

7 As a number of social commentators have noted, the Zionist pioneering ethos has not disappeared, but has been taken up and revamped by the religious-nationalist right in its efforts to gain national legitimation for its colonization project in the West Bank (see Ben-Eliezer, 1998; Ram, 2008; Shafir and Peled, 2002).

8 The biblical Hebrew word *shlichut*, which originally referred to emissaries carrying another person or God's mission, has deep Zionist connotations, as it is commonly used to refer to dedication to the achievement of the goals of Zionism. Like *hagshama*, it denotes unselfish work for the sake of the nation.

9 Haim's therapeutic approach to the Israeli-Palestinian conflict is in fact not original, as the practice of fostering unmediated open and empathetic dialogue between Israelis and Palestinians is a long-time feature of the 'peace industry' (as its detractors call it) that developed around the conflict.

References

Almog, O. 2000. *The Sabra: The Creation of the New Jew*. Berkeley: University of California Press.

Almog, O. 2001. Shifting the centre from nation to individual and universe: The new 'democratic faith' of Israel. *Israel Affairs 8*:1–2, 31–42.

Aubry, T. & T. Travis. (cds) 2015. *Rethinking Therapeutic Culture*. Chicago: University of Chicago Press.

Beit-Hallahmi, B. 1992. *Despair and Deliverance: Private Salvation in Contemporary Israel*. Albany: Suny Press.

Ben-Eliezer, U. 1998. State versus civil society? A non-binary model of domination through the example of Israel. *Journal of Historical Sociology 11*:3, 370–396.

Binkley, S. 2009. The work of neoliberal governmentality: Temporality and ethical substance in the tale of two dads. *Foucault Studies 6*, 60–78.

Binkley, S. 2011a. Happiness, positive psychology and the program of neoliberal governmentality. *Subjectivity 4*:4, 371–394.

Binkley, S. 2011b. Psychological life as enterprise: Social practice and the government of neo-liberal interiority. *History of the Human Sciences 24*:3, 83–102.

Binkley, S. 2014. *Happiness as Enterprise: An Essay on Neoliberal Life*. Albany: Suny Press.

Brady, M. 2014. Ethnographies of neoliberal governmentalities: From the neoliberal apparatus to neoliberalism and governmental assemblages. *Foucault Studies 18*, 11–33.

Du Gay, P. 1996. *Consumption and Identity at Work*. London: Sage.

Foucault, M. 1991. Governmentality. In *The Foucault Effect: Studies in Governmentality*, edited by G. Burchell, C. Gordon & P. Miller. Chicago: University of Chicago Press, 87–104.

Foucault, M. 2008. *The Birth of Biopolitics: Lectures at the Collège de France, 1978–1979*, translated by G. Burchell. New York: Palgrave Macmillan.

George, M. 2013. Seeking legitimacy: The professionalization of life coaching. *Sociological Inquiry 83*:2, 179–208.

Gill, R. & S. Orgad. 2015. The confidence cult(ure). *Australian Feminist Studies 30*:86, 324–344.

Hartmann, M. & A. Honneth. 2006. Paradoxes of capitalism. *Constellations 13*:1, 41–58.

Hemment, J. 2012. Redefining need, reconfiguring expectations: The rise of state-run youth voluntarism programs in Russia. *Anthropological Quarterly 85*:2, 519–554.

Herzog, H. 2008. Re/visioning the women's movement in Israel. *Citizenship Studies 12*:3, 265–282.

Higgins, V. & W. Larner. (eds) 2017. *Assembling Neoliberalism: Expertise, Practices, Subjects*. New York: Palgrave Macmillan.

Hoffman, L. 2006. Autonomous choices and patriotic professionalism: On governmentality in late-socialist China. *Economy and Society 35*:4, 550–570.

Illouz, E. 2008. *Saving the Modern Soul: Therapy, Emotions, and the Culture of Self-Help*. Berkeley: University of California Press.

Kaneh-Shalit, T. 2017. 'The goal is not to cheer you up': Empathetic care in Israeli life coaching. *Ethos 45*:1, 98–115.

Katriel, T. 2004. *Dialogic Moments: From Soul Talks to Talk Radio in Israeli Culture*. Detroit: Wayne State University Press.

Kimmerling, B. 2005. *The Invention and Decline of Israeliness: State, Society, and the Military*. Berkeley: University of California Press.

Klin-Oron, A. 2014. The end begins in me: New forms of political action in Israeli channeling. *Israel Studies Review 29*:2, 39–56.

McGee, M. 2005. *Self-Help, Inc.: Makeover Culture in American Life*. Oxford: Oxford University Press.

McNay, L. 2009. Self as enterprise: Dilemmas of control and resistance in Foucault's the birth of biopolitics. *Theory, Culture & Society 26*:6, 55–77.

Mäkinen, K. 2012. *Becoming Valuable Selves: Self-Promotion, Gender and Individuality in Late Capitalism*. Tampere: University of Tampere.

Mäkinen, K. 2014. The individualization of class: A case of working life coaching. *The Sociological Review 62*:4, 821–842.

Maman, D. & Z. Rosenhek. 2012. The institutional dynamics of a developmental state: Change and continuity in state–economy relations in Israel. *Studies in Comparative International Development 47*:3, 342–363.

Matza, T. 2009. Moscow's echo: Technologies of the self, publics, and politics on the Russian talk show. *Cultural Anthropology 24*:3, 489–522.

Nehring, D., D. Kerrigan, E. C. Hendriks & E. Alvarado. 2016. *Transnational Popular Psychology and the Global Self-Help Industry: The Politics of Contemporary Social Change*. London: Palgrave Macmillan.

Ong, A. & S. J. Collier. (eds) 2008. *Global Assemblages: Technology, Politics, and Ethics as Anthropological Problems*. London: Blackwell.

Pagis, M. 2016. Fashioning futures: Life coaching and the self-made identity paradox. *Sociological Forum 31*:4, 1083–1103.

Ram, U. 2000. The promised land of business opportunities: Liberal post-Zionism in the glocal age. In *The New Israel: Peacemaking and Liberalization*, edited by G. Shafir & Y. Peled. Boulder, CO: Westview Press, 217–242.

Ram, U. 2008. *The Globalization of Israel: McWorld in Tel Aviv, Jihad in Jerusalem*. New York: Routledge.

Roniger, L. & M. Feige. 1992. From pioneer to freier: The changing models of generalized exchange in Israel. *European Journal of Sociology/Archives Européennes De Sociologie 33*:2, 280–307.

Rose, N. 1996. *Inventing Ourselves: Psychology, Power, and Personhood*. Cambridge: Cambridge University Press.

Rozin, O. 2011. *The Rise of the Individual in 1950s Israel: A Challenge to Collectivism*. Waltham, MA: Brandeis University Press.

Salmenniemi, S. 2012. Post-soviet khoziain: Class, self and morality in Russian self-help literature. In *Rethinking Class in Russia*, edited by S. Salmenniemi. Farnham, UK: Ashgate, 67–84.

Sasson-Levy, O. 2013. A different kind of whiteness: Marking and unmarking of social boundaries in the construction of hegemonic ethnicity. *Sociological Forum 28*:1, 27–50.

Scharff, C. 2016. The psychic life of neoliberalism: Mapping the contours of entrepreneurial subjectivity. *Theory, Culture & Society 33*:6, 107–122.

Shafir, G. & Y. Peled. 2002. *Being Israeli: The Dynamics of Multiple Citizenship*. Cambridge: Cambridge University Press.

Shalev, M. 2000. Liberalization and the transformation of the political economy. In *The New Israel: Peacemaking and Liberalization*, edited by G. Shafir & Y. Peled. Boulder, CO: Westview Press, 129–159.

Zigon, J. 2010. Moral and ethical assemblages. *Anthropological Theory 10*:1–2, 3–15.

Zigon, J. 2011. A moral and ethical assemblage in Russian orthodox drug rehabilitation. *Ethos 39*:1, 30–50.

7 The datafication of therapeutic life management

Assembling the self in control society

Harley Bergroth and Ilpo Helén

For people who are willing or obliged to reflect on and proactively modify their personal conduct, a plethora of self-tracking devices are now widely available. By self-tracking devices we refer to near-body gadgets and related software applications that provide measurements of the rhythms and patterns of everyday life – for example, step counts, heart rate, walking distances and sleeping patterns. By providing quantitative data about vital functions or behavioural patterns, these technologies aim at helping people to enhance their self-knowledge, to adjust their behaviour and/or to accomplish self-improvement. As such, self-tracking technologies are entering and altering the domain of the 'therapeutic' that emerged and was consolidated during the 20th century (see Madsen, 2014, 2015; Moskowitz, 2001). Instead of approaching self-tracking as merely an instantiation of an overarching and static 'therapy culture', in this chapter we study more closely the therapeutic imaginaries and functions of self-tracking in everyday life, and situate the phenomenon as part of always-emergent therapeutic assemblages.

Self-tracking has emerged in conjunction with sociotechnical trajectories that are characterised by the terms 'data-driven' and 'datafication' in recent discussions (see Pentland, 2013; Ruckenstein & Schüll, 2017). The terms 'data-driven' and 'datafication' refer to the collection and mining of masses of digital data by high-performance computers. Such practices are expanding to all walks of life, from healthcare to traffic and from energy production to mass entertainment. Advocates of data-driven technologies attach great expectations to their capability to provide precise and predictive control and steering of complex technical systems, including social organisations as well as individual human lives and behaviour (e.g. Mayer-Schönberger & Cukier, 2013; Pentland, 2013; Topol, 2012, 2015). Self-tracking is undoubtedly an important dimension of this development, as it is essentially about the collection and analysis of cumulative data on bodies and personal lives. As self-tracking technologies increasingly saturate well-being-related retail contexts and cultural imaginaries of self-care, self-tracking can well be conceived of as a mode of datafication of everyday life (Lupton, 2016; Ruckenstein & Schüll, 2017).

In order to grasp the formation of therapeutic regimes of action within this data-driven practice, we approach self-tracking and its therapeutic functions with the help of two concepts. First, we deploy the idea of assemblage (*agencement*)

(Deleuze & Guattari, 1987; Marcus & Saka, 2006), which enables an analysis of self-tracking as a mode of action taking shape within and through networks and collections of things and discourses. We focus on how bodies, (technological) objects and political ideas of self-development and self-care come together in self-tracking and form therapeutic assemblages that 'hang together' (Mol, 2002) by and through the practice of gathering and analysing data about oneself. Furthermore, the concept of assemblage entails that the assemblage as a whole as well as its parts are in a constant state of emergence (Bennett, 2010; Latour, 2005). This enables us to situate the phenomenon of self-tracking within a global therapeutic assemblage while being sensitive to the possibilities, affordances and relations through which the idea of the 'therapeutic' itself becomes a meaningful concept in and through these practices. Second, we lean on Gilles Deleuze's (1995a, 1995b) ideas of control society and, more specifically, of 'dividualisation', which are particularly relevant as regards the therapeutic and political functioning of self-tracking. The concept of the dividual enables us to focus on the data-driven character of self-tracking, that is, how the practice of self-tracking becomes functional by and through data. It also helps us to situate self-tracking in current biopolitical assemblages in which individuals, their lives and their experienced selves increasingly become reduced to, as well as lived by and through, quantification-based haptic and visual information.

Drawing from qualitative analysis of promotional Internet material and interviews with Finnish self-trackers, we focus on the questions of how self-tracking becomes a therapeutic practice and what the idea of the 'therapeutic' might mean in the context of such a data-driven practice. We also ask how self-tracking, with its data-driven character, possibly shapes our understanding of the therapeutic. By studying self-tracking practices in this way, we are able to pinpoint contradictions that problematise a straightforward relationship between datafied life management and the therapeutic ethos.

This chapter proceeds as follows. First, we consider self-tracking in relation to the current therapeutic ethos and as an embodiment of dividualisation (Deleuze, 1995b). Then we present our data and methods. After this, we commence our analysis; first, we focus on the framing of self-tracking as a holistic therapeutic practice by technology developers, and show how self-tracking is reflective of what we call fragmentary holism. Secondly, we draw on interviews with Finnish self-trackers to elaborate on how self-tracking becomes a therapeutic practice in action and promotes regimes of perpetual self-assembly. Finally, we discuss briefly the political dimensions of self-tracking as self-control, and provide some concluding remarks.

Proactive self-tracking and the therapeutic ethos

People have used analogue technologies for self-measurement and lifelogging (Crawford et al., 2015; Lupton, 2016), for various reasons, for centuries. However, it may be argued that the rise of a 'therapy culture' – the relatively recent success of various forms of therapeutic life-management products and services which often involve some sort of reflective tracking practices (see McGee, 2005; Madsen, 2015) – has also driven the design, marketing and hype around contemporary digital self-tracking technologies. Whereas such technologies originally occupied quite specific domains such as (clinical) healthcare and competitive sports,[1] the therapeutic idea of pursuing a better life through holistic self-improvement combined with the cultural power of metrics and data (Ruckenstein, 2014: 77; Beer, 2016) has paved the way for the adoption of quantification-driven self-tracking technologies in various spheres of everyday life. Today, consumers certainly find these technologies an integral part of wellness-related retail contexts, and digital self-tracking has consolidated its position as a mundane way of making sense of – and possibly transforming – the body and the self.

Although the variety of regimens of self-help and self-improvement is vast in Western therapy culture (Illouz, 2008; Madsen, 2015), it is quite common in the therapeutic landscape to see that such therapeutic hermeneutics of the self (Foucault, 1993) take place in a reflexive dialogue. In it, a therapeutic instance – a psychotherapist, spiritual guide, peer group, self-help manual or a website – functions as a mirror or an echo that enables the person to acquire insights about who s/he actually is and what s/he can become. It is tempting to think of self-tracking technologies as such mirrors since self-tracking may be thought of as a practice of negotiation with 'data doubles' (Ruckenstein, 2014; Lupton, 2013; also Lomborg & Frandsen, 2016) that serve as a basis for investigating one's own life. Sociologist Deborah Lupton (2013, 2016: 39) associates self-tracking more clearly with contemporary self-help, as she links the proliferation of self-monitoring practices to the rise of popular psychology discourses that offer individualised solutions to personal problems. She analyses self-tracking as self-help-like responsibilisation of citizens on their own health and well-being. Lupton's arguments are congruent with critical studies that approach the Anglo-American therapeutic self-help as a field of neoliberal self-optimisation and governing. Such critical studies often see therapeutic self-help as a depoliticizing force as it may effectively hide structural and political problems by endorsing the management of personal qualities, traits or personality (e.g. Rimke, 2000; McGee, 2005; Madsen, 2015). However, the idea of an assemblage helps us to see that while self-tracking as a field of action is no doubt influenced and shaped by other forms of therapy culture, a focus on how the 'self' becomes enacted in practice within everyday self-tracking assemblages reveals a logic of *dividualisation rather than that of individualisation.* We argue that self-tracking reflects the interplay of the therapeutic ethos and contemporary, dividualising mechanisms of *control*, which also inverts the focus on the self/person as a coherent whole found in much 20th-century self-help.

Dividualisation is a term employed by the French philosopher Gilles Deleuze (1995a, 1995b). With an eye on the proliferation of information technologies at the dawn of the digital Internet age in the 1990s, he presented an outline of control society. He claimed that corrective and normalising interventions by public authorities and experts are increasingly being replaced by practices of control that divide its objects into ever smaller elements, parameters and action-units. Deleuze considered dividualisation as a basic requirement of the functioning of control in 'societies that no longer operate by confining people but through continuous control and instant communication' (Deleuze, 1995a: 174). The rise of digital systems would bring about practices and technologies of monitoring and modulation that work within the flows and transactions between the forces and capacities of living human beings, the environments they live in and the practices in which they participate. For Deleuze, control is continuous and anticipatory, and it works with the help of predictive and prognostic information. The objects of control are conceived of as 'factors' or 'variables', and their interaction and conjugations are assessable as 'risks' and open to modification by meticulous operations and interventions. As a consequence, living human beings as communities, persons and organisms – as units typically conceived of as *in*dividuals – as well as the environments they live in, become transformed and fragmented into *dividuals* within the matrices of control. In short, dividualization refers to the construction of clear-cut variables, dividing 'everything' – vital functions, life events, mood changes, the person, etc. – according to these variables, gathering data about these variables, and looking for patterns, trends or deviations by aggregating the data. Dividualisation pertains to all levels of human existence: to populations as well as to basic biological processes on the cellular and molecular level. It is in connection to dividualisation that we begin to see the logic of holistic self-understanding or holistic transformation, often emphasised in therapeutic parlance, giving way to a more fragmentary understanding of therapeutic life-management.

Data and methods

Our analysis is based on a variety of qualitative research material. In order to examine how self-tracking is presented within the cultural imaginary, we collected textual material from webpages of individuals and organisations that promote and endorse everyday self-tracking. These materials include Quantified Self-related website publications, public blog posts as well as promotional materials of private enterprises that manufacture self-tracking devices. Furthermore, to grasp the experiences related to the therapeutic regimes of action in everyday self-tracking practices, we employed 15 semi-structured interviews conducted with Finnish self-trackers. The interviews were gathered during 2015–2016. Of the interviewees, six were men and nine were women, all of them were employed, studying or both at the time of the interviews. During the last few years, the first author has engaged in diverse self-tracking practices, including an eight-month period of consistently wearing a popular, consumer-grade activity tracking wristband (FitBit Charge HR). This, we feel, has enabled tacit knowledge on the studied field and the 'workings' of personal self-tracking assemblages in everyday life.

In order to investigate our overarching research questions, we conducted a close reading of our research material through two main themes. First, we looked into how self-tracking technologies and the data they produce are presented as being useful and meaningful for people in self-discovery, self-adjustment and self-improvement. Second, we investigated how the data serve – and how they are narrated as serving – the pursuit of a good life. Our analysis is not focused on human-device relations, and we do not try to individuate patterns of use for the deployment of self-tracking devices. Instead, we study self-tracking as a practice and technology of the self (Foucault, 1988). This means that we have analysed how self-tracking as a regime of action springs from, mediates and shapes *one's relation to the self*, and how the self becomes examined, understood and enacted through self-tracking. In addition, the concept of assemblage works as a methodological stance that enables us to focus on constant change rather than stability. This is to say that our analysis is sensitive to the premise that things – such as 'the self', the 'therapeutic' or the practice of 'self-tracking' – are constantly put together from diverse elements and are in a constant flux rather than fixed in place through notions of static 'essences' or 'cultures'. In relation to self-tracking as a proliferating practice of life-management, then, our aim is to show that there is no unequivocal way in which self-tracking 'is' a therapeutic practice of self-care. Rather, self-tracking 'becomes' therapeutic relationally, that is, in relation to the sociotechnical and political context in which it is practised.

The fragmentary holism of self-tracking

Self-tracking technologies are often implemented in everyday life and social imaginaries in manners that resonate with the therapeutic ethos of self-discovery and the pursuit of a self that is somehow 'whole'. Perhaps already due to the term *self*-tracking, the practice often becomes associated with the management of an undeniable uniqueness and wholeness of the person that an idea of the 'self' stands for. Yet, through general calls for 'self-knowledge through numbers', as the Quantified Self movement's popular slogan goes, people are encouraged to assemble self-knowledge through a wide variety of quantified data (Lupton 2016; Berg 2017). Different instances of and devices for self-tracking measure different and often very limited aspects of personal being – such as a step count or a heart rate. Therefore, self-tracking attracts very specific modes of knowing about personal existence. In being specific in this way, the activity already builds on a quite special notion of selfhood that steers away from looking at 'unique' life conditions and settings. In this section, we examine how self-tracking is framed as a therapeutic practice of making sense of the self, and how it is presented as a means for self-improvement. Through this analysis, we shed light on a contradictory tension internal to the dynamics of self-tracking, that we call fragmentary holism.

Our research materials show a plethora of ways by which technology developers narrate self-tracking devices' holistic capacities. Take, for example, Polar Electro Ltd., the manufacturer of popular fitness tracking wristbands that gather data on daily step counts and patterns of sleep. The company claims that monitoring by the wristband helps the person to become physically more active which, in turn, reduces health risks, increases personal well-being and improves general vitality. In the developer's promotional words, the device provides a 'complete' and 'truly holistic' picture of daily activity and 'highlights the importance of every movement'.[2] Similarly, the Finnish wellness ring manufacturer Oura claims that '[w]ith Oura, you learn *your* optimal times to move, eat and take a break to get that restorative sleep'.[3] The ring collects data on, for example, heart rates and nightly heart rate variability to inform users of their sleep quality. The developers call this a 'holistic method [...] built on years of experience in human perfor-mance and the study of circadian rhythms of the body'. Taking another example, HeartMath Inc. is a technology developer that focuses on stress reduction via the measurement of heart rate patterns. The company promotes devices such as the 'inner balance' sensor, and a method for constant monitoring of the changes of the heartbeat by claiming that such tracking leads one towards a state of coherence as long as one 'stays with it'.[4] It further claims that measuring heart rate helps the person to 'incorporate the heart's intelligence into their day-to-day experience of life' and to 'become the best version [of oneself] more often'. As anthropologist Natascha Dow Schüll (2016) noted in her ethnographic study of health tech exhi-bitions in the US, the self-tracking industry's marketing constantly implies that the choices we make (in terms of attaining activity, good sleep, relaxation, etc.) reflect something crucial about who we really are.

In the above examples we see an adaptation of the therapeutic language of holistic self-understanding brought into the domain of digital self-tracking. The developers' claims often imply that the person may become something else *as a whole* through permanent tracking. For example, the individual is supposed to increase personal 'general vitality' and become 'physically more active' through step-focused activity tracking, or find 'coherence' and 'inner balance' via heart-beat data. Yet the tension between a holistic approach to personal life (referring to transformation of the individual as a whole) and 'fragmentary holism' (refer-ring to linear optimisation of nuanced functions of the body) becomes evident in the marketing language. The developers paradoxically encourage a better holistic version of oneself (e.g. a more 'vital' or 'balanced' self) by focusing on an algo-rithmically predefined functionality (such as a step count or heart rate) or neces-sarily limited combinations of such functionalities.[5] In addition, by encouraging people to become an improved version of themselves *more often* – for instance *daily* – the self-tracking imaginaries refer to an *ongoing struggle* of transforma-tion. Thus, Polar, Oura and HeartMath end up presenting self-improvement as a linear and ongoing *process* (see Bode & Kristensen, 2015) that is about constant monitoring and constant *potentiality* rather than about actuality.

Fragmentary holism highlights the idea that the 'self' is brought forth as an assemblage – disassembled and put back together through data – in self-tracking practices. First, the self consists of limited 'functions' or 'parameters' such as heartbeats or body movements, which are fragments of living that can be meas-ured – and importantly, separated and combined – by means of self-tracking. In the case of an activity tracker, for example, a seemingly general picture of 'healthiness' or 'vitality' can be assembled by combining measurements on, for example, movement, heart rate and sleep quality. Second, through longitudinal measurement of any specific fragment or vital function, the self is *enacted as a data assemblage*. Several scholars point out the relational character of tracking as a practice that requires assembly work on separate yet entangled data points or data nodes (Ruckenstein, 2014; Day & Lury, 2016; Schüll, 2016). This means that in order to make sense of and indicate progress or regress, any individual measurement (e.g. a step count) needs to be related to other similar measurements at different points in time.

We can illustrate the idea of the self as a data assemblage through the typical features of self-tracking software. Most self-tracking software visualises self-related data as graphs and charts that can be employed for self-development purposes. For example, the Polar Loop wristband gathers individual steps into longitudinal (daily and weekly) indicators of activity. In this way, the individual is disassembled into individual units of movement by the device's three-dimensional accelerometer, and re-assembled by the software. For example, depending on the device and software, a daily step assemblage on the application screen can take the form of a loop that gradually closes as one gathers steps and nears the daily goal, or a bar that fills up accordingly. A weekly activity assemblage may be visually presented e.g. as a bar chart. Similar logic pertains to measurements of heart rate, sleep, etc.; individual beats or movements are assembled into daily/nightly stats, which are then further assembled into longitudinal graphs. It is also typical that a simple number indicates the tracked self in a moral sense. For example, a self-tracking application may make complimentary claims about the person based on their total number of daily or weekly steps, or offer an 'efficiency percentage' for daily/weekly activity or sleep. Achieving high numbers or hitting 100 percent are then often virtually rewarded with animations, colour codes, trophies, etc. Here individual measurements or measurement combinations are algorithmically assembled into an *evaluation*. It is typical that such 'holistic' indicators of the self can again be disassembled into smaller-scale information in order to get more nuanced data on the specific function, for instance, to see the distribution of steps on a daily or hourly basis. However, in everyday use, to see the 'importance of every movement', as Polar mentions as a goal, is to ultimately trust the algorithm that assembles a personal evaluation. However, completion of a single evaluative checkpoint (e.g. a single day) is never really a completion at all. For example, in the Polar Loop activity tracking software, the person is implicitly encouraged to reach 100% activity (i.e. enough movement) daily. However, the weekly visualisation of one's activity shows a 'daily goal completion average', which groups together daily evaluations and offers a different number, the average.

Considering the self as a data assemblage also means that individual measurements of different functions could or should also ideally be related to each other. For example, according to Polar, when combined with a heart rate monitor, the activity wristband can become an even more precise indicator of 'activity', as it can then offer more accurate quantification-based insight on the intensity of activity conducted, calories burned, etc. It can be argued that the more elements the assemblage has, the more 'holistic' the image of the self it paints. However, the more elements there are, the more data there are on separate functions that can, or need to, be tied together and related to other measurement data.

The point here is that as the tracked self is enacted as a data assemblage, self-tracking as a way of working upon the self always feeds back to the user *through its limitations*. Data could always be more complete and more saturated through relations, references and repetition. Therefore, the practice is in principle opposed to the idea of a 'holistic' understanding of the self. Of course, we do not deny that self-trackers often pay attention to qualitative data – for example, their experiences and sensations – in order to make deeper sense of the quantitative data (see e.g. Ruckenstein, 2014; Lupton, 2016). However, while we grant that people may well experience the gaining of insights into their lives by contextualising the data, we think that holistic humanism and reflexive hermeneutics of the self often tend to be eclipsed or even be made redundant by the technical affordances of self-tracking: the precision of measurement of a specific function or activity at a specific point in time. Polar, for example, directly presents the process of 'becoming a more active person' as a project in which the person becomes conscious of her/his step-based physical movement within a day in specific ways and adjusts her/his behaviour to modify these specific modes of action. Such awareness and a trajectory of personal action are induced by the measurement because physical movement (or lack of it) is what the devices and algorithms recognise, react to and respond to by producing data that then provide feedback for the user.

To sum up, from the viewpoint of assemblages of control at work in self-tracking, individuals become increasingly conceived of as compounds of functions, parameters, capacities and resources to be regulated and operated upon. Such control as a mode of governing people and their lives sits uneasily with the holism that nevertheless surfaces as an emic emphasis in the imaginaries of the capacities of self-tracking. For holistic therapeutic practices, the individual person and her/his 'unique' life, experiences and aspirations are the focus of practices to govern and modify people, whereas control and dividualisation reach beyond and below the personal by means of the collection and aggregation of masses of data. We claim that while many therapeutic practices are concerned with encouraging people to discover their unique modes of action for self-improvement, digital self-tracking today becomes functional by focusing on self-control and by improving modes of action already predetermined in the devices' code. In what follows, we will take a closer look at everyday experiences of self-tracking and discuss these experiences as reflective of anticipatory regimes of action.

Self-tracking as a therapeutic regime of anticipation

So far we have seen that self-tracking is often presented as a holistic means of self-inspection despite its tendency to disassemble the self into (longitudinal collections of) functions and variables, which encourages further self-inspection rather than 'holistic' self-knowledge. In this section, we focus on the ways in which self-tracking assemblages are narrated to facilitate the idea and ongoing pursuit of a good – or, rather, *better* – life. We thus show how the data assemblages gathered in self-tracking practices unfold into therapeutic regimes of action in everyday lives.

When people speak of their self-tracking practices they usually say that self-tracking makes aspects of the self (activity levels, sleep quality, etc.) 'more real'. Sari, a woman in her late forties, speaks about how the Polar Loop device enables her to convince herself that she is 'really doing something' in the sense of daily activity. Specifically, she has tried to fight against a *risk* of type 2 diabetes that has been brought to her attention by medical professionals. When Timo (male, 26) talks about tracking daily movement and calorie consumption, he readily recognises the very limited employability of individual measurements and says that he does not necessarily check on the measurements on a daily but rather on a weekly basis. Despite this, he points out that the accumulation of data reveals patterns and creates a very tangible or 'real' history, evident in the repository of numbers and graphs. Through this timeline he can then reflect on and analyse 'how things have been going' in his life in a more general sense. It can be argued that self-tracking usually makes sense to people as a practice of acquiring knowledge about developments in terms of specific functions, which is also thought to reveal a bigger picture of one's own life through futures and histories of potential health, physical fitness and wellbeing.

However, despite such experiences, what is characteristic of interviewees' narratives is the pervasive tension between becoming a self-informed subject and constantly pushing the boundaries of self-knowledge further. In many cases, then, self-tracking in practice becomes anticipatory (see e.g. Adams et al., 2009) rather than evidentiary. Many interviewees acknowledge that self-tracking may provide quite a lot of self-awareness and promote joy and delightful moments when the self is actualised as 'active', for example, by reaching 10,000 steps or by producing a good sleep score daily or, even better, *consistently*, but they also reflect that it may easily turn into a repetitive practice, the main attraction of which is to predict and control. As the 'tracks' always lead on, self-tracking can spark ever further interest in the self, which makes the idea of the self as an experience of something 'whole' quite questionable. For example, Veli, a 28-year-old male, reflects that it is really 'quite silly' to engage in sleep tracking because in a sense one already knows how one sleeps. Nevertheless, he self-tracks because the data logs 'provide motivation for improvement'; that is, the logs and linear graphs psychologically move him to develop himself. This highlights the tendency of self-tracking to produce a processual regime of action in terms of datafied self-mapping.

It is our claim that through fragmentary holism, the purpose of self-tracking often becomes the process of self-assembly itself, as a sense of self-control is pursued. Relating to dividualisation, it seems that self-tracking as a therapeutic assemblage engenders a mode of action that enables not holistic self-awareness *per se* but rather an information-deprived relation to the self on pre-established scales. In other words, the self becomes highlighted as *potential*. This relates to how, in the context of border security, Amoore (2011: 28) speaks of algorithmically forged 'data derivatives' that do not centre on 'who we are, not even on what our data says about us, but what can be imagined and inferred about who we might be'. Self-tracking data derivatives are another example of how improvement is linked with attempted control of potential futures and threats.

In terms of specific threats, our analysis of the promotional material points out that self-tracking devices are often framed as quasimedical devices that are supposed to lead individuals towards health, longevity and regeneration. As such, they both answer to and produce what anthropologist Joseph Dumit (2012; see also Schüll, 2016) calls a 'double insecurity' that the medical industry enacts: not knowing whether one is already ill and never knowing enough about illness prevention. The person is thus always potentially ill. Perhaps the clearest example of this in our interviews comes from Sakari, a 50-year-old male who is a very active self-tracker and describes himself as a scientist of his own life (cf. Heyen, 2016). For example, he makes an effort to track his weight and relaxation (via heart rate) daily, his blood pressure regularly once a year, and occasionally he goes to a nearby laboratory to gain data on various biomarkers of his choice. All this provides him with 'more data' in his ever-expanding database of himself. In addition to quantitative data, he also carefully notes any events that may be symptoms of illness. (One example that he provided us with is '12th March, nose-bleed, short duration, left nostril'.) He describes self-tracking as 'at its best a very therapeutic practice' in the sense of producing a 'peace of mind' and feelings of 'self-confidence'. However, he also states that a central product of self-tracking is the feeling of 'panic' or 'terror', especially when one sees results that deviate from normal reference values and seem unexplained to him. When asked about whether self-tracking has served his well-being or not, Sakari said that a sense of control provides him with a really 'healthy feeling'. Explaining the negative side of tracking in more detail, Sakari specified his ideas on control:

> It is really about an experience of control... because you cannot really control life, but you can feel that you are in control... and the negative comes from the kind of terror, especially in the face of [measurement] results that are somehow... unexplained [...] and it seems hard for me to grasp what could be negative about [self-tracking]... like if you think that people get all hypochondriac and they increasingly go to the doctor, well I think that's a good thing in a way. Because this is preventive health care, and it's better that you go early [to the doctor] to check up on some fine nuance, than going when you're already sick.

For Sakari, self-tracking seems to become functional as self-control and an ongoing struggle against illness. However, as his life and body are now spatially and temporally divided into ever-expanding data sets by and through self-tracking technologies, it is also quite likely that he will encounter situations in which the feeling of a loss of control, in the form of unexplained data, becomes tangible. He explicitly connects such scenarios with emotions of terror. Here we can see self-tracking as a therapeutic assemblage at work: self-tracking becomes therapeutic as a practice of continuous and preventive health-related control through the dividualising and fragmentary logic of the system. This fragmentation and production of self-related data derivatives mean that a sense of full control often remains elusive. In Sakari's case, this is implied in the curious sense that self-tracking seems both a vitally important and therapeutic task, but also, in the long run, a battle one cannot win, because 'you cannot really control life'. Thus, the therapeutic assemblage of self-tracking produces its own purpose by opening up the self and the body as potential and as an object of continuous control. The self becomes a data assemblage that is not, in fact, approached as a whole individual but as dividualised into trajectories of functions, traits and biomarkers, through monitoring of which a sense of control may be pursued.

As control of potential, self-tracking may be thought of as a constant struggle against the 'deviant' within (Bode & Kristensen, 2015). While Sakari wages war on various fronts against ill health, in another example we see the struggle against the disorder and social ill of 'laziness' or 'idleness', familiar from mainstream wellness- and efficiency-related activation discourses.[6] Aino is a 39-year-old female, a mother of three children who works in an executive role. She has a background in competitive sports so she has long been familiar with heart rate monitors and other gadgets by which one can optimise physical performance via metrics. For Aino, such techniques have now become a part of coping with the demands of working life. She says that an activity wristband motivates her to move more, and she feels that if she did not exercise she 'would not have the energy to cope with [the] damn tough demands' of a stressful job. Here, as with Sakari, the way in which self-tracking comes to serve as a useful technology of the self (Foucault, 1988) is by control of vital potential, although in this case self-tracking is more explicitly connected to the maintenance of one's productive energy. Aino speaks about self-tracking as an ongoing process of avoidance of the lazy self always lurking in the shadows. She says that the whole point is to 'give yourself a kick up the ass' and 'avoid the days when [my] activity is basically zero'. She wants to avoid inactivity, which she explicitly associates with 'laziness'. In a quote Aino reveals how the device cooperates *daily* in establishing a sense of self-control:

> Of course it was nice when in the summer I went golfing and I got a huge amount of steps… of course it was nice [smiles widely], like WOW, so many steps. But in normal life it is enough for me that the wristband vibrates [haptic vibration, a signal of achieving 10,000 steps] at some point of the day, that I've been active.

It goes without saying that a life with an activity tracking wristband that counts steps and measures sleep via movement of the body may enable different modes and patterns of self-control than a life with a weighing scale or with access to high-end laboratory testing. However, the logic of dividualisation in any case frames one's relation to the self as a relation of control, because the production of the self as data assemblage highlights the self as potential. This is evident in Sakari's and Aino's cases. Sakari is potentially always in ill health, even (or perhaps especially) when there are no obvious indications of illness (see Dumit, 2012). The complex assemblages of technical devices, laboratories and biographical notes seemingly enable the person to control this insecurity, although such assemblages also produce the self as an object of 'tinkering' (Pols, 2010) with fine-grained nuances. In a similar manner, Aino is potentially always 'lazy', since every day is another struggle against 'laziness' and 'low energy', which in her case is determined primarily via step count. The process of self-management manifests itself as permanent avoidance of the illness of 'zero' activity.

We suggest that while everyday proactive self-tracking is often narrated in terms of the typical therapeutic parlance of self-discovery, self-exploration or self-improvement, interview narratives show that dividualisation and fragmentation of the self are the primary characteristics of self-tracking. Although it may be said that self-tracking enables a process of self-discovery through the longitudinal measurement of fragmented vital functions or activities, in functioning it also creates interests that tie individuals into these sociotechnical regimes of control. The functions of the data as therapeutic life management ultimately become anticipatory rather than evidentiary, as any individual event of tracking does not so much generate self-knowledge as position the self in a continuum of measurements through which future (and past) selves can be imagined and potentially realised. Self-tracking thus persistently produces knowledge-craving subjects whom it supposedly serves, and the self as a 'whole' remains persistently unattainable. Self-tracking assemblages, then, present vivid instantiations of control through anticipation because, as we have seen, from marketing rhetoric to everyday experiences these technologies reveal the self as process and as potential, as something to be acted upon consistently in order to actualise a better life. Inasmuch as self-tracking assemblages are articulated as producing knowledge of something 'real' about the self, they create a *need to know* by dividing a complex whole of life into trajectories and functions that extend indefinitely. This is fragmentary holism in action.

Therapeutic self-assembly and the politics of self-control

Deleuze (1995b: 179) wrote that whereas life in disciplinary societies is characterised by completions and new beginnings, like trajectories from families to schools, and from schools to work, 'in control societies you never finish anything'. In this chapter, we have shown how self-tracking as a technology of the self often drives fragmentation rather than unity, and anticipation rather than knowledge. Self-tracking enacts the self, through a focus on linear scales, as an ongoing process and potentiality rather than as something to be found as a whole and coherent. An important consequence is that self-tracking assemblages bring to everyday life a modality of being characterised by perpetual alteration. From the consumer perspective, the therapeutic ethos of holism and stability thus appears appealing and welcome as it promises control, yet it is ultimately futile within the assemblages that produce their *raison d'être* through producing a metastable existence – an existence that is constantly subject to change. Acting to manage this metastability associates self-tracking as a therapeutic regime with the anticipatory control and regulation of potentiality in political regimes. In the last section of our chapter, we probe briefly this political aspect of self-tracking as control.

Our analysis of self-trackers' narratives brought up struggles against ill health and laziness, both of which are identifiable as long-running trajectories of struggle in Western ethics. Considering these struggles further along with Deleuze's ideas of control society we may connect them with sociotechnical visions and programmes of 'perpetual education' and 'personalised medicine' which rely on processes of dividualisation. If we consider self-tracking, on a general level, as perpetual education – resonant with what Fotopoulou and O'Riordan (2017) call 'biopedagogy' – we can connect it with social programmes of *activation*. In critical social policy literature and in public discourse, 'activation' has typically referred to a variety of local and international policies, hugely influential across OECD countries, through which the unemployed or the 'excluded' have been made responsible for managing their labour power, working abilities and personal life in general (Eversberg, 2015: 173; Clarke, 2005: 448). Yet, as a programme or an assemblage, activation is itself contingent; it takes shape in relation to neoliberal market rationale and the logics of restructuring of the welfare state, through which the state and public powers seemingly withdraw from securing individual lives and from interfering with them. Furthermore, 'activation' may work as an umbrella term that covers a variety of traits and qualities such as, for example, education, the utilisation of prior work experience, health, well-being, mental awareness or aesthetic appearance. All of these are closely intertwined with the ability to *self-manage and maintain the social and economic utility – that is, labour capacity and productivity – of one's own body*. In this context, the point of self-tracking is to educate people not on their daily step counts or heart rates during sleep *per se*, but mainly on caring for and managing personal 'vitality' by themselves in order to reduce the 'deadweight' in the productive system (see Eversberg, 2015). Activation is thus a programme that is actualised through mundane technologies far beyond its rhetorical target population, that is, the unemployed, the precariat and the 'excluded' who are typically not the target group for self-tracking devices. We see how activation becomes actual with Aino, who worries about – and finds therapeutic functions in – managing her energies and capacities, that is, her labour power, through a struggle against laziness in a demanding and stressful work environment. In Virve Peteri's chapter in this book, we see spatial arrangements of the office space as a new mode of activation and mobilisation of workers and their labour power within organisations; in this chapter, we see parallel strategies of activation with self-tracking technologies in everyday life and outside organisational contexts.

Self-tracking as an assemblage of control also has an affinity, and perhaps a more concrete one, with a major imaginary of future healthcare envisaged as 'personalised, predictive, preventive, and participatory' (Hood & Friend, 2011). The advocates of 'personalised medicine' conceive of it as being embedded in advanced biomedicine like genomics and stem cell technology and claim that it will improve clinical care and shift the emphasis of health care to prevention with the help of more precise and patient-centred medical knowledge (for an overview, see Tutton, 2014). In addition, personalised medicine is expected to considerably reduce the costs of healthcare. Over the past few years, visions of personalised medicine have re-focused on the collection and appropriation of masses of health-related personal data (Prainsack, 2017; Ruckenstein & Schüll, 2017). According to the promoters, data-driven medicine would enable anticipatory health monitoring and preventive interventions, as well as medication and other therapies, targeted far more precisely at specific risk groups or individuals (e.g. NAS, 2011; Hood & Friend, 2011).

Self-tracking works in congruence with the data-driven personalised medicine that is expected to revolutionise modern medicine, health policy and society (NAS, 2011; Hood & Friend, 2011; Mayer-Schönberger & Cukier, 2013; Pentland, 2013; Topol, 2015). This congruence builds through the logics of control and dividualisation, both of which are embedded in massive data sets and have a focus on individual parameters and malleable patterns (see Sharon, 2017). Personalised medicine is often seen as a frame for preventive lifestyle and proactive medical interventions, supported by perpetual self-monitoring and control. As seen in our examples, many companies promoting self-tracking – as well as self-trackers themselves, such as Sakari – focus on the measurement of health-related parameters of vital functions and behaviour and narrate self-optimisation by digital tracking devices in a manner similar to preventive healthcare.

Personalised medicine is expected to have effects across populations, societies and even globally. The dividualisation taking place in such practices also lays the ground for the pervasiveness of 'therapy cultures' as personal lives are perpetually in need of preventive interventions: for example, always rather potentially ill (metastable) than healthy organisms (stable). Personalised medicine is thus another political programme that lays the ground for the sociotechnical instantiations and alterations that are shaping current therapy cultures towards a focus on ongoing self-control and metastability rather than healing, wholeness and stability.

Conclusion

In this chapter, we argue that while self-tracking can be theorised in terms of its connections to the general therapeutic ethos of self-discovery and self-improvement, it is a data-driven practice of dividualisation. As such, it creates regimes of action that build on the idea of perpetual self-assembly and which thus fit uneasily with any overarching characterisation of 'therapeutic cultures'. Instead of holistic and reflexive self-inspection we often see the fragmentation of the individuals and their lives into 'functions' and 'qualities' presented by graphs and charts, and in ways that focus on the self as a process that should be worked upon consistently. So, in terms of how these technologies come to serve life, they serve not as holistic actualisation of the self but as a means of ongoing control and management of potential. As life-management techniques, these technologies have a tendency to actively produce the kinds of regimes of perpetual action that they promise to dissolve. Furthermore, self-tracking as a technology of the self exemplifies how current therapeutic assemblages can also intertwine with political programmes and discourses such as citizen activation and personalised medicine. We see self-tracking as to some degree pertaining to the emergence of societies of control as sketched by Deleuze, especially through a focus on increasing complexity and persistent incompleteness, which both attract endless monitoring.

Acknowledgements

The authors wish to thank the Academy of Finland (grant number 292408, grant number 313703, grant number 289004) and Kone Foundation (Crossing Borders for Health and Well-being) for supporting this work.

Notes

1 Mika Pantzar (2012: 133) has noted that when Finnish technology developers such as Polar Electro tried to introduce and sell heart rate monitors to American consumers at the end of the 20th century, they faced resistance as it was thought unclear why the average consumer should need one.
2 https://www.polar.com/us-en/about_polar/press_room/polar_launches_polar_loop and https://support.polar.com/fi/support/the_what_and_how_of_polar_24_7_activity_tracking?product_id=64271&category=faqs [accessed on March 23, 2018].
3 https://ouraring.com/ [accessed on March 28, 2018, italic as in original source].
4 https://store.heartmath.com/innerbalance [accessed on March 28, 2018].
5 For example, a measurement of sleep quality may be based on a simple parameter, such as movement, or it may be based on a combination of parameters, such as movement data, heart rate data and data on breathing rhythms.
6 For example, these discourses now frame sitting as a public health threat (Peteri, 2017) and manifest themselves in various campaigns in workplaces encouraging people to be physically active during workdays.

References

Adams, V., Murphy, M. & Clarke, A. 2009. Anticipation: Technoscience, life, affect, temporality. *Subjectivity 28*, 246–265.

Amoore, L. 2011. Data derivatives: On the emergence of a security risk calculus for our times. *Theory, Culture & Society 28*:6, 24–43.

Beer, D. 2016. *Metric Power*. London: Palgrave MacMillan.

Bennett, J. 2010. *Vibrant Matter: A Political Ecology of Things*. Durham: Duke University Press.

Berg, M. 2017. Making sense with sensors: Self-tracking and the temporality of wellbeing. *Digital Health 3*, 1–11.

Bode, M. & Kristensen, D. B. 2015. The digital doppelgänger within: A study on self-tracking and the quantified self movement. In *Assembling Consumption: Researching Actors, Networks and Markets*, edited by R. Canniford & D. Bajde. London: Routledge, 119–135.

Clarke, J. 2005. New labour's citizens: Activated, empowered, responsibilized, abandoned? *Critical Social Policy 25*:4, 447–463.

Crawford, K., Lingel, J. & Karppi, T. 2015. Our metrics, ourselves: A hundred years of self-tracking from the weight scale to the wrist wearable device. *European Journal of Cultural Studies 18*:4–5, 479–496.

Day, S. & Lury, C. 2016. Biosensing: Tracking persons. In *Quantified: Biosensing Technologies in Everyday Life*, edited by D. Nafus. Cambridge: MIT Press, 43–66.

Deleuze, G. 1995a. 'Control and becoming'. In *Negotiations, 1972–1990*. New York: Columbia University Press, 169–176.

Deleuze, G. 1995b. 'Postscript on control societies'. In *Negotiations, 1972–1990*. New York: Columbia University Press, 177–182.

Deleuze, G. & Guattari, F. 1987. *A Thousand Plateaus*. Minneapolis: University of Minnesota Press.

Dumit, J. 2012. *Drugs for Life: How Pharmaceutical Companies Define Our Health*. Durham & London: Duke University Press.

Eversberg, D. 2015. Beyond individualisation: The German 'activation toolbox'. *Critical Social Policy 36*:2, 167–186.

Fotopoulou, A. & O'Riordan, K. 2017. Training to self-care: Fitness tracking, biopedagogy and the healthy consumer. *Health Sociology Review 26*:1, 54–68.

Foucault, M. 1988. Technologies of the self. In *Technologies of the Self: A Seminar with Michel Foucault*, edited by M. Gutman & P. Hutton. London: Tavistock, 16–49.

Foucault, M. 1993. About the beginnings of the hermeneutics of the self. *Political Theory 21*, 198–227.

Heyen, N. B. 2016. Self-tracking as knowledge production: Quantified self between prosumption and citizen science. In *Lifelogging*, edited by S. Selke. Wiesbaden: Springer VS.

Hood, L. & Friend, S. 2011. Predictive, personalized, preventive, participatory (P4) cancer medicine. *Nature Reviews Clinical Oncology 8*:3, 184–187.

Illouz, E. 2008. *Saving the Modern Soul: Therapy, Emotions, and the Culture of Self-Help*. Berkeley: University of California Press.

Latour, B. 2005. *Reassembling the Social: An Introduction to Actor-Network Theory*. Oxford: Oxford University Press.

Lomborg, S. & Frandsen, K. 2016. Self-tracking as communication. *Information, Communication & Society 19*:7, 1015–1027.

Lupton, D. 2013. Understanding the human machine. *IEEE Technology and Society Magazine 32*:4, 25–30.

Lupton, D. 2016. *The Quantified Self: A Sociology of Self-Tracking*. Cambridge: Polity Press.

Madsen, O. J. 2014. *The Therapeutic Turn: How Psychology Altered Western Culture*. London & New York: Routledge.

Madsen, O. J. 2015. *Optimizing the Self: Social Representations of Self-Help*. London: Routledge.

Marcus, George E. & Saka, E. 2006. Assemblage. *Theory, Culture & Society 23*:2–3, 101–109.

Mayer-Schönberger, V. & Cukier, K. 2013. *Big Data: A Revolution That Will Transform How We Live, Work and Think*. London: John Murray.

McGee, M. 2005. *Self-Help Inc. Makeover Culture in American Life*. Oxford: Oxford University Press.

Mol, A. 2002. *The Body Multiple: Ontology in Medical Practice*. Durham: Duke University Press.

Moskowitz, Eva. 2001. *In Therapy We Trust: America's Obsession with Self-Fulfillment*. Baltimore: The Johns Hopkins University Press.

National Academy of Sciences [NAS]. 2011. *Toward Precision Medicine*. Washington, DC: The National Academies Press.

Pantzar, M. 2012. Arjen uudet kartastot ja rytmit: Big data ja small data. In *Arjen kartat ja rytmit*, edited by M. Lammi, M. Pantzar & T. Koivunen. Kuluttajatutkimuksen vuosikirja 2012. Helsinki: Kuluttajatutkimuskeskus, 128–151.

Pentland, A. 2013. The data-driven society. *Scientific American 309*:4, 78–83.

Peteri, V. 2017. Tuolin imu: kansanterveys, kansallinen kilpailukyky ja istumisen vaarat. *Kulttuurintutkimus 34*:1, 15–27.

Pols, J. 2010. Telecare: What patients care about. In *Care in Practice. On Tinkering in Clinics, Homes and Farms*, edited by A. Mol, I. Moser & J. Pols. Bielefeld: Transcript Verlag, 171–194.

Prainsack, B. 2017. *Personalized Medicine: Empowered Patients in the 21st Century*. New York, NY: New York University Press.

Rimke, H. 2000. Governing citizens through self-help literature. *Cultural Studies 14*:1, 61–78.

Ruckenstein, M. 2014. Visualized and interacted life: Personal analytics and engagements with data doubles. *Societies 4*:1, 68–84.

Ruckenstein, M. & Schüll, N. D. 2017. The datafication of health. *Annual Review of Anthropology 46*, 261–278.

Schüll, N. D. 2016. Data for life: Wearable technology and the design of self-care. *BioSocieties 11*:3, 317–333.

Sharon, T. 2017. Self-tracking for health and the quantified self: Re-articulating autonomy, solidarity and authenticity in the age of personalized healthcare. *Philosophy & Technology 30*:1, 93–121.

Topol, E. 2012. *The Creative Destruction of Medicine*. New York: Basic Books.

Topol, E. 2015. *The Patient Will See You Now: The Future of Medicine Is in Your Hands*. New York: Basic Books.

Tutton, R. 2014. *Genomics and the Reimagining of Personalized Medicine*. Surrey: Ashgate.

8 The lure of self-disclosure

App-assisted quantification of mood as therapeutic companionship

Felix Freigang

It's an early afternoon when my phone prompts me to enter into a conversation in its preferred way of nudging: vibration. 'How are you feeling?' it reads on the display. Feeling overwhelmed by a week's workload ahead and glad for the excuse to take a break from writing, I willingly agree to our casual dialogue. Upon swiping the textbox, a ruler shows up, inviting me to choose from 'really bad' on the left to 'very good' on the right. Each nuance is represented by a specific emoji. I settle on the middle, slightly tilted to the right, and press accept. The app notifies me that I'm ready and I would now have to submit my entry. Upon completion, the app congratulates me by presenting a digital trophy; the message below reads: 'Well done! We're looking forward to seeing you again. In the meantime, feel free to explore the app and WE plan your happiness'. (Author's field notes, 5th November 2017)

Mood-tracking applications ('apps') have seen a tremendous flourishing in recent years and are recognised as part of an overall 'applification of mental wellbeing' (Gaggioli & Riva, 2013). They resemble digital mood journals designed to provide a proactive quantification, control and presentation of mood fluctuations through the simple swiping and tapping on a mobile device touchscreen. Most of these apps are marketed as supplements for Cognitive-Behavioural Therapy (CBT) of mental illnesses, such as depression, anxiety or bipolar disorder. At the same time, nearly all of them are promoted and distributed as efficient tools of empowerment and self-improvement that aim at strengthening the respective users' reflexive engagement with their everyday conduct by way of 'making emotions count' (Pritz, 2016).

While social scientists and cultural analysts have started to draw attention to this newly emerging technology (Belli, 2016; Davies, 2017; Pritz, 2016), there is a paucity of critical perspectives that address the multifarious engagements with these new information and communication technologies (ICTs) and their role in people's daily lives (but see Bergroth and Helén in this book). This chapter sheds light on some ways in which people aim to obtain orientation with regard to the relationship one wants to have with oneself and with others (Foucault, 1988) through mood-tracking apps. Such a search for an ethical disposition – the struggling and striving for self-actualisation and transformation – lies at the core of what various authors have identified as therapeutic cultures and self-help ideologies (Aubry & Travis, 2015; Furedi, 2004; Illouz, 2008; Nehring et al., 2016; Madsen, 2014; McGee, 2005; Rimke, 2017; Wright, 2008). What lends mood-tracking apps an aura of therapeutic applicability is their promise of positing, through the work on and of the self, a rational managing subject that is capable of observing, measuring and learning to anticipate its own pursuits of happiness and well-being by way of self-disclosure (see Weiner, 2011: 452). However, mood-tracking apps are not simply black-boxed software media, but can be viewed as 'sociocultural artefacts' (Lupton, 2014) into which different aspirations, circuits of societal discourses, economic interests and meanings are being inscribed.

Based on six months of ethnographic research centring on one particularly popular mood-tracking app in Germany, the chapter examines various contexts in which this digital technology becomes both a meaningful and alluring, as well as a contested, part of people's lives, thereby addressing an aspect that is frequently overlooked in the existing literature on self-help and therapeutic cultures: that of human and non-human companionships (Pyyhtinen, 2016; Latour, 2005) and the social worlds that emerge from such entanglements. To this end, I employ the Deleuzian–Guattarian notion of assemblage (Deleuze & Guattari, 2013 [1987]; see also DeLanda, 2006). Assemblage thinking is particularly helpful because it allows tracing of modes of arranging heterogeneous elements that become productive for a certain time before they potentially dissolve and disperse again (Müller & Schurr, 2016; Marcus & Saka, 2006). In this sense, assemblage thinking is attentive both to the active labour of pulling elements together and to the intrinsic capacities of (human as well as non-human) components to exceed their place in the assemblage: the hardware of the mobile device and software program at play; the data produced; startup entrepreneurs participating in the app's production; social networks as well as media outlets and their discursive potentials; individual selves engaging with these technologies as part of the fabric of everyday life. Following Müller's (2015: 35) conceptual work on the notion of assemblage, I suggest that it is different affective forces and intensities that serve as the assemblage's *'tertium quid'*, which make the socio-material components of mood-tracking apps stay together or fall apart. As will be demonstrated, certain expectations may be temporarily projected onto mood-tracking apps and prompt people to practically invest hope in them. At the same time, the very investment in and emotional experience of using these apps intensifies the affective flows that become constitutive of an app's assemblage.

From writing to swiping: locating mobile app-assisted quantification of mood

Taking the measure of one's mood is not a novel practice of self-disclosure: Pen-and-paper based mood-charts have had a long tradition dating back to the 18th century (Martin, 2007: 177–96) and have become an integral part in the emergence of CBT and research (Ekkekakis, 2013). Arguably, the change 'from writing to swiping' that occurred with the widespread circulation of mood-tracking apps has not entirely changed the basic philosophical and ideological premises involved in measuring one's mood. Sociologist Miriam Pritz (2016) suggests that tracking one's mood is best conceived of as a heuristic practice of self-examination (*Selbstthematisierung*) that bears upon and feeds back into other forms of institutionalised 'technologies of the self' (Foucault, 1988), such as autobiographical accounts, diaries or confessions. For Pritz, the practice of confession – viewed through its religiously connoted nexus of guilt, self-disclosure and self-control – is a particular case in point since it has 'led to a specific kind of socialisation of feelings and emotions and an increased awareness of one's own subjectivity' (Pritz, 2016: 180; see also Wright, 2008); an awareness that is based upon a cathartic teleology of salvation and purification (Pritz, 2016). Hence, disclosing one's inner self, feelings and emotions in a confessional manner can be understood as an exertion of self-discipline that aims at easing guilt or shame, also by making private concerns public.

At the same time, the self-disciplining of emotional experience (see, for example, Hochschild, 1983) has given way to an intensified acceptance of emotional expressiveness (Neckel, 2014). This convergence can be regarded as a characteristic feature of contemporary emotion cultures (Illouz, 2008) with which mobile app-assisted quantification of mood intersects: A rationalisation of life-conduct in the Weberian sense, which involves a calculating self enmeshed in a heightened awareness of and means of expressing one's own moods, feelings and emotions. Pritz concludes that

> [...] the implicit concepts of emotions underpinning emotional self-tracking techniques are characterized by a materialistic-rationalistic understanding of emotions [...]. Emotions are treated as phenomena that can be ordered, regulated and normalized. They are objectified by processes of observation and classification [...] and are remade into phenomena that can be willfully regulated and purposively shaped. At the same time, emotions are held in high esteem as personal resources of self-knowledge and self-fulfilment. A 'better' understanding, which always means better 'management' of one's own emotions and those of others, is supposed to bring about happiness and success in nearly every aspect of life.
>
> (Pritz, 2016: 184)

The rationalisation and expressiveness of emotional experiences resonates with what scholars have identified as the therapeutic self-management paradigm of mental illness (Weiner, 2011). This paradigm aligns with an overall rise of psy-disciplines (Rose, 1998) and propagates work on and of the self, positing the powerful idea of subjectivity as a possible object for rational management and systematic governing, while at the same time one's rationality is called into question (Weiner, 2011). A person needs to not merely speak and think, but is also required to assess his or her condition against the background of desired objectives – whether it be authority, efficiency, happiness or well-being (Rose, 1998, 1990). Self-management practices thereby reinforce 'therapeutic orthodoxies'

(Ecclestone & Hayes, 2009: 9) that draw from an eclectic alloy of behavioural science (e.g., James Gross' process model of emotion regulation), Freudian and Jungian analysis, as well as Rogerian counselling, but first and foremost make reflexivity a pivotal constituent of knowledge production.

In mood-tracking, quantified logic lies at the core of reflecting one's emotional experiences: by charting the daily ups and downs of our moods upon a scale, people translate subjective, bodily, and at times ephemeral experiences into symbolic sets of supposedly stable and manageable data. Once quantified, distinct feelings become comparable to those of others through a supposedly shared understanding of these metrics. This process of deploying numerical representations to create relations between experiences, that is, the transformation of qualitative into quantitative distinctions, can be identified as 'commensuration' (Espeland & Stevens, 1998: 316). In order to illustrate the commensuration of mood, anthropologist Emily Martin (2007: 187) recounts a scene from a mood disorder support group, in which people introduced themselves not only by name, but also by giving an oral mood-chart, ranging from −5 to +5 and thereby indicating a spectrum of moods from depressed to manic. In this example, the numbers produce new categories of understanding mental states. At the same time, however, the numbers also enact the complex experiences they set out to measure; in other words, mood quantification makes the 'unseen' aspects of emotional life visible and points to a formalisation of the work on the self, which transcends less formalised, situational forms of expression or 'gut feeling' and thus becomes authoritative in its own right by lending an objective aura to the messiness of life – not only individually, but also collectively.

On the other hand, the alleged capacity to objectively compare different qualities and actors can unleash an oppressive language of 'normality' and 'norm transgression'. Illouz (2008: 138–9) states that '[o]nce numerical metaphors are used [...], "balancing" emotions becomes akin to establishing a "mean" or average on a numerical scale. Numbers are metaphors for the idea that emotions and personality traits can be averaged out'. Dissolving emotions into numbers, mood-tracking may thus become vehicular to datafied processes of 'dividualisation' within a 'society of control' (Deleuze, 1992 [1990]; see also Bergroth and Helén in this book).

Assembling mood-tracking apps for depression: the affective economies of *DepressApp*

In the following sections I will focus on a single, yet intricate question: How do mood-tracking apps invoke the lure of self-disclosure? In order to approach this question, I will analyse the affective intensities constitutive of one particularly popular mood-tracking app in Germany, here called *DepressApp*.[1]

DepressApp is a free-to-use app introduced to Apple's iOS in 2015 (with Android following in 2016) and is envisioned and marketed as 'the ultimate mobile tool to assist' the therapy of mental illness, with a focus on people suffering from depression. With the aid of a coloured emoji-scale, users can rate their moods, jot diary-like journal entries and document their bodily sensations. As for the upcoming iterations, the app will automatically send the journal data to an authorised therapist, reach out to predefined phone contacts whenever the user data points to an episode of depression and will passively learn from the data patterns in order to propose 'wellbeing activities', such as taking a walk or a nap, listening to music or cooking a meal. In addition, psychotherapists will be equipped with a dashboard to receive, administer and assess a client's data, communicate through *DepressApp* and monitor the client – upon her/his approval – even after completing treatment, in order to prevent relapses. By 2017, the app has become successful enough to support a small company with three employees, having received funding from a prestigious German investment and consulting company that financially supports the app's route to a CE-marking, which is required in order to promote a medical device in the European Union.[2] Alongside the increase of financial backup, the app's media attention has grown rapidly since its launch, corresponding to a general increase in public awareness of ICT and mental health care in Germany.

The app is assembled – that is, imagined and promoted, as well as frequently understood and used – as a *therapeutic companion*[3] that accumulates meaning and momentum by way of circulation in an 'affective economy' (Ahmed, 2004a: 44–9):

> the more they [objects] circulate, the more affective they become, and the more they appear to 'contain' affect. Another way to theorize this process would be to describe 'feelings' via an analogy with 'commodity fetishism': feelings appear in objects, or indeed *as* objects with a life of their own, only by the concealment of how they are shaped by histories, including histories of production [...], as well as circulation or exchange.
>
> (Ahmed 2004b: 120–1, emphasis in the original)

The therapeutic companion can thus be seen as an object in which certain feelings and emotions are invested. This object is both shaped by and actively shaping its own enactment: on the one hand, people are drawn to it for specific reasons, with specific motivations and expectations. At the same time, the app actively produces and sustains these expectations. *DepressApp* is thus always caught up in the processes of becoming: it is a mobile technology that can be deployed, fiddled with for a while or deleted when its time has come; but it may also become productive by shaping different modes of perception, responsiveness and desires.

Analysing affect is a slippery slope. For some authors, the power of 'affect' as an analytical tool lies exactly in its 'presocial' and 'preconscious' qualities (see, e.g., Massumi, 2002) that are said to account for the non-representational 'zones of the intimately impersonal and the impersonally intimate' (Mazzaralla, 2017). Research projects that involve such an understanding of affect frequently seek to investigate the forces that work on and through bodies rather than analysing their discursive articulations. However, when engaging with digital environments, one has to rely chiefly on 'textuality' – written and spoken representations of feelings, experiences and expectations – in order to make sense of the ways in which circulation unfolds in an affective economy. The analytical approach employed here draws inspiration from studies that interrogate the entanglements of narrative, discourse and affect (Oikkonen, 2017; Wetherell, 2013; Wetherell et al., 2015) and that also aim to bring concepts of emotion and affectivity into a fruitful dialogue (see also Stanley and Kortelainen and Kolehmainen in this book). In her research on the role of affective dynamics in newspaper articulations of the technoscientific constructions of the 'Zika epidemic', Venla Oikkonen suggests:

> While affective intensities may give rise to emotions (in the sense that they precede emotion), […] emotions shape how we may become (or fail to become) attuned to affective intensities. In this sense, affective intensities and […] emotions co-constitute the preconditions of experience.
>
> (Oikkonen, 2017: 683)

By focusing on the discursive construction of the therapeutic companion and the users' articulations of their expectations and experiential engagements, I wish to examine how the app 'invites us to be affected' (ibid.), thereby revealing its affective value. Like Oikkonen, I aim to do so by analysing 'narratives' (Riessman, 2008) surrounding *DepressApp*'s construction and circulation. According to Oikkonen, this method highlights ways in which 'narrative organization produces a sense of movement, anticipation or closure':

> Crucially, narrative is more than a mode of representation; narratives condition how we orientate in time and space. Narrative organization produces a sense of movement and temporal orientation that exceeds (and sometimes even contradicts) the explicit words on the page.
>
> (Oikkonen, 2017: 686)

Apart from the emotional impact that texts produce through their language and content, textual representations of emotions influence readers through their structural, largely non-discursive orientations and connect phenomena or events 'through the fabric of circulating images, tropes, and metaphors' that are often affectively charged (ibid.).

In the following analysis, I will therefore pay close attention to recurring images and metaphors in people's articulations of *DepressApp*'s imaginaries: I will first describe how *DepressApp* becomes conveyed and engaged with as a therapeutic companion. Second, I will show how the app is perceived as a symbolic vehicle to regaining voice against stigmatising perceptions of mental illness. The empirical data was mainly produced through several semi-structured interviews – both online and offline – with the producers of *DepressApp* and a total of twelve app users[4] as well as three CBT therapists. In addition, I have examined entries in social media channels that either refer to *DepressApp* or to mobile mental health in Germany and attended startup events, conferences on digital health and developers' co-working spaces.

Therapeutic companionship and its technological imagination

> My name is Maria and I'm a person suffering from depression. For most of
> the time I have been completely alone with this topic, because I just did not
> find any peers. But I'm actually not alone because in Germany there are about
> five million people diagnosed with depression. Once I decided that I needed
> therapy, I faced a waiting time of three to six months. [...] Then most people
> are finding themselves in CBT – and to put it short: the core of CBT is to
> improve negative behaviour patterns into positive behaviour patterns. This
> means that actually the therapy is not necessarily only taking place behind the
> closed doors of the therapist; actually it is taking place in daily life and right
> here and now, whenever I need something to calm down…. We have been
> sitting together, thinking about how we can improve this problem, [...] and
> we decided that our mission is to empower people suffering from depression
> to reclaim their lives as an important process of healing (Excerpt of an oral
> presentation).

…the ticking of a clock starts floating through the surrounding speakers while music
begins to play, growing increasingly louder: 'Time goes by…so slowly'. Maria fin-
ishes her last sentence against the rising volume of the music and then quickly heads
off the stage. She had just presented *DepressApp* to an audience of psychologists,
psychiatrists, health insurance agents and entrepreneurs at the peripheries of a mental health care congress in 2017. The ticking of the clock and the music were both
part of a meticulously scripted and performed startup slam pitch.

The developers position their 'product' against the limits of access to psychotherapy and constraints of outpatient care in Germany. According to a 2017 survey
by the German Association for Psychiatry, Psychotherapy and Psychosomatics,
the average waiting time for an initial consultation adds up to 12.5 weeks. To
enter regular ambulatory psychotherapeutic care, the waiting times are estimated
to be even higher.[5] Not only is the app supposed to bridge these waiting times,
but also once the patient has entered therapy foster communication between a
therapist and a patient by providing a dashboard that allows a patient's assessment
at a spatial distance. Therapeutic engagements also take place outside 'the closed
doors of the therapist' throughout the daily life – 'right here and now', in Maria's
words. *DepressApp* is thus designed to serve as a faithful companion that people
can consult and use whenever the need for instant soothing orientation arises.

The way *DepressApp* was envisioned, designed and pitched as an everyday
companion against the structural constraints of access to psychotherapeutic
care in Germany can be referred to as the workings of 'technological imagination' (Balsamo, 2011), that is, the ways in which designers and entrepreneurs
think with technology in order to transform current modes of mental health care.
DepressApp, run on a mobile phone, enters through the user's hand into an intimate and habitual everyday relationship that might also alter the way it is perceived as an object 'always at hand to being almost always in the hand and close
to the body' (Lasen, 2004, cited in Richardson, 2007: 210).

While it was common for my interlocutors to deploy the app at home, most of them also used it in public, for example, when waiting for the bus or for appointments, sitting in restaurants or when taking walks. One participant stressed that using an app had the great advantage of being less visible than analogue writing on mood protocol sheets, given the ordinariness of smartphones usage in public life:

> I fiddle around with my smartphone all the time, playing games or just chatting with friends. People are not able to tell the difference between this casual kind of usage and me tracking my mood. […] With mood charts on paper it would be a whole different story. I would be ashamed if other people could see me doing this.

Another advantage that has been stressed by some participants lies in the degrees of practicability and functionality: instead of filling in tonnes and tonnes of paper sheets that might get lost or be forgotten, an app saves the data for later use and keeps them locked with a security code. An integrated, time-adjustable push-notification reminds users to log their moods. According to one participant, who was already familiar with analogue mood diaries during CBT:

> Every time I feel my phone vibrating in my pocket and see the reminder urging me to make another mood log sets a moment of introspection in motion […] this external stimulus is so helpful. […] When I was instructed by my therapist to document my ups and downs manually on paper sheets, I tended to forget or even get nervous about it, because I had to hide the sheets from my roommates and was not orderly enough to archive them properly.

As the user explained, the built-in vibration alarm prompted 'introspection'; for him, it felt as 'if a therapist was kindly, but emphatically urging me to do my homework'. The app, understood as an everyday therapeutic companion, allowed him to tacitly comply with a self-constructed regime of mood-management and -control, thereby keeping his emotional well-being in check. This has been seen as particularly helpful when one is desperately waiting for access to regular therapeutic treatment.

Overcoming constraints of time and space constitute one powerful discursive motive in assembling *DepressApp* as a therapeutic companion. This is reflected in the app's portrayal as a '24-hours therapist' or a 'pocket therapist' (see Figure 8.1). It is this perceived potential of being used as a standalone therapeutic solution that makes the technology alluring, yet – as will be shown – also problematic.

One interviewee, Sebastian, for instance, perceived *DepressApp* as a form of therapeutic treatment in itself: 'I've began to administer treatment with *DepressApp* in November 2016 […]. I can't say much about the therapeutic effect on my depression since the actual effects are supposed to kick in just three or four weeks from now [that is, around February 2017]'. Sebastian's expectations were high: after losing his long-time job during his mid-thirties, he sank into a 'deep hole', and although he got diagnosed with depression, for more than three months he was desperately searching for a place to start psychotherapy. During this time,

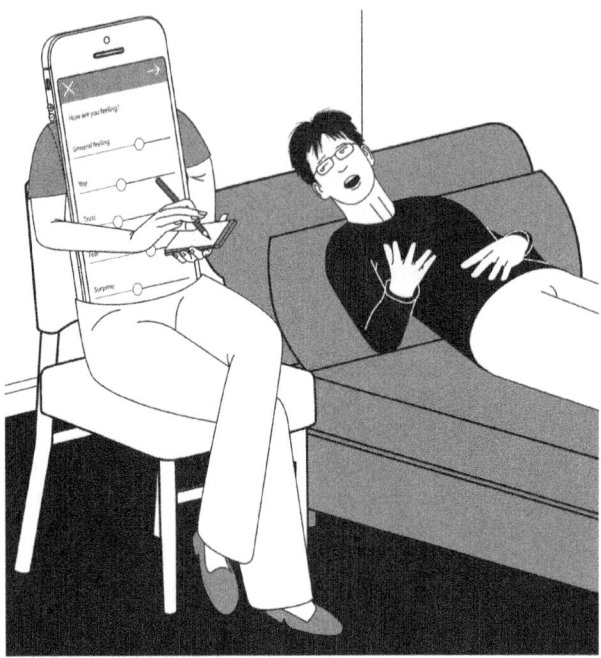

Figure 8.1 Depiction of a mood-tracking app in a popular German psychology magazine.
          © joergdommel.com

he was introduced to *DepressApp* by a fellow self-help group member and began
to use it several times every day to assuage his longing for alleviation. During our
first conversations he stressed that he at least had the app to guide him through
these times of affliction: 'It's relieving to have the app. It feels like a personal
therapist who teaches me awareness with regard to my emotions, with the only
difference, that it is available all the time'. Yet Sebastian, who was initially enthusiastic about the app, soon became dissatisfied with it:

> Although I can consult the app at any time, I have the impression that I don't
> learn much anymore. […] I still track my mood three-times a day, but just
> following the graph, my ups and downs on the chart, does not alone help me.
> It's like a one-way street: You have your digital diary with all the data and
> some information about depression, but in the end, it is up to me to decide
> what the data means. This often overwhelms me.

Sebastian's symptoms worsened rapidly and he quit using *DepressApp* after being
admitted to a psychiatric hospital.

Another interlocutor who expressed disappointment over the therapeutic effects that *DepressApp* purports to bring, referred to the app as if it were a

psychotherapeutic drug: 'I've not learnt much. But perhaps I was just not long enough *on it* [*nicht lang genug genommen*]. I guess, if I would be *on the app* for one or two years, then I would also have experienced therapeutic effects'. When she used the app, she was also proactively searching for a therapist, and again, at a time of longing for regular psychotherapeutic treatment, *DepressApp* was conceived of as a powerful vehicle for alleviation, one rhetorically, though perhaps unconsciously linked to psychopharmaceutic drugs.

While the majority of the users I interviewed did not expect the app to become a substitute to regular psychotherapeutic treatment, people who were desperately looking for help tended to have high expectations when integrating *DepressApp* into their day-to-day life, even perceiving the use of *DepressApp* as therapeutic itself. However, the app's conditions of use explicitly warn against its adoption in severe depression when unaccompanied by psychotherapeutic treatment. This warning can be understood as a 'therapeutic disclaimer': although the promotion of the therapeutic companion insinuates notions of 'quasi-therapeutic' effects by way of self-help practices, the developers relativise its efficacy as a standalone technology. As has been briefly demonstrated by the two cases above, the therapeutic disclaimer creates a paradoxical impression of the app's potentials and its use. *DepressApp* presents itself in terms of a desired proximate technology that one can carry along and consult at anytime and anywhere – this is the vision of the therapeutic companion; at the same time the app is questioned and perceived of as a distant technology that evokes powerful expectations, which it is perhaps unable to meet.

Regaining voice

DepressApp's popularity can also be linked to aspirations of empowerment. As has been shown in the pitch quoted above, Maria often utilises her experiences of suffering in order to contextualise and promote the app in public speeches, as well as across diverse media outlets. In her understanding, empowerment means overcoming constraints of space and time in the treatment of depression by assembling a therapeutic technology for the work on and of the self either outside or in support of regular psychotherapy; but it also entails the intention of working collectively towards societal destigmatisation of mental illness in general.

One 2016 TV report on Maria's struggle with depression became a focal point of discussion for many of the app's adopters. The report portrayed Maria as she went about her everyday life and was partly presented as a self-documented video diary, in which she also filmed herself in moments of emotional turmoil, crying and anxious to leave her home. At the same time, the report showed the entrepreneurial self – Maria who makes informed decisions, has to manage financial investments and becomes productive in the creation of *DepressApp*. These impressions 'stuck' with some of the app's early adopters. When asked for her motivation to use the app, one interlocutor, Claudia, stated:

> I've watched Maria's TV report and immediately became enthusiastic about the app. Maria's openness was contagious and – being a person afflicted

by depression myself – I decided to do something. For one, with regard to improving my own management of life. But more importantly, to actively support others by listening and consoling.

Claudia began to comment regularly on articles disseminated on *DepressApp*'s Facebook page. The page itself – whose number of members had reached nearly 6,000 in August 2018 – serves the app-developers as a crucial medium to post psycho-educational resources (e.g., popular scientific articles on depression and mental health care in Germany), online media like YouTube clips and photos, as well as news on technical updates. Over time, certain motives have been established: the *DepressApp* team often explicitly addresses community members, calling for feedback or participation, for instance by asking members to send pictures of their particular 'feel-good-moments' or by sharing their experiences with regard to access to therapeutic care; under the slogan 'Happy Mondays', the app-team posts revelatory and meaningful aphorisms accompanied by soothing stock photographs. *DepressApp*'s Facebook community has thus become an important site for the circulation of the 'promise of happiness' (Ahmed, 2010; see also Garde-Hansen & Gorton, 2013). At the same time, it also serves as the foundation of particular kinds of attachment and sociality, based on a shared critique of the structural conditions of therapeutic care in Germany and on 'speaking out' one's experiences with depression. One interlocutor emphasised that:

> the Facebook community feels like one big self-help group; a group where one can chat with and support each other. And I also like that this is happening publicly. […] This way people who do not have any experiences with depression can get an impression of what it really feels like. This is the difference to small private self-help groups, which gather behind closed doors.

Besides mutual support, which is expressed through consoling and the sharing of personal stories, 'speaking out' in this way also means challenging prevalent stereotypes associated with mental illness in public. In relation to depression, a recurrent trope among the interlocutors is the image of the passive victim versus an active challenger. Maria herself once said in an interview that one of her incipient entrepreneurial motivations to develop the app was to 'stop being the victim' and to make this the liberating perspective of the millions of other people suffering from depression. This potential was also widely recognised by *DepressApp*'s Facebook community members: several interlocutors poignantly criticised the societal biases in perceptions of depression. One participant stressed that depression is commonly associated with being immobilised:

> This is what annoys me most – everyone thinks that once you're suffering from depression you are prone to being paralysed. As if I were just tacitly accepting my destiny or would not even be willing to change something. […] Of course, often it's hard to work against it [depression], but using such things [apps] and interacting in the community really proves the contrary,

doesn't it? I mean, I really want to change something and even if I may not be able to get rid of my illness, then at least I learn to live and actively deal with it. [...] This is the message that I'm spreading on Facebook and I really like that others are doing the same.

Within *DepressApp*'s affective economy, the Facebook community functions as an important platform for the users' struggle against victimising identity attributions commonly associated with depression. Several scholars have asserted that being afflicted by depression implies that 'one's status as a rational person is thrown into question' (Martin, 2007: 37; see also Cvetkovich, 2012; Ehrenberg, 2010). As has been shown, some users at least emphasised app usage and engaging in the community as strategies to actively challenge and eventually overcome these attributions. For them, mood-tracking practices represented one way to make visible proactive and highly 'rationalised' coping strategies in order to tackle the societal stigma associated with depression so as to eventually overcome their own shame and embarrassment.

The societal and structural biases towards depression were also mentioned in other circumstances. One interlocutor who had been diagnosed with depression began using the app while she was still in CBT treatment. After her statutory health insurance-funded 80 sessions had ended, she still felt a need for therapy and continued to use the app three times a day in order to provide an objective document of her suffering and thereby make it visible (see also Bergroth and Helén in this book):

I have been using the app every day for nearly one year [...], primarily to understand myself and my moods [*Stimmungen*] better, but I also use the data to prove that I am actually sick. [...] People would not assume that I'm sick, because it is not as easy to recognise as a broken leg or flu. But having the data shows how I really feel [...] it also becomes recognisable for others. For example, if I would have troubles with public authorities that don't approve for my suffering, I could show them this document, so that they understand. At least, I hope so.

This account demonstrates the pressures of legitimising one's suffering from depression against its 'politics of visibility'. Comparison with other – somatic – illnesses serves as a way to account for the specific biases towards depression. Depression being not as visible as other afflictions, this participant felt the need to produce an authoritative document that would, on the one hand, enable her to gain a resource for self-knowledge (in order to understand her mood fluctuations and thus also herself better), but could also, on the other hand, potentially become representative of her experiences in its own right. The app, situated in Facebook's discursive realm, can thus be understood as a tool to challenge 'victimizing' biases by way of 'rational' self-examination and self-management of mood fluctuations, but also as a vehicle of empowerment that can 'give voice' to those who feel not heard otherwise.

In addition, Maria's moments of 'speaking out' alongside her close ties to the app often caused conflations of her own experiential narratives with those of others and – by extension – the overall workings of *DepressApp*. Following the above mentioned 2016 TV report, *DepressApp*'s download numbers escalated and some of the subsequent App Store reviews by adopters read like the following:

> Dear Maria, the feeling you're describing is very well known to me... It is such a complex illness, which receives far too little attention. I think your app can help to get to know yourself and the disease better.

By making her everyday life with depression visible and being perceived as a courageous role model who propagates the significance of self-management, Maria lends credence to the app, which makes it also appear like a trustworthy space for self-disclosure. This is particularly noticeable in some users' reflections on their potential data exposure. For example, in an online conversation about the importance of *DepressApp*'s data security policies one interlocutor, Heiko, stated that '[data security] is very important because of their [his data sets] intimate qualities. But I trust the staff at *DepressApp* – Maria is one of us'. Maria's moments of 'speaking out' create an imagined bond between users and developers that blurs the boundaries between producers and consumers and generates a sense of trust from which *DepressApp* directly benefits as it is downloaded and consumed despite the risk of processing intimate data.

The technological imaginaries of therapeutic cultures

While people's striving for well-being increasingly connects with new ICTs, the wide-ranging entanglements of human and non-human actors yet remain underrepresented in the studies of therapeutic cultures. Based upon that premise, this chapter aimed to provide an analytical avenue into the affectively charged imaginaries and socio-material intertwinements of therapeutic technologies; namely by introducing mood-tracking apps through the lens of assemblage thinking and affect theory to sketch out how certain expectations are being invested in this kind of digital technology and how these investments, in turn, may become constitutive of such a technology.

As has been shown, mood-tracking apps augment analogue therapeutic self-management techniques and thereby afford self-reflexive engagements by way of 'making emotions count' (Pritz, 2016). Analysing recurrent images and metaphors in people's articulations of one German app's technological imaginaries, I have described how *DepressApp* is presented and engaged with as a therapeutic companion that encompasses affective value. The therapeutic companion aims to compensate for structural constraints of psychotherapeutic and outpatient care in Germany. At times, this has led to projections of *DepressApp* as a 'pockettherapist', which engenders powerful expectations that sometimes cannot be fulfilled. Furthermore, I have shown that the app's entanglement with social media sites, such as Facebook, narratives of 'speaking out' (Wright, 2008: 328) and the tackling of the societal stigma associated with depression have also become elements within *DepressApp*'s affective economy.

This makes *DepressApp* an interesting case for the study of therapeutic cultures: serving, on the one hand, as a technology that propagates the work on the individual self by taking one's emotional life seriously and recognising subjective experience as a valid source of knowledge (Lears, 2015) and being situated, on the other hand, in a discursive ecosystem in which the appeal of self-disclosure blends with a collective problematisation of mental health care in Germany. *DepressApp* thus depicts a 'happy object' (Ahmed, 2010) that purports the genuine impression of a personalised and comforting technology; it emerges as a 'trustful and friendly other' that helps to navigate, often times, unsettling periods of life in order to get well. At the same time, it can also be understood as a political device in people's struggles against negative perceptions of depression.

Notes

1 The app's name as well as the names of participants are pseudonyms.
2 The CE-marking is considered a prerequisite for a product to be finally put into clinical operation. It ensures conformity with all legal regulations, clinical and diagnostic relevance and the safety of a medical device. On their route to such a marking, digital health companies have to be creative: The team of *DepressApp*, for instance, conducts efficacy trials at a hospital for medical weight loss because of the lack of adoption and testing from practicing psychotherapists.
3 The term *therapeutic companion* strongly resonates with Deborah Lupton's (2016) commentary on Donna Haraway's notion of companion species.
4 Among the participants were five men and seven women, ranging from age 19 to 45; nine of them had already been treated for mental health issues, one person was treated during the time of the research and two participants have not received psychotherapeutic treatment at all.
5 This imbalance, however, is not a matter of a lack of psychotherapists in Germany, but is due to the expensive process of gaining health insurance approval for beginning psychotherapists. In order to tackle the shortage in supply and to reduce costs, German health insurance companies also invest in clinical evaluations of digital health technologies, such as mood-tracking apps.

References

Ahmed, S. 2004a. *The Cultural Politics of Emotion*. Edinburgh: Edinburgh University Press.

Ahmed, S. 2004b. Affective Economies. *Social Text 22*:2, 117–139.

Ahmed, S. 2010. *The Promise of Happiness*. Durham & London: Duke University Press.

Aubry, T. & Travis, T. (eds) 2015. *Rethinking Therapeutic Culture*. Chicago & London: University of Chicago Press.

Balsamo, A. 2011. *Designing Culture: The Technological Imagination at Work*. Durham & London: Duke University Press.

Belli, J. 2016. Unhappy? There's an App for That. Tracking Well-Being through the Quantified Self. *Digital Culture and Society 2*:1, 89–103.

Cvetkovich, A. 2012. *Depression. A Public Feeling*. Durham & London: Duke University Press.

Davies, W. 2017. How Are We Now? Real-Time Mood-Monitoring as Valuation. *Journal of Cultural Economy 10*:1, 34–48.

DeLanda, M. 2006. *A New Philosophy of Society: Assemblage Theory and Social*. London & New York: Continuum.

Deleuze, G. 1992 [1990]. Postscript on the Societies of Control. *October 59*, 3–7.

Deleuze, G. & Guattari, F. 2013 [1987]. *A Thousand Plateaus: Capitalism and Schizophrenia*. London & New York: Bloomsbury Academic.

Ecclestone, K. & Hayes, D. 2009. *The Dangerous Rise of Therapeutic Education*. London & New York: Routledge.

Ehrenberg, A. 2010. *The Weariness of the Self: Diagnosing the History of Depression in the Contemporary Age*. Montreal: McGill-Queen's University Press.

Ekkekakis, P. 2013. *The Measurement of Affect, Mood, and Emotion. A Guide for Health-Behavioral Research*. Cambridge: Cambridge University Press.

Espeland, W. N. & Stevens, M. 1998. Commensuration as a Social Process. *Annual Review of Sociology 24*, 313–343.

Foucault, M. 1988. Technologies of the Self. In *Technologies of the Self: A Seminar with Michel Foucault*, edited by M. Luther, H. Gutman & P. H. Hutton. Amherst: University of Massachusetts Press, 16–49.

Furedi, F. 2004. *Therapy Culture: Cultivating Vulnerability in an Uncertain Age*. London & New York: Routledge.

Gaggioli, A. & Riva, G. 2013. From Mobile Mental Health to Mobile Wellbeing: Opportunities and Challenges. *Studies in Health Technology and Informatics 184*, 141–147.

Garde-Hansen, J. & Gorton, K. 2013. *Emotion Online: Theorizing Affect on the Internet*. Houndsmill: Palgrave Macmillan.

Hochschild, A. R. 1983. *The Managed Heart. Commercialization of Human Feeling*. Los Angeles & Berkeley, CA: University of California Press.

Illouz, E. 2008. *Saving the Modern Soul: Therapy, Emotions, and the Culture of Self-Help*. Berkeley, CA: University of California Press.

Latour, B. 2005. *Reassembling the Social: An Introduction to Actor-Network-Theory*. New York: Oxford University Press.

Lears, J. 2015. Afterword. In *Rethinking Therapeutic Culture*, edited by T. Aubry & T. Travis. Chicago & London: University of Chicago Press, 211–215.

Lupton, D. 2014. Apps as Artefacts: Towards a Critical Perspective on Mobile Health and Medical Apps. *Societies 4*, 606–622.

Lupton, D. 2016. Digital Companion Species and Eating Data: Implications for Theorising Digital Data-Human Assemblages. *Big Data & Society 3*:1, 1–5.

Madsen, O. J. 2014. *The Therapeutic Turn: How Psychology Altered Western Culture*. London & New York: Routledge.

Marcus, G. & Saka, E. 2006. Assemblage. *Theory, Culture & Society 23*:2–3, 101–109.

Martin, E. 2007. *Bipolar Expeditions: Mania and Depression in American Culture*. Princeton & Oxford: Princeton University Press.

Massumi, B. 2002. *Parables of the Virtual: Movement, Affect, Sensation*. Durham & London: Duke University Press.

Mazzarella, W. 2017. Sense Out of Sense: Notes on the Affect/Ethics Impasse. *Cultural Anthropology 32*:2, 199–208.

McGee, M. 2005. *Self-Help, Inc.: Makeover Culture in American Life*. New York: Oxford University Press.

Müller, M. 2015. Assemblages and Actor-Networks: Rethinking Socio-Material Power, Politics and Space. *Geography Compass 9*:1, 27–41.

Müller, M. & Schurr, C. 2016. Assemblage Thinking and Actor-Network Theory: Conjunctions, Disjunctions, Cross-Fertilisations. *Transactions of the Institute of British Geographers 41*:3, 217–229.

Neckel, S. 2014. Emotionale Reflexivität – Paradoxien der Emotionalisierung. In *Systemzwang und Akteurswissen – Theorie und Empirie von Autonomiegewinnen,* edited by T. Fehmel, S. Lessenich & J. Preunkert. Frankfurt a. M.: Campus.

Nehring, D., Alvarado, E., Hendriks, E. C. & Kerrigan, D. 2016. *Transnational Popular Psychology and the Global Self-Help Industry: The Politics of Contemporary Social Change.* Houndmills: Palgrave Macmillan.

Oikkonen, V. 2017. Affect, Technoscience and Textual Analysis: Interrogating the Affective Dynamics of the Zika Epidemic through Media Texts. *Social Studies of Science 47*:5, 681–702.

Pritz, S. M. 2016. Making Emotions Count: The Self-Tracking of Feelings. In *Lifelogging,* edited by S. Selke. Wiesbaden: Springer VS, 179–187.

Pyyhtinen, O. 2016. *More-Than-Human Sociology A New Sociological Imagination.* New York: Palgrave Pivot.

Richardson, I. 2007. Pocket Technospaces: The Bodily Incorporation of Mobile Media. *Continuum 21*:2, 205–215.

Riessman, C. K. 2008. *Narrative Methods for the Human Sciences.* Thousand Oaks, CA: Sage.

Rimke, H. 2017. Self-Help Ideology. In *The SAGE Encyclopedia of Political Behavior,* edited by F. M. Moghaddam. Thousand Oaks: Sage.

Rose, N. 1990. *Governing the Soul: The Shaping of the Private Self.* London & New York: Routledge.

Rose, N. 1998. *Inventing Ourselves: Psychology, Power, and Personhood.* Cambridge, MA: Cambridge University Press.

Weiner, T. 2011. The (Un)managed Self: Paradoxical Forms of Agency in Self-Management of Bipolar Disorder. *Culture, Medicine, Psychiatry 35,* 448–483.

Wetherell, M. 2013. Affect and Discourse – What's the Problem? From Affect as Excess to Affective/Discursive Practice. *Subjectivity 6*:4, 349–368.

Wetherell, M., McCreanor, T., McConville, A., Moewaka Barnes, H. & le Grice, J. 2015. Settling Space and Covering the Nation: Some Conceptual Considerations in Analysing Affect and Discourse. *Emotion, Space and Society 16*:1, 56–64.

Wright, K. 2008. Theorizing Therapeutic Culture: Past Influences, Future Directions. *Journal of Sociology 44*:4, 321–336.

9 No negative vibes

Organizational fun as a practice of social control

Virve Peteri

It is quite possible, then, that my employer fully expects me to respond to his bantering in a like manner, and considers my failure to do so a form of negligence. This is, as I say, a matter which has given me much concern. But I must say this business of bantering is not a duty I feel I can ever discharge with enthusiasm. It is all very well, in these changing times, to adapt one's work to take duties not traditionally within one's realm; but bantering is of another dimension altogether. For one thing, how would one know for sure that at any given moment a response of the bantering sort is truly what is expected? One need hardly dwell on the catastrophic possibility of uttering a bantering remark only to discover it wholly inappropriate.

(Kazuo Ishiguro: *The Remains of the Day*, p.16)

I never thought that during my ethnographic journey in the 2010s in two organizations carrying out big organizational changes I would identify so strongly with an old English butler from the 1950s. A butler struggling to understand how to respond to his new lord of the manor. The new lord masters the making of playful small talk, and the old butler struggles to follow this new form of social interaction. There is something oddly recognizable here. My informants discussed how they felt there was something puzzling about the organizational change seeking to promote 'fun culture' in the workplace. Although the directors would tell the employees that the changes would bring more fun into the workplace and free them from their offices, they still felt, at times, less liberated and more awkward. Occasionally, I was also perplexed by the strangeness of some situations which were described as liberating for the employees. What was creating this uneasiness?

This chapter is an attempt to make sense of those aforementioned experiences. I am interested in analysing what kind of assemblages of bodies, materials and spaces the organizational fun culture promotes, and, through ethnographic documentation, the contrary and complex meanings or 'ideological dilemmas' (Billig, 1988) this fun culture and its assemblages may produce. The ideological dilemmas perspective underlines the idea that ideologies, whether they are philosophical, political or everyday notions, comprise contrary themes. Thus, the different elements of an assemblage may construct and promote contradictory and inconsistent tendencies. Assemblage thinking emphasizes the intertwined nature of spatiality and power, because it examines why certain orders emerge in specific ways, and how these orders shape socio-materiality and spaces. The perspective underlines that assemblages are always productive. They produce new behaviours, new expressions, new actors and realities (Müller, 2015).

The ethnographic data for this study was gathered from two workplaces that have adopted an activity-based office model. An activity-based office most commonly includes an open-plan office space, meeting rooms and a few separate spaces for work requiring more concentration. An activity-based office rests on the idea that people do not have their own workstation but can choose a fitting workstation depending on their mood and work tasks and even change their place several times a day, when they move on to a new activity. The central idea behind the activity-based office is that productivity will increase through the stimulation of interaction, mobility and communication (Appel-Meulenbroek et al., 2011).

The emphasis on fun, happiness and emotions in general has, from the beginning, been central to the development of the activity-based office concept, although, in the official strategies and documents, it is considered to be more about rational calculations between different work activities. Less than ten years ago, Microsoft launched new business premises in Finland. At first, these premises were called 'Meeting Spaces'. Later, the office was reconceptualised and renamed as an 'activity-based office'. The idea was that these new premises would eventually evolve into a global office concept, a paradigm for innovative office design. Instead of fixed workstations, the workplace consisted of different spaces of encounter, with a variety of ambiance alternatives such as 'beach', 'inspiration', 'nature', 'home' or 'bistro'. These spaces were presented as places where employees, objects and information move effortlessly, without hierarchies, limits or unnecessary controls. The idea was that employees would identify their task and mood for the day in the morning and choose the space that best fitted their state of mind and jobs. I argue that this kind of office design establishes a form of a 'therapeutic space', which mixes rationality and emotionality by creating subjects who are encouraged to act like 'one-man businesses', private entrepreneurs who consider their tasks rationally meanwhile always reflecting on their current mood or emotion. The workers may choose to match their mood with the atmosphere of a certain space, but, nevertheless, they are *forced to choose*, and the chosen space directs the way they may move, communicate and feel. The office produces subjects whose duty is to start each day by contemplating which ambiance is pleasant and suitable for them that day.

The chapter is organized as follows. Firstly, I will explore the existing research and cultural analysis on fun and playfulness in organizations and discuss my empirical and theoretical contribution to the subject. Secondly, I will present my data and the methodology utilized in the chapter. Thirdly, I will analyse the data and finally, discuss my findings.

Offices as therapeutic spaces

In his *Manifesto For a Ludic Century*, Eric Zimmerman (2015) notes that 'In the last few decades, information has taken a playful turn', and this change will require new skills, as it is not enough to 'understand systems in an analytic sense.

We must also learn to be playful in them'. Zimmerman writes mostly about digital games but broadens his scope as he suggests that the playful turn is also intertwined with how we work, communicate, socialize and love. He firmly connects playfulness with the ability to be innovative and creative.

In a somewhat similar vein, in recent decades, the positive psychology movement has highlighted the need to show more interest in studying the positive and playful aspects of human life (Seligman & Csikszentmihalyi, 2014). The psychological theory by Csikszentmihalyi which emphasizes the notion of flow has been highly influential. Positive psychologists suggest that working life can be organized around playfulness, thus, creating new innovations and value by stimulating employees' imagination and adding more fun into working life. For example, Glynn and Webster (1992) have identified a need for more in-depth study of adult playfulness to understand its role in the workplace. Positive psychologists suggest that play and associated positive emotions augment individuals' intellectual and other personal and social resources (Barnett, 2007; Fredrickson, 1998; Fredrickson et al., 2000), which, at the very least, implies that fostering positive emotions at the workplace might generate more innovative employees. Since the 1980s, management gurus have emphasized that adopting a fun culture at the workplace will promote a playful and pleasurable atmosphere, which will produce more productive and dedicated employees. Interestingly, the idea of organizational fun has gone a long way considering the usually short life cycle of management and business trends (Fleming, 2005). Redman and Mathews (2002) maintain that there is even a 'well-developed "fun industry" offering would-be funsters with advice, workshops and consultancy on making work more fun', which shows that the business of creating fun is a truly serious business (see Fleming, 2005: 288).

However, organizational fun cultures are not static but in constant flux as are the organizations themselves. Fun cultures have existed even before the fun industry, in the form of joking and workplace humour. Power and resistance have been part of fun culture even before the more official fun cultures emerged. Sexual harassment in the form of innuendo, jokes, so-called 'girl calendars' and unwanted touching are ancient forms of 'fun culture' that have traditionally suppressed women (Ackroyd & Thompson, 1999). Moreover, the present organizational fun culture may reproduce and reformulate novel forms of control and subjectivities.

The reproduction and reformulation of control and subjectivities is linked with what can be called soft capitalism. The rhetoric of soft capitalism is concerned with playfulness, beauty and emotions (Chugh & Hancock, 2009: 465). This rhetoric identifies that the success of an organization lies in the narratives and creativity rather than with rationality, technologies and cost-benefit calculations even though its practices have a strong utilitarian dimension, and it is basically an attempt, as Heelas (2002: 81–82) notes, to instrumentalize these soft values for economic ends (see also Costea et al., 2005; Peteri, 2017). Furthermore, one form of soft capitalism is to promote new kinds of office environments that materialize and demonstrate the new flexible organization usually by trying to activate emotions and to maximize social interaction and mobility to produce innovations

(Thrift, 2005: 33–45). Kantola (2014: 9–11) calls this 'enthusiastic individualism' where playful informality and personal passion have become the new normative emotions of soft capitalism.

The literature concerning soft capitalism has some important resonances with the work of Boltanski and Chiapello (2007) on the new spirit of capitalism and Illouz's (2007, 2008) work on emotional capitalism. All of these emphasize the role of social critique and academic research on reinventing capitalism and organizational cultures. The solution to improving working conditions and removing faceless bureaucracy and the 'men in grey flannel suits' is, according to Boltanski and Chiapello, to produce organizations that are more flexible, innovative and mobile. The new spirit expects employees to manage themselves meanwhile their companies can offer them self-help resources. The activity-based office model can be regarded as a form of 'therapeutic space' (Gorman, 2017a, 2017b) and 'organized self-help' that offers material elements inviting happier employees and producing networking opportunities, mobility and playfulness to promote innovations. This involves recognizing space as an active agent that is capable of transforming and shaping our experiences and emotions. This connects with the therapeutic call to maintain positive thoughts about oneself and the co-workers and to keep up positive energy and enthusiastic mentality. Thus, the therapeutic ethos makes emotions central to self-work (Illouz, 2008) and enhances organizational control by controlling and directing employees' emotions.

Soft capitalism draws its ideas and legitimation from a number of sources. Its themes and vocabularies have become an important part of both the business world and academia. In a similar manner, as demonstrated previously, the culture of fun is not outside academia. In fact, its central mechanism is to 'playfully' mix and adopt ideas from a variety of sources: academic literature, popular self-help books, TV series, business media and tabloids. Even though some research has more or less accepted playfulness and happiness as the key elements of innovative organizational life, there is also plenty of research that raises more critical questions and analyses the fun culture and playfulness as providing a means for managerial control (e.g., Alexandersson & Kalonaityte, 2018; Baldry & Hallier, 2010; Costea et al., 2005; Fleming, 2005). Play is part of a wider turn to subjectivity (Costea et al., 2005), and thus, it is important to analyse what it adds to contemporary subjectivity.

The ethnographic data

I gathered data from two workplaces (in 2010 and 2014). One is a public organization with more than 2,500 members of staff and the other a private enterprise employing over 7,000 people. The work in these organizations could be characterized as knowledge work as it involves managing and organizing information and producing knowledge in different forms. During my ethnography, I also visited four other organizations that have adopted the activity-based office model. As I went to give talks in open seminars, I met people who invited me to visit their workplaces so that they could show me their new office premises and share their experiences on moving to an activity-based office. These visits are not included in the primary data, but certainly have deepened my analysis, as I have been able to discuss my findings with people who have first-hand experience of the activity-based office model.

The organizations in my data had already adopted the activity-based office model. Although the official strategies concerning the activity-based office do not mention fun culture or playfulness, all the organizations I visited included elements that can be identified as promoting the culture of fun. This might be interpreted as a signal that the elements of fun, at least at the moment, in themselves signify or mark the 'new' in office decoration and spatial design, so much so that they have to be included in official strategies without a reference to them. The material has been obtained through interviews, observations, discussions and the gathering of documents. The documents include, for example, the *Proposed Government Premises Strategy* (2014) and the *Government's Decision in Principle on Premises Strategy* (2014) as well as different research reports and brochures on the activity-based office model (e.g., Haapamäki et al., 2011; Nenonen et al., 2012; Nenonen & Niemi, 2013; Sandberg, 2012). I have also collected newspaper and magazine articles that deal with activity-based offices.

The material has been anonymized by changing the names of the workers and removing information that risks identifying the organizations. Workers who could have been compromised by the research have had the opportunity to check the text and make comments on it before publication. Furthermore, some examples of the organizations' interiors presented in the analysis have been edited. For example, if I describe a wallpaper, its details and theme may have been changed to resemble the original while not being identical with it. However, there are plenty of examples that I could easily use because equivalent elements could be found in all of the organizations I visited and also in the media texts.

During my fieldwork, I enjoyed rereading Lefebvre's *The Production of Space*. Lefebvre writes about 'representations of space', that refer to existing ways of conceptualizing spaces. These representations are produced and implemented by architects, political decision-makers, officials, planners and engineers. Lefebvre also mentions 'social engineers' (Lefebvre, 2015: 38), who would today include consultants, interior designers, and 'change managers' hired to execute pre-planned organizational changes. Lefebvre suggests that analysing representations of space is a specific form of critique, equivalent to literary critique, a critique of space that recognizes dominant representations of space and shows how space is not just a frame or background for action. Human agency, social practices and spatial arrangements are intertwined so closely that they cannot really be understood as separate entities. Each can be understood through the other, as Foucault (2003: 372) notes. According to Lefebvre, a critique of space or 'spatial imagination' has to start with a *lived space*, the embodied users' experiences of power, tensions and resistance working with and through space (Soja, 1996: 68). These conceptualizations seemed to speak directly about the experiences I had when talking with the employees at their newly decorated office spaces, and they made me realize that I could not just do research on them, but I had to also do it *for* them.

In the private sector, many office employees have moved from their own workrooms to open-plan offices where they 'hot-desk' or use shared workstations. A working lounge, office hoteling and hub-type spaces are also becoming more common. It seems that a spatial shift is taking place in office settings in general. In Finland, *Proposed Government Premises Strategy* (2014) expresses that all ministries, government agencies and departments will be transformed into activity-based offices by 2020. Many private enterprises have already adopted the same model. Thus, my article is a critique of a certain kind of hegemonic space that is officially recognized and accepted by the Finnish government, even though its first adaptations were found in private companies.

My ethnographic field notes and the critique of space based on them may come at times close to absurd drama or even tragicomedy. Every so often, the fun culture itself might seem like a joke. According to Cate Watson (2015), before modernity put the emphasis on rationality, laughter and humour were actually seen as having a deep philosophical meaning. The absurd and the irrational were considered as inherent parts of human existence and thus humour had an essential role in revealing something that rational means could not. During my fieldwork, there were quite a few occasions where the employees and I laughed at the changes. You could say that we were constructing a hidden form of fun culture, resisting the official one with the employees' own take on fun. After all, finding humour in difficult situations can sometimes be a liberating force (Mulkay, 1988), and at its best, it provides a means for challenging the status quo and makes people feel more at ease (Nilsen, 1994).

The spatiality of fun

In the data, officially created 'fun culture' is evident in the way offices incorporate playful elements: shared spaces may include board games or a PlayStation. Also, shared areas may have Fatboy beanbags or similar floor-level seating. One of the organizations I studied had seating that resembles huge Lego blocks. The furniture in both organizations was bright coloured. The more traditional chairs in the open office areas echoed hotel lobby furniture. This type of furniture promotes mobility among the employees: puts them on the move, ready to encounter others (Peteri, 2017).

In practice, activity-based offices consist mainly of open-plan spaces without partition screens. In both organizations, big plants were used to provide visual obstruction. Strikingly, bright green was a prominent colour in the decor. In meeting rooms, photographic wallpaper depicting images of a jungle, space ship or motor racing signals playfulness and offers a visual illusion of being in another place or dimension. The office fun culture is also evident in the new names given to different departments. The departments still have doors and walls, albeit made of glass, and the names of specific departments are still on display on the doors. The font is playful, colourful and cartoonish. Often the name does not clearly reveal the function of the department, and it is impossible to discern any single logic from which the names were derived. One name reminded me of a specific children's fairy tale, another name resembled a management consultancy buzzword and a third one seemed to refer to a certain state of mind.

> I met up with Anne first thing in the morning, as she knew the managers would not be in and would not see us talking. We went to see the chill-out area. The area reminded me of my child's day care, with similar kinds of bright colours, big cushions and board games. Anne noted that nowadays it was very difficult to try to concentrate at work, as the chill-out area was right in the middle of the office space, and the young guys were often playing PlayStation games and being very loud. Some people had complained about the noise, but the managers had said that you either live with it or you leave. She told me that she and a few of her older colleagues had once suggested that they would arrange a lecture and conversations on some topic in the chill-out area. One of the bosses had said that the space is not meant for that kind of activity. (Field notes, September 2010)

While talking with Anne I noticed a laminated poster on the wall of the chill-out area. It stated: 'Everybody is Welcome here. Everybody Belongs'. The message was written in English making me wonder how welcome non-English speaking people were. Anne and her older colleagues did not feel welcome (although that had nothing to do with their language skills). The material assemblages associated with 'playbour' clearly influence how inviting different employees find the workplace. The ideal subject for these spaces seems to be a young man of a certain type. The new materials and furniture in the open-space areas are attractive for youthful bodies that can actually sit down as well as get up again from the Lego blocks or Fatboy beanbags. Wearing a dress or a top with a low neckline also make it trickier to lounge and properly relax on these beanbags. The material assemblages derive artefacts from worlds that are traditionally associated with masculinity (e.g., car racing or PlayStation games). Although emotional expression and aesthetics have traditionally been associated with femininity, they are now perceived as new resources for everyone in the workplace (Adkins, 2005; Swan, 2008). Thus, the new organizational fun culture might appear feminine with its emphasis on aesthetics and expressions of emotions. Instead, however, it may reproduce the old hierarchies in novel ways. Work cultures emphasizing informality often end up creating a 'laddish culture' (Gill, 2002) without any explicitly stated criteria why the aesthetic staging derives ideas from the world of motor racing rather than from the world of pony stables. This is not clear-cut, of course, as there were, for example, a few women who expressed that they enjoyed PlayStation games, but not at work, not at this chill-out area. It shows that it is not about who likes ponies and who likes PlayStation games, but rather of the assemblage of bodies, materials, spaces and staging.

In the official strategy (*Proposed Government Premises Strategy*, 2014), the activity-based office is introduced as a flexible environment for different kinds of tasks and people, bearing in mind, for example, ageing workers and increasing multiculturalism. The central idea behind the activity-based office is choosing a workstation and working area according to current mood and the activity at hand. In the morning, employees find a desk where they can work, and quite often they have to do so again after a meeting or lunch break. Employees seem keen to find a workstation near their closest colleagues, rather than trying to figure out which workstation would fit their activities best. They appear to choose intentionally or unintentionally ignoring the basic premise of the activity-based office.

Some workers described how, over time, they started 'deliberately' forgetting their things on certain desks, even though the directors tried to prevent this and even removed the stuff. In time, this 'misbehaviour' (Ackroyd & Thompson, 1999) developed into tacit knowledge about which workstation 'really' belonged to whom. Officially, nobody had assigned workstations, but unofficially every employee knew where their colleagues preferred to sit and work. In the other organization, the directors discussed the possibility to use an electronic system to monitor how often employees used a certain workstation. If an employee tried to use the same workstation more than twice a week, the workstation would not allow it. This electronic control would break conventional habits and force people to spend time with people they would not deliberately choose to sit next to. This spatial design seems to imply that innovations are born when unfamiliar people get close to each other, not through historical connections.

The organization of a space is conceived as activity-oriented, rather than taking into account historically developed skills and relationships in the workplace. The organization takes into account emotions, but only the fleeting ones such as moods and feelings, but ignores or even tries to remove more stable and long-term emotions of loyalty, friendship and solidarity between the employees. In both organizations, the directors encouraged staff to destroy all the 'old stuff' (papers, folders, books, etc.) and adopt a new line of thinking, which meant working mostly without paper and print media. However, in both organizations, several members of staff took those things home or to their summer cottages without informing the employer. Now that the archived work documents and books have been moved to domestic settings, a large proportion of the employees' competence and work-related information has moved off the company's premises. When I talked to the employees, they justified this by saying that the things were not just any old stuff but a very concrete part of their expertise. It seemed evident that they had interpreted the request to get rid of 'old stuff' as a signal that historical understanding of work processes was not appreciated anymore. The documents consist of information on how their special expertise has developed over time and what the expertise includes. Thus, the new office design seems to reject historical knowledge, materials, relationships and developments.

The ideological dilemmas of play and work

Huizinga (1980) observes fun and pure play in his book *Homo Ludens* as 'one of the main bases of civilization'. Huizinga defines play as a voluntary activity. If play is artificially generated or people are ordered to play, it is no longer play. It is just 'a forcible imitation' of play (Huizinga, 1980: 5–7). Here, I might add, lies one of the most obvious ideological dilemmas of generating fun and playfulness in work organizations. According to Huizinga, play is a free activity that cannot be tamed. Thus, it cannot be turned into business. This does not mean that it cannot inspire attempts to capitalize play and fun (Alexandersson & Kalonaityte, 2018).

While the playful office aims to enrich a certain leisure mentality, it simultaneously decreases spaces where one can concentrate in peace. Thus, the concept of increasing open-space areas promotes the idea that concentration is an individually created state of mind. Although playful offices aim to make people more mobile and social, they also mean that people must be able to find an intensely peaceful place inside their heads so that they rarely need quiet spaces for working.

> We were having coffee together. Seven employees and I. Someone suggested we go to a meeting room to talk more privately. The actual coffee room was an open space next to the working area, so you could not really have a private conversation there. Once we had settled, the employees started to reminisce about a meeting where the directors of the company had presented 'six theses' which the whole organization was supposed to agree on and commit to. One of the theses was 'no negative vibes'. One director explained that this slogan was from a reality TV show. According to the director's story, one of the stars of that show had confessed that there was just too much relationship drama in her life, and she wanted 'no more negative vibes'. We had a laugh. After a while, one of the employees exclaimed, 'this activity-based office thing is like an ideology!' Several of the workers murmured approvingly or laughed and an older man added that it actually reminded him of his youth; of the Maoism in the seventies. You just had to obey and not question the ideology in any way. The employees agreed that the directors seemed more thin-skinned about this organizational change than of any previous ones. (Field notes, June 2014)

One form of play is the way the managers adopt and mix ideas and slogans from very different sources; TV shows, self-help books, academic literature and tabloids. *No negative vibes* was adopted from a reality TV show and its emerging new star who had already gained some notorious fame for her colourful private life. Rejecting criticism from the employees by adopting this slogan and turning it into one of the theses produces a dilemma for the employees. The aforementioned thesis is disguised as humour, but the employees are expected to obey the rule all the same. Any criticism is regarded as breaking the rule, but also as a sign that the employee lacks a sense of humour. You disregard the central idea of having fun if you do not 'play' along and obey the joke.

Playfulness is linked with the idea of wellness and specifically with happiness and the ethos of self-work; keeping oneself happy at work is a new duty for employees (Costea et al., 2005). Although the traditional boundaries between play and work are modified, they are not reinvented. While the employees need to work on their proper 'jobs' and on their positive selves, they also have to be productive and obey the managers, in this case, by offering *no negative vibes*.

> We sat down in the colourful entrance hall area with the manager. We sat on two blocks that reminded me of jigsaw puzzle pieces. The manager stated that the new organizational change meant that the organization was now a story-telling organization, 'a narrative organization', she emphasized with pride in her voice. She explained that this was actually only the beginning of a bigger change. There is no need to inform the employees yet, she pointed out to me. I was bewildered that she told me, an outsider she had only known for a few days, about the upcoming change. I asked how the employees experienced these on-going changes. She sighed and admitted that it was not easy. She explained that people are so old-fashioned, and it is not easy giving up your personal workstation and room. She shared with me a story of a female worker who wanted to keep a picture of her dog on her desk. She imitated their conversation about the employee having to give up the picture and her having to tell the person that nobody in that department had their own work-station and thus, no one could keep their things on the desks. Her voice – when she was imitating herself – was like that of a parent when talking to a toddler. She portrayed the employee and her wishes and motivations as childish. I thought that the story was probably not a real story but rather an exaggeration that tried to emphasize a certain point or an ideal story to dem-onstrate something. After the story, she told me that the next step would be an authentic nomadic organization, which would complete the plans to increase the mobility and interaction of employees. She told me that she imagined this change as the bound of a giant tiger. (Field notes, September 2014)

The organizational change can also be experienced as exciting and liberating, especially for a manager. From a management viewpoint, the change seems to offer opportunities to take pleasure in experiencing a 'paradigm change', the excitement of creating a new organizational culture. In addition, management has the information on how the processes will proceed, which makes it easier to enjoy the change without anxieties. While I talked to the manager, she repeatedly referred to the organizational change as 'the bound of a tiger'. Only afterwards, I realized that she had most likely adopted the metaphor from a self-help book on organizational changes (Manka, 2010). The book introduces the metaphor of 'the bound of a tiger', which refers to a change that 'demands creating structures that prevent routines and make room for free interaction' and demands an understand-ing that 'we are prisoners of the past and thus blinded' (Manka, 2010: 283). The book is based on the idea that the past has nothing to teach us – it is just 'bureau-cratic skeletons in the closet' (Manka, 2010: 280) – and that organizations must embrace radical changes.

The culture of fun and its material and narrative assemblages promote the idea that employees will regain their inner child. However, there is a thin line between childlike behaviour and the *right kind* of childlike behaviour. In both organizations, the management told stories of employees wanting to keep their personal things. The punchline of these stories was that the employees were 'endearing' in their desire to 'mark' their own place with a photo of a loved one or with piles of paper. In these stories, the managers always mentioned that the piles of papers were *old* and sometimes even dusty. The tone of the stories was ironical. The employees seemed to have infantile wishes and no genuine understanding of 'the real world'. The employees were like aboriginals who have to 'mark' their territory. The management would start the stories by stating that they understood that change was difficult. Thus, the moral of these stories is that change is fundamentally not about office spaces, but really about people and their need to change.

By interpreting stories as potentially exaggerated, I do not mean that the managers were telling 'untrue' stories. Real life events do not organize themselves neatly in a narrative form. Thus, stories are something told, not just a description of how something was lived. In everyday life, we use stories to make sense of the world, as instruments to highlight something or create new information (Carr, 1986). For example, the aforementioned stories could be interpreted as an attempt to invite me to take part in a playful conversation. Hyperbole is sometimes a means to create playful talk or introduce a play frame. In spite of my view on the narrative, which dispels the difference between real and fictive elements in talk, I have to point out the ideological nature of the stories.

By sheer chance or not, the principal characters in these stories were all women. As noted before, the new organizational fun culture might appear feminine with its emphasis on aesthetics and emotions. Instead, however, it may reproduce the old hierarchies in novel ways. Those who revealed that they did not feel comfortable with the organizational fun culture were both men and women. However, the new emotional culture still reproduces stories where the women are the ones constructed as overemotional and even hysterical. As Swan (2008) suggests, men can increase their cultural capital at work by adopting feminized emotional performances in ways that are not possible for women.

Considering the stories told by the managers, women's position in the culture of fun might also be more fragile. The aforementioned stories may carry on and make use of the old idea that women do not really know how to have fun. Fun often involves humour and jokes (Fine & Corte, 2017), which are highly gendered by nature. For example, recent research has shown that cultural ideas of humour or 'talk as play' are based more on a male norm about what is considered funny. Typically, in social situations, men have preferred more formulaic joking and women share funny stories of their everyday life to create solidarity (Coates, 2007). Thus, it is more difficult for women to increase their cultural capital by expressing emotions, and with regards to the organizational fun culture, they seem to be in a bigger danger of coming across as humourless or even killjoys (see also Gill, 2016). More formulaic joking is a safer technique when the spatial and material order encourages people to mingle with new people. Sharing stories of your everyday life often demands a certain kind of familiarity with the people the stories are shared with.

Furthermore, the previous passage from the field notes is a good illustration of the 'linguistic turn' of the business community (Thrift, 2005). The manager uses metaphors like 'narrative organization' and 'nomadic organization', which are familiar also from academic texts. Ironically, the manager describes their organization as a story-telling organization in a context where she tells me not to share a piece of information with the employees. Soon afterwards, she shares a story of a woman who wishes to keep a picture of her dog on her desk. A story that I interpreted as potentially not true but rather a narrative that tries to make a point more visible by exaggerating certain features. These narratives allow the managers to exaggerate some features to the point of absurdity. The stories of the pictures of loved ones and ridiculously old, dusty and heavy piles of paper construct the women employees as infantile and the situations as somehow hilarious, yet in conflict with the new culture of fun.

The office premises in both organizations included a lot of open space and many glass walls, and that made some employees more reluctant to talk to me. 'If I criticize the new order, I'll get the chop,' commented one employee with whom I ended up talking in a storeroom among old furniture and partition screens. In this shadowy room, we were able to talk peacefully in a safe place. Thus, sometimes, the 'hidden injuries' (Sennett, 1972) were very concretely hidden, but taking part in the research was clearly an effort to preserve some sense of dignity. Many of those who took part highlighted that it was important for their story to be told.

Conclusions

I do not want to deny the possibility that a fun organizational culture could exist. I am also prepared to entertain the idea that fun could be consciously created and organized. However, as Fleming (2005) notes, the organizational fun culture needs to be rethought in terms of dignity, democracy and respect. The fun culture I encountered reminded me of situations where parents want their children to play with children their children do not particularly want to play with. As a child, I realized that parents thought that play was the same for every child when in fact it meant so many different things for different children. 'You go and play with them *now*', my mother insisted when I tried to explain that I do not know how to play with them. I went and sometimes we eventually found a form of play that we understood in a similar fashion, but other times it did not work out. I think the possibility of creating a fun culture for adults would demand recognizing that fun still does not mean the same for everyone. To put it bluntly, one man's fun culture is another woman's #metoo campaign. Fun has to do with hierarchies, gender, age, ethnicity, sexuality and social class, and therefore, a uniform and single fun culture is an impossibility. Even in my ethnographic material, different kinds of fun cultures could be identified; those that legitimized and those that tried to resist the official fun culture.

This chapter has aimed to shed light on how new forms of office decoration and spatial planning connect with the therapeutic ethos that has brought emotions to the core of organizational culture. I have considered the activity-based office model as a form of 'therapeutic space' (Gorman, 2017a) and organized self-help (Boltanski & Chiapello, 2005) that offers material elements which try to shape happier, more mobile workers ready to network with new people while being more playful and positive. I have shown how the emphasis on positive emotions produces new forms of organizational control. The fun culture encourages subjects to find their 'inner child' and to free themselves. This invites the employees to a new landscape where they have to try to recognize and learn what that 'fun' actually means. The fun culture infantilizes the employees, and thus, they risk positioning themselves as childish. Once they have embraced their inner child, they have entered a place where they are potentially considered more innovative but have a more fragile position as they no longer have all the chips to gain a place in the adult world.

The new spaces of work may in some ways be more flexible, as promised, but they still produce social relations and power and renew old gender hierarchies (see also Salmenniemi et al. in this book). The fun culture emphasizes aesthetics and emotions, which are traditionally considered as belonging to the feminine sphere. However, the fun itself seems to invite more traditionally masculine fun practices and invites certain kinds of male bodies to enjoy the 'laid-back' chill-out areas. The rhetoric in official documents, in media texts and managers' stories is about increasing the freedom of employees. The freedom means that in the mornings you act like a 'private entrepreneur' who is forced to reflect on which space suits your mood best instead of just walking to your own space, to your own desk. This emotional culture invites subjectivities that define fleeting emotions and ambiances as essential to work but underestimate more long-term emotions.

References

Ackroyd, S. & P. Thompson. 1999. *Organizational Misbehavior*. London: Sage.

Adkins, L. 2005. The new economy, property and personhood. *Theory, Culture & Society* 22:1, 111–130.

Alexandersson, A. & V. Kalonaityte. 2018. Playing to dissent: The aesthetics and politics of playful office design. *Organisation Studies*, 39:2–3, 297–317.

Appel-Meulenbroek, R., Groenen, P. & Janssen, I. 2011. An end-user's perspective on activity-based office concepts. *Journal of Corporate Real Estate* 13:2, 122–135.

Baldry, C. & J. Hallier. 2010. Welcome to the house of fun: Work space and social identity. *Economic and Industrial Democracy* 31:1, 150–172.

Barnett, L. A. 2007. The nature of playfulness in young adults. *Personality and Individual Differences* 43:4, 949–958.

Billig, M., Condor, S., Edwards, D., Gane, M., Middleton, D., & Radley, A. 1988. *Ideological Dilemmas: A Social Psychology of Everyday Thinking*. Thousand Oaks, CA: Sage.

Boltanski, L. & E. Chiapello. 2005. The new spirit of capitalism. *International Journal of Politics, Culture, and Society* 18:3–4, 161–188.

Boltanski, L. & Chiapello, E. 2007. *The New Spirit of Capitalism*. London: Verso.

Carr, D. 1986. Narrative and the real world: An argument for continuity. *History and Theory* 25:2, 117–131.

Chugh, S. & Hancock, P. 2009. Networks of aestheticization: The architecture, artefacts and embodiment of hairdressing salons. *Work, Employment and Society 23*:3, 460–476.

Coates, J. 2007. Talk in a play frame: More on laughter and intimacy. *Journal of Pragmatics 39*:1, 29–49.

Costea, B., N. Crump & J. Holm. 2005. Dionysus at work? The ethos of play and the ethos of management. *Culture and Organisation 11*:2, 139–151.

Ehdotus valtion toimitilastrategiaksi. 2014. Valtion toimitilastrategian päivittämistyöryhmän muistio. [The Proposed Government Premises Strategy] Valtionvarainministeriön julkaisuja, February/2014, http://vm.fi/documents/10623/307565/Toimitilastrategia+ 2020/964fa234-3698-4b74-aadf 5c15aa6cdb4d.

Fine, G. A. & Corte, U. 2017. Group pleasures: Collaborative commitments, shared narrative, and the sociology of fun. *Sociological theory 35*:1, 64–86.

Fleming, P. 2005. Workers' playtime? Boundaries and cynicism in a 'culture of fun' program. *The Journal of Applied Behavioral Science 41*:3, 285–303.

Fredrickson, B. L. 1998. What good are positive emotions? *Review of General Psychology 2*:3, 300–319.

Fredrickson, B. L., R. A. Mancuso, C. Branigan & M. M. Tugade. 2000. The undoing effect of positive emotions. *Motivation and Emotion 24*:4, 237–258.

Foucault, M. 2003. Space, knowledge and power. In *Rethinking Architecture: A Reader in Cultural Theory*, edited by N. Leach. London: Routledge, 367–380.

Gill, R. 2002. Cool, creative and egalitarian? Exploring gender in project-based new media work in Euro. *Information, Communication & Society 5*:1, 70–89.

Gill, R. 2016. Post-postfeminism?: New feminist visibilities in postfeminist times. *Feminist Media Studies 16*:4, 610–630.

Glynn, M. A. & J. Webster. 1992. The adult playfulness scale: An initial assessment. *Psychological Reports 71*:1, 83–103.

Gorman, R. 2017a. Smelling therapeutic landscapes: Embodied encounters within spaces of care farming. *Health & Place 47*, 22–28.

Gorman, R. 2017b. Therapeutic landscapes and non-human animals: The roles and contested positions of animals within care farming assemblages. *Social & Cultural Geography 18*:3, 315–335.

Haapamäki ym. 2011. Käyttäjälähtöiset tilat. Helsinki: Tekes, December/2011. [User centered spaces] http://www.tekes.fi/globalassets/julkaisut/kayttajalahtoiset_tilat.pdf.

Heelas, P. 2002. Work ethics, soft capitalism and the turn to life. *Cultural Economy: Cultural Analysis and Commercial Life*, edited by P. Du Gay & M. Pryke. London, England: Sage, 78–96.

Huizinga, J. 1980. *Homo Ludens: A Study of the Play-Element in Culture*. London: Routledge and K Paul.

Illouz, E. 2007. *Cold Intimacies: The Making of Emotional Capitalism*. Cambridge: Polity Press.

Illouz, E. 2008. *Saving the Modern Soul: Therapy, Emotions, and the Culture of Self-Help*. Berkeley: University of California Press.

Kantola, A. 2014. Emotional styles of power: Corporation leaders in Finnish business media. *Media, Culture & Society 36*:5, 578–594.

Lefebvre, H. 2015. *The Production of Space*. Oxford: Blackwell.

Manka, M.-L. 2010. *Tiikerinloikka työniloon ja menestykseen*. Helsinki: Talentum.

Mulkay, M. J. 1988. *On Humor: Its Nature and Its Place in Modern Society*. Cambridge: Polity Press.

Müller, M. 2015. Assemblages and actor-networks: Rethinking socio-material power, politics and space. *Geography Compass 9*:1, 27–41.

Nenonen, S. & O. Niemi. 2013. Tilat ja työympäristö – näkökulmia monitilatoimistoon. [Spaces and workplaces – perspectives on the activity-based office] Rakennustieto. https://www.rakennustieto.fi/Downloads/RK/RK130302.pdf.

Nenonen, S., U. Hyrkkänen, H. Rasila, W. Hongisto, J. Keränen, H. Koskela & E. Sandberg. 2012. Monitilatoimisto. Ohjeita käyttöön ja suunnitteluun. [Activity-based office. User's and designer's manual] http://www.ttl.fi/fi/tutkimus/hankkeet/toti/Documents/monitilatoimiston_suunnitteluohje_toti_03092012.pdf.

Nilsen, A. P. 1994. In defense of humor. *College English 56*:8, 928–933.

Peteri, V. 2017. Bad enough ergonomics: A case study of an office chair. *SAGE Open 7*:1, 1–11.

Redman, T. & B. P. Mathews. 2002. Managing services: Should we be having fun? *Service Industries Journal 22*:3, 51–62.

Seligman, M. E., & Csikszentmihalyi, M. 2014. Positive psychology: An introduction. *Flow and the Foundations of Positive Psychology*, edited by M. Csikszentmihalyi & R. Larson. Dordrecht: Springer, 279–298.

Sennett, R. 1972. *The Hidden Injuries of Class*. New York: Alfred A Knopf Inc.

Soja, E. W. 1996. *Thirdspace. Journeys to Los Angeles and Other Real-and-Imagined Places*. Cambridge, MA: Blackwell.

Swan, E. 2008. 'You make me feel like a woman': Therapeutic cultures and the contagion of femininity. *Gender, Work & Organization 15*:1, 88–107.

Thrift, N. 2005. *Knowing Capitalism*. London: Sage.

Valtioneuvoston periaatepäätös valtion toimitilastrategiaksi. 2014. [The Government's Decision in Principle on Premises Strategy] http://vm.fi/documents/10623/307565/Valtioneuvoston+periaatep%C3%A4%C3%A4t%C3%B6s+valtion+toimitilastrategiaksi/0a92ff49-8d57-43fe-b49a-ae911c98b59d.

Watson, C. 2015. A sociologist walks into a bar (and other academic challenges): Towards a methodology of humour. *Sociology 49*:3, 407–421.

Zimmerman, E. 2015. Manifesto for a ludic century. *The Gameful World: Approaches, Issues, Applications*, edited by S. P. Walz & S. Deterding. Cambridge, MA: MIT Press, 19–22.

10 'Living on a razor blade'

Work and alienation in the narratives of therapeutic engagements

*Suvi Salmenniemi, Johanna Nurmi
and Joni Jaakola*

[T]he contemporary psychological discourse summons the individual to a highly autonomous task of psychological self-optimization within a distinctively individualistic therapeutic regime. In short, this is a vision of psychological life as enterprise, one centred on the individual pursuit of well-being as one of calculating self-interest, and a project of repudiation centered on the inherited dependencies of social government.

(Binkley, 2011: 94)

The available cultural scripts, such as 'self-help' discourse, reinforce the messages of self-reliance and personal responsibility that are deeply rooted in the trials of individual experience, and hence serve as a therapeutic ethos that hides real economic and social failure and disappointment behind a projected fantasy of individual self-reliance through careful emotional self-management.

(Foster, 2016: 112)

As in the quotations above, much of the literature on therapeutic culture and neoliberalism suggests that therapeutic knowledges and practices have been successfully harnessed to serve neoliberal projects seeking to cultivate self-governing, enterprising and self-reliant subjects (Cloud, 1998; Madsen, 2014; Ouellette & Hay, 2008; Salmenniemi & Adamson, 2015). Therapeutic techniques are argued to operate as powerful instruments to manage subjectivity across social domains, casting structural issues of power as individual psychopathologies, and thus masking and legitimising capitalist exploitation (Foster, 2015). While this interpretation undoubtedly captures important dimensions of therapeutics in neoliberalism, this chapter suggests that the relationship between the two may be more complex. Drawing on fieldwork among practitioners of alternative therapeutic practices in Finland, we argue that rather than being directed merely towards strategic self-optimisation and entrepreneurial self-management, therapeutic practices may also be mobilised to critique, contest and disengage from the destructive and exploitative effects of neoliberalism. Thus, they are neither inevitably nor necessarily allied with neoliberalism, but may have different effects and functions depending on the assemblage they become part of. They can be assembled both to reinforce regulation of subjectivity for the capitalist production of value (Davies, 2015; Mäkinen, 2014; Ehrenreich, 2009; Peteri in this book) and to foster resistance to alienating and dehumanising aspects of neoliberal work.

Working life was not initially at the core of our research, but in the course of fieldwork we were alerted to its centrality in narratives of therapeutic engagements. Although we did come across a number of therapeutic training activities and practitioners preaching strategic self-management as a prerequisite for success, these were overshadowed by countless stories of work-related exhaustion, depression, burnout, disillusionment and disappointment. These stories articulated a deeply felt and embodied sense of contradiction between ideological interpellations and the lived realities of work. They invited us to delve more deeply into relationships between work, therapeutics and neoliberalism in our research materials. Accordingly, in this chapter we trace how working life is experienced and made sense of by therapeutic practitioners, and the meanings and functions acquired by therapeutic forms of knowledge and practice in this context. We suggest that the interview narratives convey a profound experience of alienation, articulated through the tropes of 'loss of the self' and 'refusal of subjectivity'. In dialogue with assemblage thinking, we show how the practitioners seek to contest and alleviate this alienation by assembling a package of therapeutic self-care practices with which to distance and disengage themselves from the ethic of constant performance and efficiency and the valorisation of waged work. We approach such therapeutic assemblages as a generative force (Newman, 2017: 89) and a form of everyday resistance (Scott, 1989), organised not as publicly visible contestation, but rather as individualised and small-scale acts of non-compliance and subversion in the everyday.

Whereas much previous research has focused on tracing dominant interpellations of therapeutic discourse and how it operates as an oppressive ideology or a form of governmentality (Furedi, 2004; Madsen, 2014; Cloud, 1998; Ouellette & Hay, 2008), this chapter zooms in on the lived experience of therapeutic practices. Echoing Illouz's (2008: 18) call for studies of 'what people actually *do* with certain forms of knowledge' and what these knowledges are 'good for', we explore how therapeutic practices are assembled and mobilised to tackle the experience of alienation. Our analysis draws on materials gathered from an ethnographic study among practitioners of popular self-help psychology, complementary and alternative medicine and new spiritualities in various parts of Finland, conducted by the first author, Suvi, between 2015 and 2017. The fieldwork was informed by a multi-sited fieldwork methodology, with the central principle of 'following' as a mode for defining the objects of study (Marcus, 1998: 84). The research circulated across diverse sites of the therapeutic field, following the participants and the types of practices they were engaged in, as well as metaphors and storylines, such as belief in the power of thought and interconnections between body, mind and spirit.

In this chapter, we draw on interviews with 32 research participants who were professional healers or practised therapeutic activities as part of their everyday lives, as well as materials from participant observations of therapeutic events (fairs, training sessions, workshops, lectures, etc.). The interviews mapped practitioners' life stories, as well as their experiences of therapeutic engagements and the meanings attached to them. The overwhelming majority of the research participants (29) were women. This reflects the overall gender profile of the therapeutic field, which continues to be femininely marked and utilised by women more than men (Swan, 2008; Sointu, 2013). The participants ranged in age from their early thirties to their seventies. Only six had a university education, while the others had intermediate or little formal education. Sixteen worked either full-time or part-time as professional healers or therapists. The rest worked in some form of care work or office work, or as teachers, HR managers, salespeople, bookkeepers, entrepreneurs or school assistants, or were unemployed, on pensions or studying. In our analysis, we focus on the interview narratives, with ethnographic observations providing crucial contextual sensitivity for the interpretative work.

In what follows, we first discuss the connections between therapeutics and neoliberalism and the role of therapeutic practices in the workplace. We then explore experiences of alienation in the workplace, followed by an examination of how therapeutic assemblages may be mobilised to contest the destructive effects of work. The concluding section suggests that therapeutic assemblages open up a horizon of hope by creating a space to voice the hidden injuries of neoliberal capitalism and envisage alternative ways of being in and connecting with the world.

The therapeutic spirit of capitalism

Previous research has highlighted the seminal role played by the therapeutic discourse in the historical development and transformation of capitalism (Rose, 1990; McGee, 2005; Madsen, 2014; Illouz, 2008). It has been suggested that the therapeutic discourse has served as an instrument of class power by legitimating capitalist oppression, inhibiting political dissent and turning structural issues into individual psychopathologies to be remedied by commodified self-improvement regimes (MacNevin, 2003; Cloud, 1998). In particular, therapeutic knowledges and practices have been seen as being intimately entangled with neoliberal governing projects promoting a politics of self, whereby work on the self is normalised and posited as an ethical duty (Rimke, 2000; Ouellette & Hay, 2008; Foster, 2016; Salmenniemi & Adamson, 2015). According to Foster (2015), therapeutic and neoliberal discourses converge around the key categories of autonomy, personal growth, self-reliance and self-regulation, hailing individuals to understand themselves as objects of investment and repositories of capital geared to maximising material success and personal happiness (Salmenniemi, 2017). Neoliberalism emphasises the capacity to make enterprising choices and maximise one's interests as a condition of self-rule, and commodified regimes of self-improvement, self-help and life management have emerged to respond to this demand in the context of diminishing state provision of social protection (Ouellette & Hay, 2008: 476). Here, the self becomes a project that is permanently 'under construction', entangled in a never-ending project of optimising bodily and psychic dispositions (see also Bergroth and Helén in this book).

Boltanski and Chiapello's (2005) historical study tracing ideological changes in capitalism is an important theoretical contribution for making sense of this fusion of the therapeutic with neoliberalism. They argue that the legitimation narrative underpinning the capitalist system was forcefully questioned during the 1960s and 1970s, not only through traditional social critique of the labour movement, but also through what they call 'artistic' critique. This critique targets the dehumanising aspects of capitalism and criticises it for conformism, hierarchy, and the destruction of creativity, individuality and authenticity. The linking of work with self-realisation channelled the countercultural value of self-fulfilment into the workplace (McGee, 2005: 112); as Boltanski and Chiapello (2005) argue, the capitalist system assimilated the artistic and countercultural critique and turned it into a key ingredient of its new legitimation narrative. Thus, critique of capitalism was harnessed to engender a 'new spirit of capitalism', centred around the idea of work as a source of pleasure and self-realisation. According to Foster (2015), this new spirit was then imbued with intrinsically individualistic categories of psychology, offering instruments for an ever-deeper colonisation of subjectivity for the capitalist production of value. This new spirit of capitalism was accompanied by a profound reorganisation of work structures, giving rise to the process of precarisation and more flexible and insecure work (Boltanski & Chiapello, 2005).

Although 'psy' technologies have long been instrumental in the organisation of work (see Illouz, 2008), the new spirit of capitalism has paved the way for their increasing utilisation in regulating worker subjectivities (see Peteri in this book). Therapeutic practices are mobilised to make workers more productive, committed and 'resilient' (Swan, 2010), and to incite them to learn to draw pleasure from this. Workers are invited to apprehend all work as fulfilling and enjoyable and develop a positive attitude towards work. This is connected with a broader trend towards individualisation and subjectification of work, where the focus has shifted from structural conditions to individual capacities to manage work, and where subjectivity as a whole is harnessed for the production of value (Julkunen, 2008; Mäkinen, 2014). At the intersection of the individualisation of work and therapeutic culture, problems and conflicts in work tend to morph from structural problems relating to work organisation and resources into individual psychological issues to be remedied by ethical work on the self. Thus, therapeutic practices such as meditation, mindfulness, motivational seminars and yoga have been introduced into workplaces as a way to foster enthusiasm for work, improve workers' performance and help them deal with the pressures of work (Davies, 2015; Peteri in this book).

Neoliberal capitalism, with its new therapeutic spirit, has also given rise to new modalities of alienation. Rosa (2015a: 93) has called for the revival of the concept of alienation in sociology as a 'general term describing subjects' dysfunctional relation to the world'. He identifies self-estrangement from one's body, desires or personal beliefs as an important dimension of alienation. In a similar vein, Browne (2017) has developed the concept of alienation to capture the dynamics in which subjective involvement and self-realisation are promoted, yet at the same time refused and turned into instruments of normalising and disciplining power. According to Browne, alienation involves:

> ...the thwarted participation of individuals and experiences that are destructive of subjectivity. Individuals' experiences and interpretations of compelled, but limited, action expose the contradiction between institutions' normative representations and the structural conditions of their reproduction.
>
> (Browne, 2017: 61)

We suggest that the experiences of work-related suffering articulated in our research material can be productively interpreted through the concept of alienation. As Browne (2017: 80) and Rosa (2015a, b) suggest, central to the concept of alienation is damage to subjectivity, which finds expression in affective states such as dissatisfaction, frustration, burnout and depression. This resonates with Rikala's (2016) argument that increasing individualisation of the structural contradictions of work results in individual bodies and minds being turned into crucial battlefields in which the contradictions of capitalism are confronted and felt. The concept of alienation is also helpful since it underscores the centrality of the 'hidden injuries' of capitalism: the hidden weights, anxieties and feelings of inadequate control (Sennett & Cobb, 1972: 33). Our analysis foregrounds how therapeutic practices may provide a space and language through which to voice and make sense of these injuries. However, it is important to note that alienation engenders not only suffering and frustration, but also forms of resistance (Browne, 2017). Among our research participants, this resistance manifested itself in attempts to cultivate forms of life that were not entirely conducive to or subsumed to neoliberal capitalist logic (Lilja & Vinthagen, 2014).

The unbearable weight of work

Taking our cue from these ideas, we can now flesh out how alienation is articulated in our research materials. In both the interviews and the therapeutic events Suvi attended during her fieldwork, she heard many stories of neoliberal work life causing exhaustion, depression and stress. Many spoke of having felt 'completely exhausted', 'totally broken' and 'really on the bottom'. Most often, such experiences of psychic and physical overload were referred to as 'burnout'. Nearly half of the research participants had had personal experiences of burnout, and almost all the professional therapists identified burnout as a crucial reason why clients come to see them. As Rosa (2015b: 296) suggests, burnout can be seen as 'an extreme form of alienation' in which 'the world faces the subject in a rigid, harsh, cold and silent form'. Burnout generally has a distinctively gendered profile, particularly affecting women and female-dominated sectors of the labour market (Rikala, 2013).

Many of our research participants problematised the valorisation of waged work as a measure of human worth, which makes losing a job ever more threatening and makes those out of work feel worthless. The vocabularies through which they talked about working life were often quite violent. For example, Nora, who had been in a supervisory position in a large company before embarking on a career as an alternative therapist, saw in her therapy practice how people were living 'on a razor blade' with a 'constant threat of being made redundant' and that many were 'on a final burnout edge'. Pia, a politically active practitioner of meditation, echoed this in lamenting how people were forced to 'push forward at full speed and just deliver, deliver, deliver'; while Elina, a life coach in her forties, described how people were 'whipped' to make profit for companies. Tom, leading a firm offering self-improvement classes, thought that heightened demands in the workplace had resulted in growing numbers of burnouts so that people had to be regularly 'rebooted'. Maria, an alternative therapist in her forties, contemplated this as follows:

> Work life keeps spinning around quicker and quicker, and people are just catapulted from it, or they choose to leave the cogwheel voluntarily because they cannot take it anymore … Work life has become quite wretched in the sense that those who have work are just drudging so hard, and the demands are getting harder and harder all the time, you need to know and handle thousands of things, all of that at the same time. It's really stressful. And those who don't have work are stressed as well.

Similar mechanical metaphors recurred in the interviews, conveying an image of people being caught up in a Weberian 'iron cage' (Weber, 1958), or as spinning in a giant machine that also threatens to turn them into a machine, like a computer in need of 'rebooting'. There was a sense of constant forced movement: one must be on the move, out and about, running and spinning at the mercy of the machine, unable to control or influence it.

The experience of alienation that emerges from these accounts was articulated through two tropes. The first was 'loss of the self', which conveys a sense of losing touch with oneself and being estranged and disconnected from one's body. This was referred to, for example, as 'going blind' at work, not 'seeing' how tired one was and 'losing touch with who I am'. Many talked about burnout as something that 'crept in' slowly and unnoticed, making one neglect oneself. Sometimes it crept in through a heightened passion for and commitment to work, á la 'new spirit of capitalism'. This was the case for Salli, a thirty-something mother of a small baby who had trained as an angel therapist after experiencing serious burnout in her previous job as a youth worker, which she described as her vocation. She described herself as a workaholic whose work gradually took over everything in her life. As for many others, burnout appeared for her as a 'rupture':

> My physical condition collapsed, I was ill all the time and was just crying at home. Work did not give any satisfaction anymore. And I somehow realised that my relationship with work is not healthy, that I want something else in my life than just work. I want peace, I want to feel calmer and more balanced,

I want to laugh and not cry all the time. [...] I liked my work enormously, I did it for a long time. [...] but at the expense of myself. [...] Well, when your body collapses, you are forced to stop and think.

Like Salli, many research participants problematised the imperative of constant performance as 'sick', not allowing them to 'stop, rest and recuperate'. They also viewed this imperative as being amplified by a specific Finnish work ethic idealising hard work and self-sacrifice as a source of moral reward (Kortteinen, 1991; Kettunen, 2008). This articulation was challenged, for example, by Linda, an angel therapist and yoga instructor in her thirties. She felt that the Finnish work ethic was effectively harnessed to support the increasing acceleration of working life, leading to self-estrangement.

If we think about the pressures in working life, how hectic it is, so now in economic crisis people are made redundant and others have twice as much work as before. The pressure is high, and with our sense of always managing no matter what, we always try to do our best. We over-perform which means that we are soon burnt out. [...] But demands are rising all the time and we just give more all the time, show that we can do it even better and better, and we just do not stop for a moment to ask ourselves what it is that we really want or what our body is telling us.

Therapeutic practices were thus narrated as promising to deliver that which neo-liberal working life refuses to: an opportunity to slow down the movement, halt the spin, turn off the machine.

Paula, a longstanding work–life coach and energy healer in her fifties, questioned the neoliberal spirit of capitalism centred around self-governance, flexibility and autonomy. In her view, it had turned into an oppressive imperative that constantly demanded one to be more but led to a sense that nothing was ever enough. Interpellations of self-governance led to the loss of one's sense of self. As with the machine metaphors above, there was a sense of being caught in an 'iron cage':

First, there's no working time any more, in the sense of from eight to four or something like that. [...] The more creative the field you are in, or the higher in the hierarchy you go, the meaning of working time decreases. And in many workplaces you have to be self-governing. [...] It's in principle a very fine phenomenon, but I wonder if people are always really ready for that. [...]. It's an ideal, you know; we admire people who travel and are self-governing. [...] And we think that gee, what a dream job, she has a car, phone, computer and all, Burberry scarf round her neck and everything. Wow. But at the end of the day, I think many of them are lost with their work. They just simply don't get rid of their role, they don't get away from work, because they are working and self-governing all the time. There's no-one to say that 'Hey, now you can slow down, you don't need to do more'. [...] When you don't have working time, when you constantly meet new people. [...] well, then you don't neces-sarily know who you are any more. [...] Well, you really need to halt, simply because there's no one telling you anymore that your work day is over.

The second trope through which experiences of alienation were articulated was 'refusal of subjectivity', stemming from an inability to influence one's work con-ditions and a sense of being refused as a person. As discussed above, in contempo-rary working life, people are incited to invest in work and apprehend it as a source of pleasure and self-realisation; yet the narratives of work in our study repeatedly emphasised the imperatives of unconditional obedience, docility and disciplining power over personality. Many of our research participants had actively voiced problems and criticisms in their workplaces, some even in their capacity as trade union representatives, and had tried to negotiate their workloads and work organi-sation (for similar observations, see Rikala, 2016). They had sought institutional support from health and safety departments or had contacted occupational health staff to deal with their situation, but to no avail. These experiences of not being heard or allowed to express work-related discontent had often been instrumental in leading to burnout.

We illustrate this with three cases. Our first case is Tiina, a middle-aged woman who was employed in university administration for decades and had a history as a shop steward in her workplace. She had gone through a severe burnout involv-ing a period of hospitalisation in a psychiatric ward. She recounted how work had 'swallowed her completely' and 'expanded everywhere', as she was constantly checking her emails and answering phone calls after the workday had finished. Moreover, her workplace had been in a cycle of constant reorganisation, which meant that her tasks had been both changing and increasing all the time. She recounted how her autonomy at work had gradually diminished, which she felt was 'cutting off my fingers one after another'. She contemplated with a sense of disbelief how her workplace had turned from an organisation emphasising criti-cal thinking into one where 'you are no longer allowed to question or criticise, you just have to perform as you are told'. She vociferously problematised what she saw as increasing demands for obedience and 'blind submission' to work: 'Everyone should just be like the managers proclaim. They proclaim that if you're not capable of coping with the change, or if you don't accept the change, then you are automatically somehow a worse person.' Thus, Tiina felt that the structural problems at work had translated into her being dismissed as a person.

Julia, another middle-aged woman, had gone through burnout and had also served as a shop steward in her workplace. She worked in a security company and had experienced serious workplace bullying after voicing her dissatisfaction with the way the organisation was led. She felt that people were nowadays expected to 'work like robots', 'just perform and have no opinions' and 'simply obey those who have power'. Like Tiina, she had a strong sense of having been refused as a person in her workplace: 'I was not accepted in my community as a person'. This expression conveyed a strong personal sense of exclusion on the basis of subjectivity. Julia's criticism had been labelled by the leadership as 'grumbling' and 'negativity'. She described how the situation at work 'drove her to the edge of madness', which she managed to avoid by starting to read spiritual self-help books and writing down her feelings. Reading and writing had led her to a 'spiritual path' that allowed her to 'care for herself' and gave her moral strength. Unlike Tiina, Julia had stayed in her workplace as a form of resistance:

> They tried to oust me out of my job, but I decided that I'm not going away as I haven't done anything wrong. If I had gone then, I feel I would have somehow been accepting all the things that they accused me of … So, I found spirituality in my life through this kind of hell.

Our last example comes from Carita, a single mother in her forties, working in a facility for the disabled. She was suffering from prolonged ethical strain in her work. As a result of workplace bullying, lack of resources and her own precarious position as a temp, she felt she was unable to work according to her own values, but had to treat her clients in a way that she experienced as humiliating. At the time of the interview, she said she was depressed and was thinking of changing jobs. She felt dismissed and denied as a person, having to 'squeeze herself' into a mould into which she could not fit. Crucial to her sense of alienation was a clash between her enthusiasm for work and its refusal by her workplace:

> I'm the kind of person who gets excited about everything and I want to be involved, would like to develop and do things. I'm a cheerful and enthusiastic person, so I'm annoyed that I just have to keep my mouth shut and keep my thoughts to myself [at work]. I have to diminish and reduce myself there.

In her interview, she contemplated at length how a women's therapeutic self-help group that she was attending at the time of the interview had provided her with a 'new language' to make sense of her situation. The group had allowed her to apprehend her problems as stemming from power dynamics in the workplace rather than from herself, allowing her to turn her self-blame into critique against injustice experienced at work:

> They can't treat me however they like, tell me whatever they like. Before, I used to withdraw into myself and get depressed, filed for sick leave because I felt too distressed. I'm quite distressed also now. I would like not to go to my work anymore, 'cos I'm nobody there. I feel I'm not appreciated. It's so demeaning. And I think my co-workers won't change even if I change. My thinking is becoming better, and my self-esteem as well, but my co-workers will probably stay the same. They will treat me bad even if I were to change and try to defend myself. I think there's even more resistance and they slate me even more now that I try to voice my opinions. Before, I used to withdraw into myself and scold myself, but now I see that it's not necessarily my fault, that the problems do not stem from me.

The psychological discourse learnt in the self-help group had allowed Carita to see her work from a new angle and formulate criticism of the power relations at work in her organisation. Rather than individualising and psychologising problems at work, the self-help group had helped her to turn the blame away from herself and towards the work organisation. However, as the quote above reveals, she was well aware of the limits of self-transformation as a solution to workplace conflict.

These three examples illustrate how therapeutic practices had allowed the research participants to make sense of their burnout as socially produced, stemming from poor leadership and organisation of work, destructive culture and lack of necessary resources. These narratives are striking, as they reveal a deep contradiction between the neoliberal 'new spirit of capitalism' kinds of interpellation promising flexibility, self-realisation and autonomy, and the experienced realities of work 'on the ground', where work is seen as characterised by stern discipline and demands for conformism, obedience and subordination – the same characteristics that the 'new spirit of capitalism' was supposed to do away with (Boltanski & Chiapello, 2005). This contradiction leads to a deeply felt sense of alienation. In what follows, we discuss how the assembling of therapeutic packages of self-care operates as a way to try to alleviate alienation and escape the grip of neoliberal working life.

Getting out and getting away

All of our research participants were engaged in a host of therapeutic self-care practices through which they attempted to negotiate the destructive effects of working life. By assembling personalised self-care packages, they sought to refuse the norm of ever-performing and productive workers. These self-care assemblages consisted of a range of therapeutic practices (e.g. mindfulness, reiki, life coaching, angel therapy, yoga, art therapy, folk healing, Rosen therapy, acupuncture, reflexology), forms of knowledge (e.g. brain research, popular psychology, Eastern philosophies, religious bodies of thought) and objects (e.g. herbal medicine tablets, tarot cards, angel cards, crystals, flowers). In many cases, dancing, painting, photography, listening to music and writing poetry were also part of the therapeutic assemblage, as well as a range of lifestyle practices, such as following particular diets (e.g. functional nutrition, vegetarianism/veganism or consuming only organic food), ethical consumption, selective or outright refusal of vaccination, voluntary simplicity and efforts to protect the environment in the everyday.

These self-care assemblages were shifting and changing and were subject to constant labour. Many participants talked about 'roaming around in trainings', constantly plugging new practices into their personalised packages and dropping others that did not help or had served their purpose. They voiced a hunger for spiritual, alternative medical and psychological knowledge, and spoke of how they 'gobbled up' information from various sources, fitting elements of these into their therapeutic package. This process also engendered communities and new forms of sociality.

For our research participants, therapeutic self-care assemblages were not about strategic optimisation and maximisation of the self, but rather about making life more bearable under the conditions of neoliberal capitalism (see also Swan, 2008). Many had made futile efforts to influence the structures of work, so cultivating alternative dispositions and values by assembling personalised self-care packages had resulted in a more feasible strategy of resistance and survival. With these packages, they sought to harness their little remaining energy and agency to implement changes that were deemed possible 'here and now' and to try to 'unlearn' the performance imperative. For example, Tiina, whom we introduced in the previous section, had assembled a package of therapeutic practices that included psychotherapy, antidepressants, Rosen therapy, bible reading, swimming, energy healing, angel healing, psychological reflexology, yoga, goal-mapping and a women's self-care group. She certainly did not employ these practices as a way to accrue value for herself, nor to rehabilitate herself and return to the 'rat race', but rather as a way to drag herself back to life and understand what had happened to her and why. As she put it, she had 'stepped out of the river' and was contemplating whether to return to work and under what conditions.

While Tiina's therapeutic assemblage involved antidepressants and psychotherapy, many interviewees had turned to alternative therapies following disappointment with licensed psychologists and psychiatrists. For example, Katarina, an alternative therapist in her fifties who had gone through a period of depression, felt that a psychologist in a municipal mental health clinic had not given her 'a single tool with which to work on my feelings'. Although publicly-funded rehabilitative psychotherapy is available in Finland for those who can prove that their ability to work or study is impaired by mental health problems, alternative therapies appeared to many participants to be more accessible than official ones, since the latter often suffer from long queues and are unevenly accessible in different parts of the country. Moreover, the purpose of publicly funded therapy is to help people 'remain economically active, or enter or return to working life' (Kela, 2018) – the very idea against which many of our participants were protesting. For many, alternative therapies also appeared more appealing as they were seen as offering a more inclusive frame for making sense of themselves and their lives, allowing the incorporation of spiritual and religious aspects of self-care practices.

Quite often, a preference for alternative therapeutic practices also arose from critique of the medicalisation and pharmaceuticalization of mental health, which was seen as contributing to the exploitative character of neoliberal work life. The research participants felt that medication was being used to erase the suffering caused by the structural organisation of work. Rather than tackling the underlying causes, doctors were seen as prescribing medication to minimise worker absence, making them complicit in reinforcing the market logic and commodifying health. Thus, medicalisation was seen as providing the oil crucial to keeping the neoliberal mills spinning. As Lena, a life coaching client, sighed: 'I feel that in the pressures of this performance society, pills get emphasised. But I think that just giving you pills and sending you home doesn't constitute proper care. ... I think we should treat the cause, not the effect'. Aino, an alternative therapist in her fifties, thought that one should not just:

> ...work long days, stress out and try to manage everything by yourself. And when you're feeling really bad and your heart is beating like hell and you have high blood pressure and all sorts of things, you go and see the doctor, get the pills, throw a couple of them in your mouth and just continue as if nothing has happened. Well, it doesn't work that way. You need to start asking yourself why you can't sleep, what is it that is weighing on your mind so much that you can't calm down and have a normal sleep rhythm?

Thus, the research participants saw the logic of maximisation of labour productivity as underlying the structural causes of illness. They took issue with the normative ideal of the high-performing worker always being forced to get back in the saddle as quickly as possible with the help of medication. Many talked about the importance of rest, slowing down, meditation and self-reflection as meaningful alternative ways of caring for the self. While the official healthcare system was seen as merely treating symptoms, alternative therapies were seen as allowing exploration of the underlying causes. Although not solving the structural problems as such, alternative therapies at least provided ethical validation and recognition of the experience of alienation and suffering (see also Sointu, 2013), as well as tools with which to care for the self so that the destructive side of work could be kept somewhat at bay.

As we have highlighted above, while some research participants assembled therapeutic packages of self-care as a way to 'escape the system without leaving it' (De Certeau, 1984: xiii), or in other words as a way to forge a new relationship with work that would be less alienating, others mobilised such packages to sign off from waged work altogether. During fieldwork, and especially during angel evenings, Suvi came across women in their thirties and forties who had left their secure jobs to embark on 'a spiritual path'. They felt that their previous careers had been in conflict with 'who they really were' and they wished to live 'true' to their newly discovered spiritual ideals. Some were living on social assistance; others were doing occasional odd jobs or receiving economic support from their spouses or families. Some of these women told they were frustrated about constantly having to explain themselves to other people and institutions since they were not living a 'normal biography' centred around waged work.

For example, Rosa, who at the time of the interview had been out of work for three years, was in her thirties and was living with her partner in a major Finnish city. She narrated her life as one of constant 'searching'. Over the years, she had gradually moved towards a deeper involvement with angel healing and Ayurveda, leading her to quit her job in sales. At first, she had tried to continue her work part-time, but said that 'I developed such a strong resistance to it [work] and I felt so awful all the time so I couldn't overlook it'. For her, work appeared incompatible with her new, more spiritually devoted self. She said that her disengagement had been inevitable: 'I had no other choice'. For her, therapeutic practices were a way to realise herself and her values, but she felt that they were in conflict with prevailing social norms which emphasise the need to 'do as others do and run in the rat race'. We suggest that dropping out of waged work, facilitated by therapeutic engagements, can be understood as a form of resistance to the work-centred ethic of neoliberalism. Although our research participants did not articulate this as a conscious political strategy, their non-compliance with the expectation of waged work resonates with autonomous Marxist ideas emphasising refusal of work as a crucial way to protest against capitalism (Weeks, 2011).

Although Rosa was hesitant about becoming a spiritual therapist and establishing her own practice, many others had done so and become professional healers as a strategy to escape the alienation experienced in waged work. For example, Diana, a single mother with a school-aged child, had gone through a burnout and what she called a 'semi-depression' ten years earlier. Like many others, she had first sought help from occupational health services, but had been disappointed as 'they just gave me tissues and that's it'. She had subsequently turned to angel spiritualities and trained as an angel therapist. She had decided to drop out of her job in fashion and devote herself to healing work, as dropping out had become the only obvious option. Like Rosa, she tried at first to continue working, but at a slower pace; however, she soon realised that this was impossible because she felt that she was always being 'drawn back' into the hectic rhythm. Although she had been 'terrified' about leaving her job, she had decided to do so with the conviction that 'I will always survive somehow'. Indeed, for many, the decision to drop out of working life had entailed economic insecurity, living on social assistance or a lifestyle of voluntary simplicity. The economic disadvantages were less consequential than the need to 'be true to oneself' and live according to one's ethical values. Interestingly, entrepreneurship, an emblematic practice of neoliberalism, was represented here as an opportunity to escape the grip of neoliberal structures of work.

However, although becoming professional healers and establishing practices had served for some as a way to escape waged work, many faced exactly the same pressures as entrepreneurs, struggling to keep their practices productive and manage financial uncertainty. Mia's case is illustrative in this regard. At the time of the interview, she was in her thirties and had been an entrepreneur for a couple of years. Trained as an engineer and working in a big company, she had never had an interest in anything spiritual or therapeutic. This changed when she developed an anxiety and panic syndrome as a result of prolonged work stress. In her interview, she spoke of how:

> …one day my mind just collapsed. I was just crying and trembling all the time. … I was on sick leave for a while, I just couldn't go back to work. I was so terribly tired …. I was just sleeping for two years, twelve hours a day. Then I just decided that I needed to get out of that workplace.

After quitting her job, she had trained as a relaxation instructor and established her own practice. However, although this was meant to allow her to 'get away' from stressful work, constant financial problems and running her business on her own had worn her down. The practice that was supposed to liberate her from the iron cage gradually became another cage in a new disguise. She had another burnout and decided to close her practice. While some of our research participants were quite successful and content as entrepreneurs, many shared stories of economic precarity and difficulties in making ends meet through therapeutic work. Some had had to take part-time jobs, while others were confined to living with fewer resources. Some had been able to pursue therapeutic work thanks to financial support from their spouses.

Mia's interview also reveals an important tension in therapeutic entrepreneurship. Although she acknowledged the ethic of constant performance as being destructive to subjectivity and wished to avoid it in her own practice, she nevertheless relied on it when selling her therapeutic practices to companies. She talked about devising 'before and after' measurements of stress hormones as part of her meditation programme package in order to 'prove' to companies that meditation brings real benefits. Like many other research participants, she had tried to distance herself from the logic of performance, yet she was constantly pulled back to it in trying to make a living. Her predicament illustrates the intimate entanglement of resistance with the very power that it seeks to undermine.

Therapeutic assemblages and hope

This chapter has explored what it feels like to live and work under neoliberal demands for competition, productivity and performance. While therapeutic practitioners are often presented, implicitly or explicitly, as strategic self-managing subjects buying into the ethos of neoliberalism, we have sought to complicate this interpretation by showing how therapeutic assemblages may also enable and initiate contestation of the neoliberal ethic of work and its destructive effects on subjectivity. The narratives of work analysed here portray how neoliberal capitalism and its alienating effects are lived and confronted at the intimate level of subjectivity. They highlight that therapeutic practices need not automatically and seamlessly coalesce with neoliberal governing projects, but may also be used to disengage from them. Therapeutic practices may thus be 'radical in some ways and reactionary in others' (Swan, 2010: 11) and may also be translated into a form of political critique.

In assembling personalised therapeutic self-care packages, our research participants sought to renegotiate their relationships with work and express moral resistance to neoliberalism and its hidden injuries. They used these therapeutic assemblages to drag themselves back to life from the murky waters of burnout, not to rehabilitate themselves back into work and performance but to carve out possibilities for something different. This chapter highlights the complexities involved in negotiating one's relationship to work and oneself: research participants contest the dominant interpellations of neoliberal working life and seek to escape its disciplining grip with therapeutic assemblages; yet these assemblages may also draw them back into its grip in the form of exhaustion as a professional healer. This chapter also shows that while resistance tends to take the form of individualised politics, it also incorporates an aspiration for social change, as many perceived the individualised tactics, should more people adopt them, as potentially contributing to transforming the broader social formation (cf. Haenfler et al., 2012).

The interview narratives bring forth another subject from the shadow of the self-optimising subject: a fragile and exhausted subject struggling to rid herself of the alienating forces of neoliberalism. Articulation of this subject position may in itself be seen as a subversive act, destabilising the normative ideal of a heroic, self-improving and productive subject, and revealing what lies in its shadow. Therapeutic assemblages emerged as vehicles of everyday resistance, allowing things to be done 'against the grain' and expressing discontent and suffering. Seeing and acknowledging these practices as forms of resistance, or as processes that can bring about changes regardless of whether or not the actors intended them as political resistance (see Ortner, 2006: 44–45), also helps us understand what made these practices meaningful and transformative for our participants. Although many were seeking to change their lives through ethical work on the self, they nevertheless acknowledged and alluded to structural changes. Indeed, therapeutic engagements had often allowed them to understand their condition as socially produced rather than as an individual pathology.

Neoliberal individualising power in work tends to block collective resistance; therefore, as our research subjects' experiences testify, effecting structural changes at work can be far from easy. In this situation, assembling personalised packages of self-care emerges as an accessible tool to try to disengage from the alienating forces of work and envisage alternative ways of being in and connecting with the world. For many, these packages appeared as an antidote to a sense of getting stuck in the oppressive iron cage. This helps to highlight why therapeutic practices can be experienced as appealing and empowering: they can craft hope and a sense of agency under difficult life circumstances and offer resources to envisage and implement life projects irreducible to the neoliberal logic (see also Swan, 2008: 104). They convey a sense that something can be done 'here and now', and that everything is not lost. To paraphrase Sara Ahmed (2017: 2, 47), therapeutic engagements may offer hope that 'carries us through when the terrain is difficult' and helps to sustain a belief that 'the paths we follow will get us somewhere'.

Acknowledgements

The research for this chapter has been supported by the project *Tracking the Therapeutic: Ethnographies of Wellbeing, Politics and Inequality*, funded by the Academy of Finland (grant number 289004). Many thanks to the contributors of this book for helpful comments and suggestions.

References

Ahmed, S. 2017. *Living a Feminist Life*. Durham, NC: Duke University Press.
Binkley, S. 2011. Psychological Life as Enterprise: Social Practice and the Government of Neo-Liberal Interiority. *History of the Human Sciences 24*:3, 83–102.

Boltanski, L. & Chiapello, E. 2005. *The New Spirit of Capitalism*. London: Verso.

Browne, C. 2017. *Critical Social Theory*. Thousand Oaks, CA: Sage.

Cloud, D. 1998. *Control and Consolation in American Culture and Politics: Rhetoric of Therapy*. Thousand Oaks, CA: Sage.

Davies, W. 2015. *The Happiness Industry*. London: Verso.

De Certeau, M. 1984. *The Practice of Everyday Life*. Berkeley, CA: University of California Press.

Ehrenreich, B. 2009. *Bright-Sided: How the Relentless Promotion of Positive Thinking Has Undermined America*. New York: Metropolitan Books.

Foster, R. 2015. The Therapeutic Spirit of Neoliberalism. *Political Theory 44*:1, 82–105.

Foster, R. 2016. Therapeutic Culture, Authenticity and Neoliberalism. *History of the Human Sciences 29*:1, 99–116.

Furedi, F. 2004. *Therapy Culture: Cultivating Vulnerability in an Uncertain Age*. London: Routledge.

Haenfler, R., Johnson, B. & Jones, E. 2012. Lifestyle Movements: Exploring the Intersection of Lifestyle and Social Movements. *Social Movement Studies 11*:1, 1–20.

Illouz, E. 2008. *Saving the Modern Soul: Therapy, Emotions, and the Culture of Self-Help*. Berkeley, CA: University of California Press.

Julkunen, R. 2008. *Uuden Työn Paradoksit: Keskusteluja 2000-Luvun Työprosess(e)ista*. Tampere: Vastapaino.

Kela. 2018. Rehabilitative Psychotherapy. Kela [website]. https://www.kela.fi/web/en/rehabilitative-psychotherapy (accessed 24 July 2018).

Kettunen, P. 2008. *Globalisaatio ja kansallinen me*. Tampere: Vastapaino.

Kortteinen, M. 1991. *Kunnian Kenttä: Suomalainen Palkkatyö Kulttuurisena Muotona*. Helsinki: Hanki ja jää.

Lilja, M. & Vinthagen, S. 2014. Sovereign Power, Disciplinary Power and Biopower: Resisting What Power with What Resistance? *Journal of Political Power 7*:1, 107–126.

MacNevin, A. 2003. Remaining Audible to the Self: Women and Holistic Health. *Atlantis 27*:2, 16–23.

McGee, M. 2005. *Self-Help, Inc.: Makeover Culture in American Life*. Oxford: Oxford University Press.

Madsen, O. J. 2014. *The Therapeutic Turn*. London: Routledge.

Mäkinen, K. 2014. The Individualization of Class: A Case of Working Life Coaching. *The Sociological Review 62*:4, 821–842.

Marcus, G. E. 1998. *Ethnography Through Thick and Thin*. Princeton, NJ: Princeton University Press.

Newman, J. 2017. The Politics of Expertise: Neoliberalism, Governance and the Practices of Politics. In *Assembling Neoliberalism*, edited by V. Higgins & W. Larner. New York: Palgrave, 87–105.

Ortner, S. B. 2006. *Anthropology and Social Theory: Culture, Power, and the Acting Subject*. Durham, NC: Duke University Press.

Ouellette, L. & Hay, J. 2008. Makeover Television, Governmentality and the Good Citizen. *Continuum 22*:4, 471–484.

Rikala, S. 2013. *Työssä Uupuvat Naiset ja Masennus*. Tampere: Acta Universitatis Tamperensis.

Rikala, S. 2016. Työuupumus ja Vastarinnan Mahdollisuudet. In *Ruumiillisuus ja Työelämä*, edited by J. Parviainen, T. Kinnunen & I. Kortelainen. Tampere: Vastapaino, 182–198.

Rimke, H. M. 2000. Governing Citizens through Self-Help Literature. *Cultural Studies 14*:1, 61–78.

Rosa, H. 2015a. Capitalism as a Spiral of Dynamisation: Sociology as Social Critique. In *Sociology, Capitalism, Critique*, written by K. Dörre, S. Lessenich and H. Rosa. London: Verso, 67–97.

Rosa, H. 2015b. Escalation: The Crisis of Dynamic Stabilisation and the Prospect of Resonance. In *Sociology, Capitalism, Critique*, written by K. Dörre, S. Lessenich and H. Rosa. London: Verso, 280–305.

Rose, N. 1990. *Governing the Soul: The Shaping of the Private Self*. London: Routledge.

Salmenniemi, S. 2017. 'We Can't Live without Beliefs': Self and Society in Therapeutic Engagements. *The Sociological Review 65*:4, 611–627.

Salmenniemi, S. & Adamson, M. 2015. New Heroines of Labour: Domesticating Postfeminism and Neoliberal Capitalism in Russia. *Sociology 49*:1, 88–105.

Scott, J. C. 1989. Everyday Forms of Resistance. *Copenhagen Papers 4*, 33–62.

Sennett, R. & Cobb, J. 1972. *The Hidden Injuries of Class*. Cambridge: Cambridge University Press.

Sointu, E. 2013. *Theorizing Complementary and Alternative Medicines: Wellbeing, Self, Gender, Class*. Basingstoke: Palgrave Macmillan.

Swan, E. 2008. 'You Make Me Feel Like a Woman': Therapeutic Cultures and the Contagion of Femininity. *Gender, Work and Organization 15*:1, 88–107.

Swan, E. 2010. *Worked Up Selves: Personal Development Workers, Self-Work and Therapeutic Cultures*. Basingstoke: Palgrave Macmillan.

Weber, M. 1958 [original 1905]. *The Protestant Ethic and the Spirit of Capitalism*. New York: Charles Scribner's Sons.

Weeks, K. 2011. *The Problem with Work: Feminism, Marxism, Antiwork Politics and Postwork Imaginaries*. Durham, NC: Duke University Press.

11 Feminists performing the collective trauma

Inna Perheentupa

A visiting group of Finnish feminists have just presented their activist project to an audience of about 60 in St Petersburg. After the presentation, a woman in her forties stands up to ask, in Russian, how the group could admit men to feminism, 'since it is supposed to function as a shelter for women'. This question, posed in a tone of clear concern, haunted me long after my fieldwork in Russia. I had never before heard someone associate feminism with a shelter in such a direct manner. I gradually came to apprehend how vital this spatial metaphor is to understanding feminist activism in Russia, the setting for my ethnographic study. The shelter idea, I suggest, is pivotal for examining feminist activism in contemporary Russia and the root causes for the radical forms it takes, often stemming from experiences of gendered violence. The thematics scrutinised in this chapter thus resonate with the #MeToo movement and its aftermath, in which women around the world have become empowered to stand against gendered violence.[1]

Feminism has experienced a resurgence of interest in Russia in the 2010s, after a decline in popularity and public visibility that was largely due to paring back of funding for feminist projects earlier in the new millennium (Brygalina & Temkina, 2004; Hemment, 2007; Salmenniemi, 2008). While Pussy Riot is the most well-known contemporary Russian feminist group internationally, the field of feminism in Russia is multifaceted and filled with activists tirelessly seeking opportunities for publicity on the scale achieved by that group with their 'Punk Prayer' performance and subsequent imprisonment.[2] One key reason for feminism's renewed popularity in Russia, especially among young women in bigger cities, has been the rise of conservative politics. Whereas President Boris Yeltsin's regime in the 1990s largely failed to develop a 'national idea' after the collapse of the Soviet Union, President Vladimir Putin's government has sought a new basis for legitimacy in a conservative ideology closely connected to nationalist ideas (Temkina & Zdravomyslova, 2014; Sperling, 2015: 126, 274–275). This concerns feminist activists most tangibly through several proposals and laws in the 2010s for limiting reproductive rights and public discussion of non-heterosexuality.[3] Valerie Sperling (2015) has pointed out that the success of the Russian government's patriarchal politics and laws is partially due to the absence of a strong women's movement. However, the enactment of those laws has sparked a new generation of feminist activists, who at times carry out strikingly confrontational and radical actions.

As Eva Illouz (2008) has highlighted, the feminist and therapeutic discourse have similar starting points – they both encourage working on one's relationship to oneself. However, relations between the two have been turbulent and dynamic from the beginning. In the 1960s, feminists raced in to challenge sexist forms of therapy and create their own feminist versions of it, ultimately forcing mainstream therapy to update its practices too (Herman, 1995). In fact, some scholars have suggested that, because feminism was so occupied with therapeutic practices of consciousness-raising, it actually lost its political dynamic (Becker, 2005; Cloud, 1998). Others have argued to the contrary that therapeutic strategies, rather than depoliticising feminism, enabled feminists to bring in a novel way of conducting politics (Stein, 2011). I contribute to these debates here by shedding light on how feminist activism in contemporary Russia takes therapeutic and political dimensions simultaneously, forming what I call therapeutic politics. Hence, my main focus is on the way politics and therapeutics come together and manifest themselves in feminist activism produced around activists' traumatic experiences.

I will begin by discussing the relationship between the feminist and therapeutic discourses. With this background, I can then introduce the research context and material. My analysis is divided into two parts: In the first part, I examine how the 'shelter' mentioned above is narratively produced and what kinds of individuals and ideas assemble in this space. With the second part, I turn to how therapeutic elements are combined with public feminist activism.

Feminism, therapeutics, and trauma culture

Feminists were among the first political movements to draw from the therapeutic discourse, in the 20th century (Stein, 2011: 167). As therapy did, feminism offered a cultural resource that 'invited self-examination, the acknowledgment of past injuries, and the revelation of those injuries to others in order to make sense of oneself' (ibid.: 187). The feminist and therapeutic discourses shared not only the idea that self-examination liberates but also that of the private sphere and family as the ideal object for transformation aimed at fulfilling individuals' desires (Illouz, 2008: 122–123).

As Ellen Herman (1995: 302) has shown, therapeutic practice was from the beginning both a friend and a foe for feminists. Conventional modes of therapy were male-dominated and often deeply misogynist and homophobic, as were the modes of psychiatry and psychoanalysis (Staub, 2015: 107). However, in how it construed the 'female', the therapeutic establishment, in fact, helped to concretise some of feminism's main critical arguments along the way, thereby gradually forcing therapy experts to reflect on their sexist practices (Herman, 1995: 281). What may well be characterised as the finest aspects of contemporary therapeutic culture – its democratic and nonhierarchical practices – stem in large part from the advances sought by radical and feminist therapists (Staub, 2015: 107).

The coupling between feminist and therapeutic discourse grew tighter in the 1970s when feminists started politicising issues of sexual abuse. This alliance involved connecting experiences of abuse to the therapeutic concept of trauma (Illouz, 2008: 167). Feminists pointed out that people could be damaged psychically, not just physically, and that damage from traumatic events may exert effects years after the events themselves. They emphasised, further, how trauma greatly threatens self-development and a healthy psyche, to which all citizens have the same rights. Feminist activists deployed therapeutic knowledge so as to transform private trauma of abuse into a public issue (ibid.: 168–169).

One central method launched by the feminist movement in the 1960s was collective work carried out in feminist consciousness-raising (CR) groups. As Dana Becker (2005: 8) has demonstrated, CR enabled women's collective reflection on their gendered experience in both personal and political terms. The self and private experiences were taken as a starting point for politicisation and for seeking common ground among women of all stripes (ibid.: 136). The idea for CR was of women coming together in order to reach a feminist consciousness – that is, recognise the connection between their ostensibly personal problems and social structures – and, as their consciousness grew, becoming politically activated to promote social change by bringing those 'personal' problems to the public's awareness. The feminist slogan 'personal is political' encapsulates this idea of politics running through all levels from personal to political.

Numerous scholars have claimed that what ultimately transpired was quite different: therapeutic practices applied in CR ended up merely privatising social problems. Dana Cloud (1998), for example, has suggested that the CR groups, in fact, shied away from confrontation with systemic power by withdrawing to the realm of their 'therapeutic enclaves'. According to Cloud, an additional problem with CR was that it mainly attracted middle- and upper-class women, who tended not to be focused on the profound social change envisioned by radical feminists. Feminist politics has been accused also of falling back to identity politics, as it had no apparent push for moving beyond the personal (Becker, 2005: 136–137). Conversely, it has been argued that feminists of that time showed success in launching a new personal way of conducting politics (Illouz, 2008: 170). This brave approach gradually encouraged other groups to share painful feelings publicly instead of holding them back (Stein, 2011: 192) and opened a discursive political space of action for those who had previously been marginalised and lacked a public voice (ibid.: 189).

While Western feminists were politicising the personal in CR in the 1960s and the 1970s, feminism in the Soviet Union was heavily suppressed. Nonetheless, 1979 did see a dissident feminist group publish an underground paper (*Almanac: Women of Russia*) dealing with abortion, the miserable conditions of Soviet maternity hospitals, and the challenges of single parenting, although the group was soon brought under the surveillance of the State Security Committee (KGB) and some of its members were ultimately deported from the country in the early 1980s (Iukina, 2007: 456–457). As did feminism, the 'psy' disciplines occupied a relatively marginal position in Soviet society and were not popular among the masses. Instead, biomedical, physiological, and pedagogical discourses were employed to make sense of the self, emphasising correct Communist socialisation. (Matza 2010, quoted in Salmenniemi & Adamson, 2015: 90–91.)

It was with the breakdown of the Soviet system that both feminist thought and psychological knowledge started to spread in Russia. Motivated by foreign grants and funders eager to support the country's democratic development, its feminist groups began politicising the 'private' with the aid of CR (see e.g. Sperling, 1999). However, the expanding women's movement and various women's organisations were situated mostly within the academic realm and remained accessible primarily to the middle classes and elite (Salmenniemi, 2014).

Also, various forms of popular psychology were being disseminated in the 1990s via television, self-help books, and meeting groups (Honey, 2014; Lerner, 2015; Salmenniemi & Vorona, 2014). The number of therapy professionals grew rapidly, accordingly (Matza, 2009). However, the intervening years have not made them affordable for many: private psychological services are provided and consumed mostly by the middle classes and the elite (Matza, 2012). While psychology itself, especially in its popular form, has maintained its appeal among the masses, feminism was rather supplanted, with anti-feminist sentiments coming to dominate in the early 2000s. Postfeminist ideas were domesticated in Russia with self-help books directed to female audiences (Salmenniemi & Adamson, 2015) highlighting not so much the collective as the individual-oriented sides of feminine agency, intimately tied to neoliberal ideas of personal-level responsibility and self-governance (see also Gill, 2007).

With this chapter I suggest that the generation of feminist activity that has emerged in the 2010s is producing a public trauma culture. Via this concept, introduced by Ann Cvetkovich (2003), the walls often erected between therapeutic and political are brought down (see also Salmenniemi et al. and Yankellevich in this book). Here, I will follow Cvetkovich's lead in analysing trauma as a social and cultural discourse (rather than clinical) that emerges in response to struggling with the psychic consequences of historical events and 'cultural memory'. With this analysis, I explore the feminist activism produced around trauma to uncover how psychic injury and painful memories are assembled to form therapeutic politics.

The context, material, and methods

The feminist activists interviewed for this study connect their feminist politicisation with increasingly conservative state politics conducted by the Russian government in tandem with the Russian Orthodox Church. The launch of the conservative politics can be traced back to around 2005, when the government started to impose increasing regulation of sexual and reproductive rights (see for example Temkina & Zdravomyslova, 2014). It reached its climax between 2011 and 2013, when both women and non-heterosexuals encountered political limitations through limits placed on access to abortion and banning of public 'propaganda' on non-heterosexuality for minors. Russia's conservative turn has been traced to attempts to address the country's declining birth rate, which has been framed as a 'demographic crisis' (Rivkin-Fish, 2010). While similar tendencies of conservative governance exist elsewhere, there are peculiarities to the Russian conservativism. For example, embracing conservative ideology combined with a strong national sentiment has been assessed as a strategy to win back Russia's lost international status and to position the country as morally superior to an overly emancipated and liberal West that trumpets the value of human rights (Wilkinson, 2014; Stella & Nartova, 2016). The ideological distance the Russian government has built in relation to Western countries is evidenced in recently enacted laws abolishing non-governmental organisations' right to receive foreign funding, while those that do are declared foreign agents. However, this is only one example of government-level attempts to police civic activism deemed not in line with its politics. Since 2005, freedom of assembly in public places has been limited, and in the wake of the mass anti-government protests of 2011–2013, officials have been equipped with a new set of tools for limiting public use of space and demonstrating (see, for example, Gabowitsch, 2017).

Meanwhile, the promotion of conservative moral values in day-to-day life is rhetorically centred on the concept of a 'traditional family' based on heteronormative gender relations that are portrayed as natural. For example, decriminalisation of some forms of domestic violence in 2017 was introduced to 'protect the traditional family'. One of the key ideological figures in this traditional setting, positioned alongside the devoted mother, is the 'real man' (*muzhik*) who is able to protect both his family and, when necessary, the nation. Elena Gapova (2016: 36) shows how a man who cannot fulfil his duty as the head of the household and provide for his family (i.e., be a 'real man') tends to be stripped of his masculinity and honour in this configuration. Gapova goes on to point out the close link between the Russian ideal 'real man' figure and national ideas of power, militarism, violence, and the army (ibid.: 63–65), as strong men are supposed to be a manifestation of a strong and virile country. The ideological campaign surrounding masculinity, also referred to as neomasculinism, presents new obstacles to feminist activism in the 2010s (Johnson & Saarinen, 2013: 550).

This chapter draws on research material produced through four months of fieldwork in St Petersburg and Moscow, primarily in 2015. Regular follow-up visits were also conducted between 2016 and 2018 in order to visit feminist events. The ethnographically produced material consists of 42 interviews with self-identified feminists and with individuals who identified otherwise but were active on the fringes of the movement. The fieldwork for this research included both participatory and non-participatory observation during feminist events, unofficial meetings, demonstrations, self-defense classes, and theatre rehearsals. Alongside participant observation, my work has been informed by Internet observation as I analyse some key social media feminist actions. This is because social media serves as a central stage for contemporary feminist activism.

Most of the interlocutors identified as women, although there were some who identified as men or genderqueer. In addition, roughly half of my informants identified as non-heterosexual (LGBTQ). The key activists who will accompany us through this chapter are anarchofeminist Anna, radical feminist Katia, queerfeminist Sonia, and queerfeminist Zhenia.[4] Most of them discussed trauma and violence in relation to their activism, at length, in the interviews. Only Zhenia was an exception, not discussing gendered violence or trauma but, rather, contributing to the idea of feminism as a shelter for certain kinds of vulnerable subjects. Trauma is thus an emic concept deployed by the activists themselves, with the exception of Zhenia. However, among the numerous individuals interviewed for this study there were also many who avoided discussing violence or noted that it had become too big an issue within the movement. With this article, I choose to concentrate instead on the significant proportion of the activists who focused on gendered violence and/or discussed their trauma.

For example, anarchofeminist Anna mentioned not being able to ignore the theme of violence in practice even if she was already fed up with it: 'Even if you do not really want to discuss violence but do something, all the same you end up talking about violence in the end. And that is why feminism is so important in Russia: because it gives people statements about violence'.

Further, I suggest that the contemporary Russian political context invites certain radical expressions of feminism 'onstage'. In this I refer both to radical feminism and to radical forms of action. The former, which focuses on a binary gender order and often views gendered violence as a 'keystone of women's oppression' in patriarchy (MacKay, 2015), takes strikingly visible forms in Russia today. Radical forms of action, in turn, are visible in Russian feminism in its vocal disagreement with the current regime and its politics.

For Katia, who was in her late twenties, radicality in activism took on many dimensions. As she identified as a radical feminist, her activism was focused chiefly on fighting gendered violence and male supremacy over women. However, since Katia took part in confrontational street actions, radicality manifested itself in her public actions too. Katia emphasised that she was not an 'elite' feminist but a feminist politicising the situation of those she saw as holding the most vulnerable position in the society: lower-class women with limited resources. For her, feminism was thereby an issue of class. This is Katia's narration of becoming a feminist:

> I was in a new relationship. And as I still suffered from an unhappy past relationship, I started searching for psychological articles on the Internet in order to solve my problems. And it so happened that I found an [feminist] article about abuse... I started reading it, further and further, and it turns out that Katia had become a feminist!

Katia was not the only one to associate feminism intimately with psychology. In fact, I soon noticed that psychology was something the activists were often as keen for as feminism itself in their strivings to deal with painful past experiences and to initiate change in their life. Many of the feminist events I attended included sessions that drew on psychology, with titles such as 'Post-Traumatic Stress Disorder and Psychological Trauma'. I soon noticed that these sessions were often the most well-attended events held at feminist gatherings. As I will show in the analysis, the therapeutic dimension to feminism encompassed much more than merely listening to lectures on psychology for aid in tackling difficult life situations. That said, before I delve into the activist narratives about the feminist 'shelter' and therapeutic politics, I want to highlight that the therapeutic functions feminism served should be considered in context with the fact that activists such as Katia rarely had access to psychotherapeutic services or other social support structures.

Producing a mental shelter for the traumatised

Remarkably many of the activists I spoke to had a personal story to share about violence and abuse. Katia was not alone in this, and her experience was that women often came to feminism expressly because of such experiences: 'Those women who have it all good rarely become feminists', she sighed. Some activists described having faced violence while growing up, whereas others described later violence, whether in intimate relationships or in encounters with strangers. Many of the activists also mentioned popular videos spread via the Russian-speaking Internet that present gendered or sexual violence against young women without criticising this phenomenon – serving rather as a platform for young men showing off. During my fieldwork, a teenage girl was killed in a violent attack by a group of teenage boys, and various peaceful demonstrations were organised in her memory and to call attention to the issue of gendered violence.

For queerfeminist Sonia, the experience of feminist awakening was associated not only with a culture of endemic violence but also specifically with trauma:

> I, like many people in this society, had a very traumatising experience of family in childhood. My father was violent, and our family very authoritarian. This was followed by a traumatic experience as a woman. [...] with a lot of things, people, violence. Though I think almost all the women I know share my experience.

Attaching one's experience to the concept of trauma was common practice for many of the activists: the concept of trauma was employed as a collective tool for narrating past injuries and experiences, many first-hand but others indirect. For instance, anarchofeminist Anna labelled her trauma as a 'moral' injury when recounting an encounter with a stranger who had nearly raped her but whom she had dissuaded by giving him money:

> Well, I am alive and was not strongly traumatised in a physical way, rather morally. And, of course, I told everyone about it: this is what happened to me. Because it was very triggering for me – but I can talk about it, and I believe it is important. All the women I told about it, and even all the men to whom I mentioned it, then started reminiscing about how their friends had experienced something similar... It was somewhat symptomatic.

Anna highlighted that her trauma stemmed from a constant threat of violence and referred to it as 'symptomatic' of cultural ills. This echoes how Cvetkovich (2003: 18) defines trauma in the context of trauma cultures. Even if the traumas the activists narrated were different in nature, the narratives were tied together by the way the activists discussed the trauma: they did so from a collective point of view, thus building collective identity and a sense of we-ness by recalling similar kinds of threatening or violent moments in their life. Ron Eyerman (2001: 5–6), who associates memory closely with cultural trauma, has stated that a group is solidified and becomes aware of itself through reflection of a shared memory. The past becomes collectively experienced and interpreted – it is construed as a reference point for upcoming action (ibid.: 7).

I suggest that the feminists in Russia, by narrating their traumatic experiences, constructed a mental shelter to shield themselves from the 'culture of violence' even if only momentarily. The term 'shelter', in its dictionary definition, denotes a safe place or a refuge. When one feels the need for a shelter, this is because one feels vulnerable to something outside the shelter. While the metaphor is connected with a physical space of safety, that space in the context of feminist activism in Russia remains without physical walls or a roof. Indeed, feminist groups seldom had a permanent place to hold their meetings. For these activists, who were constantly on the move and on the lookout for available spaces, even only a metaphorical space of their own to which they could withdraw conveyed a relative feeling of comfort. At the same time, though, the 'shelter' notion also very concretely refers to physical havens for people who have faced gendered violence. The notion of feminism as a shelter thereby resonates with the fact that there is a great shortage of physical shelters for victims of gendered violence in Russia. With the decline of foreign funding for feminist initiatives in Russia in the first years of the 2000s, most NGO-run shelters were closed down. Today, it is mainly state-led public crisis centres that can afford physical shelter spaces (Johnson & Saarinen, 2013: 555–556). Accordingly, those shelters still available focus on a more conventional notion of violence (ibid.: 561) and are most likely not sensitive to non-normativity and feminist issues.

The narratives of finding one's path to feminism were often also narratives of non-normative gender and sexual identity cast as deviant by the conservative political discourse. Zhenia, a genderqueer feminist, discussed feeling like an outsider everywhere. Reflecting further on this outsider identification, Zhenia connected it with personal gender and the toughening public atmosphere that followed on the heels of the 'homopropaganda' law and other conservative laws limiting activists' space. While describing a complicated relationship to even the feminist community, this personal narrative at the same time seemed to identify feminists as the only community Zhenia could somewhat relate to. This was crystallised during a discussion of the police having inspected a local feminist event: while not having been there during the incident, Zhenia lamented: 'How could they invade my space?' In Zhenia's narrative, feminism featured as the community and collective coming closest to the idea of belonging, something like a home for Zhenia. The metaphor of home that Zhenia hinted at resembles, in many ways, the idea of a shelter. As Saara Jäntti (2012: 81) has pointed out, safety is a notion often associated with the home, since a home is a place that is expected to provide a shelter from the world outside. At the same time, a vast body of feminist scholarship illustrates how the reality for a significant proportion of the population is not actually safe, because of domestic violence (ibid.: 83). The idea of belonging that was articulated by Zhenia suggests that feminism offers an alternative space of belonging for those who feel at home and safe neither in the realm of the heterosexual normative family nor in a national community that depicts them as deviant outsiders and even as a threat to national unity.

I suggest that feminism has offered those coming together in its 'shelter' a resource and a refuge for momentarily detaching themselves from sticky concepts such as binary gender, most often bound up with conservative definitions of womanhood and heterosexuality. In the research material, various narratives of feminist becomings highlighted a strikingly narrow understanding of womanhood on the part of the surrounding society and its conservative context. The 'shelter' metaphor reflects an idea of the feminist collective as a space of withdrawal from that context, a space in which activists can take a 'time out', together healing their traumas and spending time with like-minded people who are not hostile towards feminist ideas and non-normativity.

Although feminism clearly took on shelter-like functions, it was connected also to ideas of publicly speaking out and making the trauma and 'culture of violence' visible. Indeed, the idea of the feminist shelter could, alongside other concepts, be discussed in dialogue with the notion of the political underground, with resonance as the place for political dissidence in the politically repressive Soviet era (see, for example, Zdravomyslova, 2011). It can be interpreted accordingly as a momentary collective refuge for those whose political demands are silenced in national politics but also as a platform from which public resistance arises.

Performing the trauma in public: being an active and responsible feminist

It has been argued in feminist research that a focus on gendered violence tends to victimise feminists and deprive them of agency by rendering them as passive objects (see, for example, Cloud, 1998; Gilson, 2016; see also Freigang in this book). However, the feminist activism I observed, even when it stemmed from traumatic memories, was connected to a new publicly active subjectivity. This was notwithstanding the fact that many of the activists did not believe they would be able to bring about social change any time soon as they felt the political situation to be too suppressive. Sonia, for example, took part in activist missions by night to highlight the problematics of gendered violence. Her group would choose a public place, take provocative pictures commenting on the thematics of violence, and publish them online the next day in hopes that the shocking stunt would attract wide attention on the Internet.

As was typical for many of the activists, Sonia discussed her activism as a moral obligation that she could not evade, even if – because she always ran the risk of being caught by the police – she did not particularly enjoy the actions themselves.

At the same time, though, Sonia discussed her public activism in tandem with dealing with her personal trauma:

> I tried to defeat my traumatic experience, sought help from books and articles. And little by little I understood... I decided to do anything [I could] to ensure that there is less of this in the society. I decided to do all that I can, so that fewer girls would have an experience similar to mine.

Sonia thus highlighted that, while aiming to aid others and ultimately help initiate social change, she also received something herself in the process. This points towards the therapeutic dimensions of public action.

Anna added her own brushstrokes to the picture. Discussing the feminist virtue of being active in relation to the growing political apathy in Russia, she pointed out that fewer and fewer activists were ready to take to the streets after the crackdowns and mass detentions following the anti-government protests of 2012. She explained that, in continuing to take part in feminist public performances and events, she now was acting 'on autopilot' in trying to do at least something in order not to surrender to political apathy. Here, feminist active subjectivity was contrasted against a passive subjectivity figuratively looming constantly behind one's back. It was also portrayed in opposition to passive acceptance of a conservative lifestyle with its normative ideas of gender and family, which she suggested that most people were leading. One had to be active so as not to surrender to passivity (i.e., the conservative, conventional life). The way Anna discussed being active not only paints a vivid picture of narrowing political prospects for all political opposition in Russia but depicts those prospects as being especially narrow for non-male activists. In the case of both Pussy Riot and the Ukrainian feminist group Femen, the group's protest was depoliticised in the government responses, with attention being paid to their gender and 'improper' public behaviour rather than to the issues they had sought to highlight, such as homophobic policies, despotism, and problematics of prostitution (Bernstein, 2013; Thomas & Stehling, 2016). In this context, Sonia and Anna appeared to be publicly 'making noise' to resist constant silencing and their political subjectivity being denied. It seemed profoundly therapeutic to be publicly active rather than surrender to apathy as others had.

One popular mode of feminist action involves theatre and other performance. An action that made waves online called 'The Road to the Temple' is an interesting example of feminists fighting the conservative imperatives of passivity and the 'culture of violence' via public performance. Pictures from the action were published in February 2016 to coincide with Defender of the Fatherland Day, which celebrates war heroes and, indirectly, all Russian men. About a dozen activists conducted the performative action, on the steps of a local cathedral. Accordingly, photographs published online portray two men dragging 'battered' and bruised-looking female activists up the stairs to the church. As to why feminist actions in Russia often draw in such ways from theatrical strategies such as performance, one of the many reasons is simply that 'culture' is still less regulated than open political action. However, these kinds of performances appeared fundamental to feminist politics also from a therapeutic standpoint: theatre provides a venue for articulating traumatic experiences without pathologising the performers; instead, their trauma is transformed into a resource (Cvetkovich, 2003). In dealing with the trauma by performing it, the activists can be interpreted as looking for dignified active agency rather than surrendering to passivity or the 'illness' often connected with trauma. Further, my observations indicate that feminist theatre, whether performed on the streets/Internet as in the above-mentioned case or in a theatre hall, was a way to deal with the traumatic memories in a delicate way for activists and audiences alike. Firstly, the mechanism of acting enabled them to create distance from possibly first-hand experiences of violence. The performances had an obvious therapeutic impact on their audiences too, with the ensuing emotions being vividly sensed during plays that dealt with gendered violence – for instance, as members of the audience quietly sobbed in the dark. It was striking how strongly emotions of sorrow could be sensed 'in the air' during performances yet were seldom discussed at feminist meetings and other gatherings (see Kolehmainen in this book). Performances thus manifested themselves as a form of dealing with the uncomfortable emotions connected with the traumas, and as a collective forum for healing.

Whereas emotions were performed rather than discussed, being responsible was dealt with at length in many of the interviews. Activists highlighted the community's task of attracting new individuals and teaching them to take responsibility – that is, to actively organise feminist public actions themselves and spread the feminist word in society. The more people take up the responsibility, the more publicly visible feminist issues such as gendered violence can become. At the same time, however, many of the activists emphasised the movement's shortage of individuals able to carry responsibility. Attention thus was turned from the social to the individual, with questions raised as to whether individual activists were responsible and moral enough to actually take part in feminist public action. Some activists even suggested that the 'not-responsible ones' simply had not yet dealt with their trauma.

Indeed, responsibility is a core therapeutic concept and has often been discussed in the neoliberal context as problematic (McRobbie, 2009; Salmenniemi & Adamson, 2015) in that it ultimately tends to burden individuals with an exhausting amount of responsibility for issues that can be resolved only socially. As Cloud (1998) points out, the pattern of discourse translating social and political problems into the language of individuals' responsibility is a powerful persuasive force: it positions the individual as both the locus of the problem and responsible for bringing change. This is emphatically problematic in the context of a trauma culture, for it easily turns into blaming the victims and causing them to suffer more instead of looking for social solutions. Just such a tendency to lay the blame at the victims' feet has been found to exist also at Russia's public crisis centres, where the discourse frequently casts women as responsible for resolving the domestic violence they themselves have suffered or are at risk of (Jäppinen, 2015: 262). While I do not want to question the importance of taking responsibility in the context of activism, I wish to point out how much more complex the issue of responsibility is when traumas of violence are involved simultaneously. The feminist virtue of 'bearing individual responsibility' that I often encountered in the interviews appeared to flirt at times with the postfeminist ethos domesticated in Russian society alongside neoliberal capitalism (Salmenniemi & Adamson, 2015). As Salmenniemi and Adamson (ibid.: 90) have pointed out, this neoliberal self-monitoring produces social hierarchies rather than eliminating them – in the feminist case, it suggests that those who have already suffered should, in addition, carry the responsibility rather than turn to collective efforts for social resolutions or demand that the perpetrators shoulder their responsibility. This pattern was visible during my fieldwork too. However, some of the feminists focusing on violence in their activism openly rejected a push for individual-level responsibility and shifted their gaze towards the perpetrators and structures.

A more recent feminist online action comments on both the trauma culture and who is to ultimately carry the responsibility: timed for 2017's Defender of the Fatherland Day, it could be viewed as a public invitation for young men to come share the trauma of violence with the women. Instead of themselves performing, female activists had invited a group of male allies to protest with them. Pictures later published on a feminist social media page showed these activist men at a local war memorial with bare backs turned to the camera. Across their backs was a message painted as if with blood: 'Happy Day of the Fatherland!' – highlighting the precarious position of young men, who are assigned the role of national 'protectors' and may be forced to join the army and go to war. I posit that this action is a manifestation of how the trauma culture is evolving and negotiated among the various activists who are weary of the increasingly militant and conservative national politics. The focus thereby was shifted publicly from women to men, with the latter being portrayed as themselves vulnerable and in need of protection. They do not have to be 'real men', always ready to protect others and, if necessary, the nation. This action, I suggest, brought gendered violence into the discussion not only at the level of private day-to-day life but also as something on the level of structures. In fact, it mounted a critique of the state system's machinery that produces one generation after another of defenders. Whereas 2016's Road to the Temple action could be seen as addressing the responsibility of the Russian Orthodox Church, because it took place on the steps of a cathedral, the more recent action could be read as a direct commentary on the state's culpability in maintaining violent structures with the aid of normative and stiff gender roles.

Conclusions: feminist activism as therapeutic politics

With this chapter, I have focused on how feminists in Russia produce a culture around their traumatic experiences. I have discovered the shelter metaphor to illuminate how individuals arrive at feminism in their efforts to combat traumas caused by experiences of gendered violence and a sense of being unsafe and outsiders. As a response to those emotions, the trauma narratives are further used as a way to build collective identity and belonging. Analysing feminism as a shelter cast into relief its dual role: I illustrated how it is produced as a mental safe space for people who feel out of place and unprotected in society at large (especially under conservative politics that stress the importance of 'traditional' values and family over human rights and safety). At the same time the shelter, far from being symbolic of pure withdrawal, exists also as a platform from which feminist activists have a footing to publicly combat a 'culture of violence' that concentrates on producing generations of defenders rather than acknowledging gendered violence as a social problem.

The trauma culture thus evolves into a wider critique of violence on all levels of Russian society, exhorting the state to carry its responsibility. This culture is both private and public, and, while it mostly brings together people who identify as women and others who do not accept the label 'male', the 'Happy Day of the Fatherland!' action in 2017 demonstrates a door gradually opening here for young men too. Their trauma arising from Russia's militant politics and the associated narrowly defined male roles is now at least partially acknowledged as a pivotal element of the trauma culture.

Tracing the feminist trauma culture has enabled me to sketch out an assemblage of feminist therapeutic politics also, addressed in terms of feminist ideals of being active and responsible as well as feminist performances as a forum for both therapeutic and political endeavours. In the activists' narratives, the therapeutic facet to the feminist virtue of being active was visible not only in relation to combating violence but also in incorporating the therapeutic idea of being publicly active despite the trauma. Along similar lines, the feminist performances presented particular stages for both politicising the issue of violence and engaging in collective therapy for cultural trauma. I suggest that both feminist action in general and the performances in particular take on therapeutic dimensions because they allow the activists to hold on to their agency despite the trauma and the increasingly repressive politics.

One key aspect of therapeutic politics is that of balancing between personal and social responsibility in the context of trauma and a 'culture of violence', with the thorny matter of negotiation: who holds responsibility at the end of the day? The aspect of responsibility brings me back to the radical dimensions of feminism that I suggest are key to therapeutic politics in this context. As this chapter has illustrated, feminist activism often has roots in profoundly personal experiences of violence and outsiderhood. I find that in a context of vast inequality in distribution of resources, it is, in fact, highly radical – and most likely therapeutic – to decline to engage with neoliberal concepts of individual-level responsibility with its associated tendency to overlook collective and societal responsibility.

The dimension of class plays a pivotal role here. Feminist radical action and identifying as a radical feminist are both connected to classed positions to some extent, as we saw in Katia's case. I suggest that the flame for both radical feminism and carrying it into action is far more likely to be lit in people with less to lose – here, women, with weaker access to resources (such as platforms for disseminating critical knowledge and money for professional counselling) and generally at greater risk of gendered violence. It is no wonder, then, that this classed activism takes strikingly radical forms in its public action and performance. After all, it often springs forth from embodied and traumatic first-hand experiences.

To conclude, feminist therapeutic politics should be read as a critique of the failure of official politics to acknowledge non-male political subjects. In addition, it should be interpreted as an indictment to the lack of support structures for those in need of shelter and safety in contemporary Russian society.

Acknowledgements

I wish to thank the Academy of Finland, project Tracking the Therapeutic: Ethnographies of Wellbeing, Politics and Inequality (grant number 289004) for funding this project and all the activists who shared their thoughts with me during the research process. I want to thank the other contributors of the book for their valuable comments concerning the chapter. I am also grateful to Alisa Zhabenko, Anna Avdeeva, Paulina Lukinmaa, Iuliia Gataulina and Laura Kemppainen for their insightful comments on this chapter.

Notes

1 Russia had its own #MeToo, a year earlier: In 2016, a similar campaign of publishing gendered experiences of violence and harassment emerged in the Russian-speaking countries and their social media after a Ukrainian feminist published her story of gendered violence for the first time. The name of this campaign (#ianeboiusskazat) meant 'I am not afraid to speak'.
2 The feminists interviewed for this study varied in their attitudes towards Pussy Riot, with some of the activists not considering Pussy Riot a feminist group and criticising their actions while others expressed respect for their bravery and support for those actions.
3 In 2011, Russia adopted a law that limits abortions, though rejecting some of the toughest restrictions backed by the Russian Orthodox Church. The new law limits abortions to the first 12 weeks of pregnancy, with certain exceptions, and requires a waiting period of two to seven days for abortions. The law on gay 'propaganda' was enacted on the federal level in 2013, following similar laws at regional level and bans on 'propagating LGBTIQ issues for minors'.
4 All names used in this chapter are pseudonyms. Radical feminism refers to a feminism that views women and men as distinct political classes (MacKay, 2015) whereas queer-feminism and anarchofeminism rather dismantle the binary understanding of gender as well as aim to challenge numerous norms such as heteronormativity. However, like Finn MacKay notes, 'definitions of any type of feminism are fraught with difficulty' (ibid.). They are defined in different and at times even in contradicting ways also by the activists interviewed for this study.

References

Becker, D. 2005. *The Myth of Empowerment: Women and the Therapeutic Culture in America*. New York: New York University Press.

Bernstein, A. 2013. An Inadvertent Sacrifice: Body Politics and Sovereign Power in the Pussy Riot Affair. *Critical Inquiry 40*:1, 220–241.

Brygalina, J., & A. Temkina. 2004. The development of feminist organisations in St Petersburg in 1985–2003. In *Between Sociology and History: Essays on Microhistory, Collective Action and Nation-Building*, edited by A.-M. Castren, M. Lonkila & M. Peltonen. Helsinki: SKS, 207–226.

Cloud, D. 1998. *Control and Consolation in American Culture and Politics: Rhetorics of Therapy*. Thousand Oaks, CA: SAGE Publications.

Cvetkovich, A. 2003. *An Archive of Feelings: Trauma, Sexuality and Lesbian Public Cultures*. Durham, NC: Duke University Press.

Eyerman, R. 2001. *Cultural Trauma: Slavery and the Formation of African American Identity*. Cambridge: Cambridge University Press.

Gabowitsch, M. 2017. *Protest in Putin's Russia*. Cambridge: Polity Press.

Gapova, E. 2016. *Klassy Natsii. Feministskaia kritika natsiostroitel'stva*. Moscow: Novoe Literaturnoe Obozrenie.

Gill, R. 2007. Postfeminist Media Culture: Elements of Sensibility. *European Journal of Cultural Studies 10*:2, 147–166.

Gilson, E.C. 2016. Vulnerability and Victimization: Rethinking Key Concepts in Feminist Discourses on Sexual Violence. *Signs: Journal of Women in Culture and Society 42*:1, 71–98.

Hemment, J. 2007. *Empowering Women in Russia: Activism, Aid and NGOs*. Bloomington, IN: Indiana University Press.

Herman, E. 1995. *The Romance of American Psychology: Political Culture in the Age of Experts*. Berkeley, CA: University of California Press.

Honey, L. 2014. Self-Help Groups in Post-Soviet Moscow: Neoliberal Discourses of the Self and Their Social Critique. *Laboratorium 6*:1, 5–29.

Illouz, E. 2008. *Saving the Modern Soul: Therapy, Emotions, and the Culture of Self-Help*. Berkeley, CA: University of California Press.

Iukina, I. 2007. *Ruskii Feminizm kak Vyzov sovremennosti*. St Petersburg: Aleteiia.

Jäntti, S. 2012. *Bringing Madness Home: The Multiple Meanings of Home in Janet Frame's Faces in the Water, Bessie Head's A Question of Power and Lauren Slater's Prozac Diary*. Jyväskylä, Finland: University of Jyväskylä.

Jäppinen, M. 2015. *Väkivaltatyön käytännöt, sukupuoli ja toimijuus. Etnografinen tutkimus lähisuhdeväkivaltaa kokeneiden naisten auttamistyöstä Venäjällä*. Helsinki: University of Helsinki.

Johnson, J.E., & A. Saarinen. 2013. Twenty-First-Century Feminisms under Repression: Gender Regime Change and the Women's Crisis Centre Movement in Russia. *Signs: Journal of Women in Culture and Society 38*:3, 543–567.

Lerner, J. 2015. The Changing Meanings of Russian Love: Emotional Socialism and Therapeutic Culture on the Post-Soviet Screen. *Sexuality & Culture 19*, 349–368.

MacKay, F. 2015. *Radical Feminism: Feminist Activism in Movement*. London: Palgrave Macmillan.

McRobbie, A. 2009. *The Aftermath of Feminism: Gender, Culture and Social Change*. Los Angeles: SAGE.

Matza, T. 2009. Moscow's Echo: Technologies of the Self, Publics, and Politics on the Russian Talk Show. *Cultural Anthropology 24*:3, 489–522.

Matza, T. 2012. 'Good Individualism?' Psychology, Ethics, and Neoliberalism in Postsocialist Russia. *American Ethnologist 39*:4, 804–818.

Rivkin-Fish, M. 2010. Pronatalism, Gender Politics, and the Renewal of Family Support in Russia: Toward a Feminist Anthropology of 'Maternity Capital'. *Slavic Review 69*:3, 701–724.

Salmenniemi, S. 2008. *Democratization and Gender in Contemporary Russia*. New York: Routledge.

Salmenniemi, S. 2014. Feminismi, naisliike ja tasa-arvon paradoksit. In *Naisia Venäjän kulttuurihistoriassa*, edited by A. Rosenholm, S. Salmenniemi, & M. Sorvari. Helsinki: Gaudeamus, 290–315.

Salmenniemi, S., & M. Adamson. 2015. New Heroines of Labour: Domesticating Postfeminism and Neoliberal Capitalism in Russia. *Sociology 49*:1, 88–105.

Salmenniemi, S., & M. Vorona. 2014. Reading Self-Help Literature in Russia: Governmentality, Psychology and Subjectivity. *British Journal of Sociology 65*:1, 43–62.

Sperling, V. 1999. *Organizing Women in Contemporary Russia: Engendering Transition*. New York: Oxford University Press.

Sperling, V. 2015. *Sex, Politics, and Putin: Political Legitimacy in Russia*. New York: Oxford University Press.

Staub, M. 2015. Radical. In *Rethinking Therapeutic Culture*, edited by T. Aubry, & T. Travis. Chicago: The University of Chicago Press, 96–107.

Stella, F., & N. Nartova. 2016. Sexual Citizenship, Nationalism and Biopolitics in Putin's Russia. In *Sexuality, Citizenship and Belonging: Trans-National and Intersectional Perspectives*, edited by F. Stella, Y. Taylor, T. Reynolds, & A. Rogers. New York: Routledge, 17–36.

Stein, A. 2011. Therapeutic Politics – An Oxymoron? *Sociological Forum 26*:1, 187–193.

Temkina, A., & E. Zdravomyslova. 2014. Gender's Crooked Path: Feminism Confronts Russian Patriarchy. *Current Sociology 62*:2, 253–270.

Thomas, T., & M. Stehling. 2016. The Communicative Construction of FEMEN: Naked Protest in Self-Mediation and German Media Discourse. *Feminist Media Studies 16*:1, 86–100.

Wilkinson, C. 2014. Putting 'Traditional Values' into Practice: The Rise and Contestation of Anti-Homopropaganda Laws in Russia. *Journal of Human Rights 13*, 363–379.

Zdravomyslova, E. 2011. Leningrad's Saigon: A Space of Negative Freedom. *Russian Studies in History 50*:1, 19–43.

12 Uncanny experiences as therapeutic events

Kia Andell, Harley Bergroth
and Marja-Liisa Honkasalo

Encounters with the 'uncanny' – or 'supernatural' as it is often labelled in Euro-American societies – are commonly conceived of as a 'premodern' (Latour, 1993) mode of experience and characteristic of cultural 'otherness' (Kapferer, 2002). However, social scientific research has shown that such experiences are also commonly reported in post-industrial, contemporary social settings (see Dein, 2012). It seems that disenchantment, as Weber (1922/1967: 139) put it, has only had a limited effect, as people's engagements with the supernatural, the magical, and the otherworldly have not vanished in technoscientific societies with highly specialised education systems (see Josephson-Storm, 2017). By uncanny experiences we refer to 'extraordinary' sensory and embodied experiences that are often unexpected, uncontrollable and quite powerful.[1] Such experiences range from premonitions and visions to encounters with spiritual or otherworldly beings, and from telepathic communication to contacts with the deceased.

This chapter draws upon a letter archive of reported encounters with the uncanny. The letters have been written by a diverse group of people living in Finland. Instead of embarking on a quest to determine the actuality or 'truth' of such experiences, as might be the objective in the fields of, for example, neuroscience or psychiatry, we draw from classical anthropology (Levi-Strauss, 1968; Mauss, 1902/2001) in investigating uncanny experiences and related practices as *social* phenomena. We approach the textual narratives through the question of *how do uncanny experiences promote therapeutic knowledge production and world making*. We start from the empirical observation that as part of autobiographical narratives uncanny experiences are often made sense of through their transformative and fundamental effects. We argue that the uncanny becomes meaningful – and thus quite 'real' – in the sense that it shapes one's actions, life paths and conceptions of oneself and the surrounding world in ways that often promote stability and healing.

Engagement with the uncanny has been intertwined with ameliorating practices in the healing traditions for ages. In the rich historical research on the topic, the ability to mediate between different worlds and to work with extraordinary forces is considered a crucial part of the healer's competence (Eliade, 1964; in

Finland e.g. Honko, 1960; Siikala, 1978). Furthermore, in healing traditions the extraordinary in its various forms appears as a crucial resource for knowledge and for strengthening the bonds between people and society; here the process of healing is not limited to a patient–healer dyad but involves a multiplicity of actors, for example, other people such as fellow villagers as an audience that confirms the evidence of the ritual efficacy. The ritual healing involving the uncanny is a mechanism for bringing the effusive, transient, and fragile qualities of social relations into the light of the visible (Turner, 1968).

Due to modern medicine's marginalisation of traditional healing practices, healing by and through the uncanny is now commonly discussed through the notion of 'therapeutic culture' – a term referring to the rise of individualistic life management discourses in Euro-American societies. In particular, discussions on new spiritualities and New Age address the topic of otherworldly connections. Sociologist James Tucker (2004) has analysed what he calls the 'therapeutic theologies' of contemporary healers in the US, arguing that modern healers practice an extreme form of self-centred and hyper-individualised therapeutic culture through which the self is elevated as its own master and the individual notion of any definitive 'truths' are ultimately rejected as one is encouraged to forge one's own path in life. By reading through the healers' conceptions of the world and their social positions and lifestyles, Tucker (2004: 167) claims that such New Age practices work unlike religion because they 'do not bind people to a larger group of people or society nor require them to submit themselves to higher authority'. However, this is not necessarily the picture we encounter in the context of this research, as it seems that such experiences need not only be about being the author of one's own life, but also very much about being led and cared for, as well as about caring for others. In addition, uncanny experiences are also not only about constant change, but also about stability in the face of unpredictability, as they appear profoundly connected to the maintenance of social relationships. In this chapter we show how the uncanny can and does become part of people's therapeutic assemblages precisely because it entrenches connections and stabilities in the middle of personal, political, local and global crises.

For our analysis of the textual data, we employ a Latour-influenced framework of actor-network theory. This enables us to treat uncanny objects (i.e. beings, voices, feelings, sensations) as 'actants' that in cooperation with other actants influence the world and contribute to (re)arranging it. We ultimately argue that uncanny experiences and the narration of these experiences can be understood as 'therapeutic events', that is, as significant sequences of truth-making in terms of the self and as sequences of actualising social (care) relations. In this chapter we will first elaborate upon our theoretical framework by relating it to the dominant neuroscientific ways of understanding uncanny experiences and by introducing the concepts of *actants* and *events*. The data and methods will then be presented in more detail. This is followed by three analytical sections, the division of which is based on our thematic reading of the letters. Finally, we will provide brief conclusions.

Uncanny experiences: cognitive anomalies or socially significant life events?

In the wake of scientific rationalism, uncanny experiences in the 20th century have been widely understood through psychiatric discourses labelling them as pathological. In recent decades, however, neuroscientific research has had a remarkable impact on cultural conceptions and representations of such experiences. Using new imaging technologies, neuroscientific research has managed to show how uncanny experiences have an actual (i.e. visible and measurable) correlation in the brain (Raij et al., 2009; Silvanto, 2015; Mobbs & Watt, 2011; Blanke & Arzy, 2005). Discussions based on such research have thus emphasised experiences such as hearing voices without a visible source and out-of-body experiences as normal instead of merely pathological. Nevertheless, the research carried out within the natural scientific paradigm still tend to treat uncanny experiences as deviant (see Schmidt, 2016) or as temporary 'error' states of an individual brain. The idea of the uncanny as an error state has been consolidated by a wide range of research within cognitive psychology (for an overview, see Rancken, 2017)[2] which has also influenced seemingly different fields of research. For example, though sympathetic to the understanding of uncanny experiences as inherent in the faculty of the human mind, the phenomenologist Matthew Ratcliffe (2017) promotes the idea of the uncanny as a disturbance of the modal structure of the mind. By constructing uncanny experiences as disturbances or errors such accounts overlook the fact that these experiences may appear as highly meaningful to the experiencer and crucially affect their life in ways that sit uneasily with the idea of a mental error that needs to be corrected (see also Luhrmann, 2018).

Setting aside the conception of mental error, we argue that the narratives of uncanny encounters often construct such experiences as therapeutic instances that serve as crucial resources for self-understanding, identity construction, healing and work on one's social relations. By this we mean that in the analysed narratives, the uncanny appears as a central building block of the cultivation and craft of one's identity and one's social surroundings, no matter whether the actual encounters or happenings themselves are described as positive or unsettling; as 'natural' or 'mysterious'. In Levi-Strauss' (1968) terms, uncanny experiences are a *bricolage*. For example in our letter data, people often make sense of these experiences by employing various modes of knowledge, such as modern science, mysticism, parapsychology and religion. Drawing from this idea of the bricolage, we further approach the uncanny through a Latourian (2005) framework which problematises clear-cut dichotomies such as science–religion, real–not-real, natural–unnatural or human–non-human, and thus attempts to question some of the basic paradigms of scientific rationalism from which mainstream scientific accounts on uncanny experiences typically draw.

Like the social scientist Latour, several anthropologists have rejected the notion of the inanimate nature of objects, a notion which deprives objects of agency and personhood (Descola, 2013; Viveiros de Castro, 2004). The so-called 'flat ontology' rejects divisions between different levels of being (e.g. social–material, real–imaginary, natural–supernatural etc.). Latour has emphasised that in order to make sense of the social world, we need to consider objects – be they technical devices, human beings, ideas or words – as active participants in the course of action (Latour, 2005: 63–86); in this view, existence is not an a priori property of any 'thing', but rather it can be claimed that things exist *only in the sense that they affect the world around them*. Any social reality can then be said to consist not only of human action, but of (material, ideal, semantic or perhaps metaphorical) objects that afford certain actions while preventing others (e.g. a door may *both* suggest and enable a passage, *and* prevent or redirect movement) and thus very concretely *act* by affecting how the world works (see Latour, 1992). In this tradition, it is typical to speak of 'actants'.[3] The concept of an actant denotes an attempt to surpass the human tendency to see agency or the ability to act as an exclusively human trait. Any 'thing' that affects the world is an actant, an actor in its own right.

This suggests that whenever the social scientist wishes to analyse a human practice (such as therapeutic world making), the practice in question should be made sense of as a collection of actants – an assemblage, as all actants within an assemblage make the practice what it is. Intuitively, it may be relatively easy to conceptualise human life coaches (see Yankellevich in this book) or digital self-tracking technologies (see Bergroth and Helén and Freigang in this book) as actants in the sense that such objects may (or may not) notably influence one's self-image and, most of all, they *really exist* in the world! However, we argue that in the sense of people's everyday therapeutic assemblages and world making, uncanny actants can be just as effective and therefore just as 'real' in shaping one's life (see also Honkasalo, 2017a).

The idea of assemblages connects to the idea that the world or reality is never fixed-in-place, but is always subject to change and becoming. Each actant in a network of actors affects the assemblage so that the assemblage contingently 'hangs together' and is, in this sense, multiple (Mol, 2002). In assemblages, different actants fall into relations with each other; they 'happen' to each other. For the purposes of this chapter, we then employ the Latourian idea of an 'event' that relates to a rupture or a happening through which the world comes to hang together in a distinct fashion. After all, everyday life is usually not characterised by a relativistic stance towards the world; human beings do constantly establish truths – or at least relatively stable conceptions – about themselves, about others, about the things they perceive and the things they practice. In Latour's (1999) philosophy of science, the concept of an event is supposed to replace the notion of a 'discovery', which implies that one could merely discover a fact – for example, a fact of nature or a fact of history – which has always been there and exists irrespective of the observer, just waiting to be found. 'Events', in contrast, refer to occurrences or sequences – possibly temporally unspecific and covering a long period of time – in which actor-networks 'set up' the world and make it known in certain ways. This is to say that 'events […] do not discover truth, but they make truth happen' (Sansi, 2013: 453).

Materials and method

Our empirical investigation is based on an archive of over 200 unsolicited letters about people's everyday uncanny experiences. They were sent to the research project *Mind and the Other* (see Honkasalo 2017b) after the project gained public visibility in the Finnish media. The letters bring forth a diverse range of experiences. Some writers mention lonely experiences of intuitive thoughts, visions and weird feelings, and others speak of vivid and powerful encounters with mysterious beings or dead relatives, friends and pets. Some people recount having the obscure sense of a presence or someone touching them when no one seems to be around.

The letters in question have been sent by people from all walks of life and with diverse educational and occupational backgrounds. In contrast to some previous work on therapeutic spiritualities (e.g. Tucker, 2004; Heelas & Woodhead, 2005), writers are often not practitioners (healers, mystics, clairvoyants, etc.) or participants in spiritual movements and well-being practices, although as will be shown through our examples, uncanny experiences have led some of them on paths of helping others. One part of the letters is from writers who are keen on finding an (scientific) explanation for particular uncanny incidents. For others the uncanny has 'always' been a part of life and the experiences are further elaborated upon in autobiographical letters. For the purposes of this chapter, we unpack three such autobiographical narratives which neatly illuminate the various therapeutic dimensions of uncanny experiences.

We read the narratives closely, combining elements of narrative studies, thematic content analysis and Latourian-inspired material semiotics. We have carried out thematic content analysis of these assemblings on a case-by-case basis, paying close attention to how different actants emerge and come together to enable therapeutic knowledge production on oneself and the world. The analysis is further informed by ethnographic studies on 'illness narratives' focusing on people's personal experiences and the subjective truths that have generally been neglected in medical accounts. Narrative approaches often draw attention to 'disruptive' (Bury, 2001) or 'exceptional' (Rancken, 2017) moments and experiences. The uncanny, especially when it occurs repeatedly, often constitutes a major instance of 'autobiographical disruption' (Bury, 1982), and thus, similarly to illness narratives, stories of uncanny experiences can be understood as narratives of disruptions which shed light on personal meanings, relations towards the world and wider cultural/societal issues (Bury, 2001, 264). Furthermore, it could be argued that uncanny experiences and their narration also serve as disruptive instances that 'make the truth happen' in terms of self-understanding and one's social reality.

We have organised the narratives analysed in this chapter under three key themes based on the idea of the therapeutic as active work one engages in: *work on the self, work on the society* and *work on social relationships*. The analysis follows this three-fold structure, and in each section we seek to illuminate one theme through one particular narrative while also seeking to link distinct narratives. Focusing on one narrator at a time enables us to concentrate on the whole of their personal narratives. This in turn allows us to grasp the processual, event-like nature of uncanny experiences and their therapeutic effects, as well as recognise transformations that take place in the narrators' relations to the self, others and the world through the assembling of uncanny and other actants.

The uncanny and work on the self

Joonas is a 33-year-old family man who self-identifies as a 'seeker'. He recounts that his childhood was spent in a religious home environment (his father was a priest), which he says provided him with a 'framework for interpretation of the world'. Later in life he has conducted university-level studies in theology and cultural studies of religion, and has had a long-standing interest in esoteric literature and mysticism. Joonas, like many other writers, reflects on his uncanny experiences as something that may and often do seem frightening or 'crazy', even to himself, and he ponders whether these experiences have been distorted or altered by his memory. Yet he assures the reader that the experiences have had significant effects on his life.

> I regard myself as a seeker and I try to find some kind of meaning in everything that I have experienced over the years. I think of myself as a relatively normal and sane person and I have an aversion towards New Age thinking, but at the same time I cannot disregard my experiences as just some kind of underlying insanity; I rather see them as one of the most significant building blocks of my identity.

In shaping the identity of a seeker, Joonas refers to something that is common across many of the writings on uncanny experiences: that one is 'attuned' towards experiencing the uncanny or that it is a trait that has *always* been a part of oneself. The adoption of the identity of a seeker also seems to function as a narrative way to balance – or overcome – the evident tension between experience-based and science-based modes of knowing, for example, the labels of 'sanity' and 'insanity' that Joonas struggles with. Joonas' time in his childhood home seems to have been a crucial, temporally unspecific and longitudinal *event* in his becoming a seeker. In addition to living with his family, he says that he also shared his childhood home with two 'beings' that he alone was able to sense. In his letter, he describes how the presence of the 'veil-being' – a veil-like figure that communicated telepathically – was always a source of comfort. For example, Joonas describes an incident in which he was hiding under the living room table because his parents were having an argument. There, the veil-being lingered beside him and spoke to him, telling him that his parents would not be divorcing but are 'learning each other'. However, in contrast to the comforting presence of the veil-being, there was also another being that appeared to him regularly, the 'spool-man', whose figure was that of a man with the head of a hammerhead shark and a torso of spools. Joonas mentions that one of these encounters with the spool-man happened while he was sitting on a potty in a room he shared with his brother. For him, the spool-man's presence was always a source of nervousness and anxiety. Here, the uncanny beings, as both comforting and distressing, surface as actants that affect the way Joonas perceives himself and produce knowledge on the world in particular situations.

However, Joonas' identity as a seeker is not only about *receiving* the uncanny, but also about actively seeking a connection with extrapersonal forces. For Joonas, such active (identity) work of a seeker has been evident in the form of the 'prayer'. Joonas' praying practice reflects his way of drawing from different knowledge and belief systems such as religion and mysticism. He has been engaged in such active work since he started seeing frightening visions in his early adolescence after reading the Book of Revelations in his childhood home. He describes the development of the practice as follows:

> Around when I was about ten years old, I developed a recurring habit of praying. My relation to the church was sceptical and even hostile, but especially when I was walking in nature, I used to constantly talk to myself, as in my own prayer.
>
> I vividly remember how I sat on a swing in the neighbouring yard on a summer day, feeling strong anxiety, and I prayed in a mantra-like fashion for tens of minutes that the things I dream about would not come true. I then felt a voice somewhere inside of me – not in my head but more like somewhere between my spine and the back of my head – and the voice said that everything that I've seen will come true in my lifetime but that I would be safe. It is now hard for me to define how much of that answer was the product of my own imagination and how the years that have since passed have affected my experience. However, the truth is that at that moment I felt the answer as real, and most of all comforting.

So for Joonas, praying is a practice that invokes answers that establish truths about the world and the future. This is reminiscent of how Mauss (1909/2003) understood prayer as a social practice, a rite that has efficacy in world making. Notably, for Joonas, the prayer connects to self-preservation not only through the reception of comforting knowledge about the future but also because the reception of answers to his prayers seems to have *required* active care for the self. For example, in Joonas' narrative, it gradually becomes evident that he has struggled with the consumption of substances such as alcohol, particularly during student years. After one of the worst months of almost non-stop binge drinking – all the while suffering from what would later be diagnosed as an ulcer – he tried praying after having not done so for several months, but could not get any answers. He writes that it was 'as if the world was sulking at me'. In his narrative, these times are characterised by frightening 'visions'; he writes that he constantly saw visions of rough and rugged 'interiors of houses', which he interpreted as places he would end up. He also writes about an incident involving a mysterious character when he was in a possibly life-threatening situation:

> I was walking home from a bar, very drunk. I stopped at the corner of a closed-down store and I felt a need to lay down into the snow just for a while.

I passed out and then woke up frightened as a tall figure in front of me shouted, 'Get up! You were not born just to die there!' I was freezing and walked home, laid down on my bed, and cried through the whole night.

We may then theorise uncanny experiences and practices as social forms or instantiations of care for – and cultivation of – the self. Uncanny experiences, such as visions of places, mysterious beings that provide comfort or traumatic experiences, and concrete, embodied 'answers' to one's prayers, are often made sense of through the effects that they impose on one's self-understanding and relation to one's actions or situations. In Joonas' narrative, uncanny experiences are therapeutic 'events' that actualise self-understanding and self-care, and by writing about himself as a 'seeker', Joonas establishes a difference to religious self-understanding (a religious person) or scientific self-understanding (a disturbed mind).

Joonas' narrative hints that uncanny experiences may be understood as a way to handle emotionally and psychologically taxing situations, to deal with fractures and turning points in one's life. In terms of comfort, what seems typical in these experiences is that they provide security in the face of the fragility of human life and insecurity about the future; for example in addition to the aforementioned examples of domestic arguments and substance abuse, Joonas' narrative of experiences connected with the uncanny involve a near-drowning incident, a decision to pursue a new line of university studies, his mother falling seriously ill and his own looming divorce, among other things. However, these experiences are not only about insecurity and uncertainty in relation to the everyday lifeworld of the individual. Uncanny experiences may also connect with wider social, political and technological frameworks and dis/continuities which induce uncertainty and chaos in relation to the future(s) of local communities, nations and even mankind as a whole. In relation to visions, Joonas writes of having seen 'chaotic nightmares' about global threats, in his words 'everything from clouds of pollution to exploding nuclear facilities'. In addition, these visions – and the accompanying anxiety – have always been partly tied to globally significant political events and ruptures such as the fall of the Soviet Union, the Gulf War, and more recently, the events in Ukraine and the Crimean Peninsula, which he says he followed almost obsessively through the media. In hindsight, Joonas writes about dreams and premonitions that have haunted him before these events actually took place. As typical in a Latourian (1999) conception of events, there is no evident causal relation between the experiences of such premonitions and actual political events (after all, it is perhaps impossible to say which comes first, the political event or the idea of related premonitions); in any case, such political upheavals are crucially connected to the sense of dis/continuity of the world as it is.

In summary, we argue that Joonas' uncanny experiences are about self-care and self-work in the face of uncertain futures and a chaotic existence. They are a social practice of coming to grips with experiences of uncertainty, powerlessness and negative states such as fear or anxiety. They may also help to handle overwhelming positive feelings and excitement. However, what sets our account of uncanny experiences apart from the basic functionalist idea of the uncanny happening in a time of crisis is the idea that the uncanny is not only a 'therapeutic tool' that serves a predetermined function but it is a 'real' actant in people's therapeutic assemblages, which include various actants from traditional beliefs to holy texts and from mysterious beings to political decisions and national armies. This is to say that uncanny actants are part of a complex network of actants which have established Joonas' identity. They are also a part of a self-care assemblage; as Joonas says, undefined forces – 'the other' – have been and will now always be present in his life, helping him to navigate the complexities of personal and political life although also at times invoking anxiety and other negative feelings. Thus, such experiences may well even become actively sought after. Furthermore, experiences of such 'guidance' may also detach one from self-centred ways of understanding social reality.

In Joonas' narrative, active work with the uncanny focuses on the self as he keeps these experiences mostly to himself. We will now move on to exemplify how such work can also focus on other people as uncanny experiences become a 'skill' that can be put to use for the good of others and the community.

The uncanny and work on the society

Elisa is a 58-year-old entrepreneur and former artist who has spent the last three decades of her career helping, healing and educating others as a professional massage therapist. Like Joonas, Elisa says that she has 'always' had a sensitivity towards the uncanny. For example, she makes a reference to a 'spiritual friend' whom she used to play with as a child. She also says that she has always been sensitive to communications with the deceased. She writes that at the age of eight she could sense that her grandfather had passed away. When her mother received the sad news on the phone, Elisa told her not to answer the call because it will make her cry. Afterwards, Elisa describes her mother as having been 'astonished' by the warning. Elisa was not really shocked by the news as she says she felt that 'grandfather had it good now'. A further instance which has affected Elisa's process of coming to terms with such abilities concerns an out-of-body experience she had in the early 1980s as a young mother. During this experience, she 'was watching [my] body from the roofline', and there was 'no fear and no evil, just an incomprehensible freedom'. In this narrative, however, the experience is interrupted by a voice commanding her to return to her body. Elisa does not want to go back, but finally gives in as the voice commands her and says that she has a purpose, that she 'still has much to do'. Elisa then writes that she felt out of breath afterwards, and that all fear of death has since vanished.

Elisa has come to understand her sensitivity to see or sense things unobservable to others as a special ability; a skill to be used to receive knowledge across the boundaries of this world and the other world. Notably, in her adult life she has come to recognise this skill can be refined, and she has developed it in order to help others. Shortly after her out-of-body experience she started to engage in therapeutic work. In the 1990s she carried out mental support work with entrepreneurs before moving on to start an association which brings people together to discuss topics 'from birth to death and afterlife'. As a massage therapist, she has been developing a holistic treatment which also incorporates uncanny elements as Elisa discusses these themes with some of her customers. In Elisa's story different medical and healing discourses emerge as notable actants; for example, contemporary discourses of holistic health affect the ways in which she taps into the uncanny in order to help others. On the other hand, as will be shown, dominant medical discourses appear as equally powerful actants since Elisa's healing work is much about fighting the pathologising effects of discourses that treat the uncanny as error states of the mind.

Within the group sessions, the group has explored the future and the past. With the group, Elisa engages in making sense of the self and the world in a similar way as Joonas in his narrative. Elisa, however, also highlights herself as a helper of others as she assists people in training their senses and forming an understanding of a world in which both the uncanny and physical reality play an essential part. For example, she says that a customer's deceased father once entered the group session situation. With Elisa's assistance, the deceased was able to get a sign to the customer who recognised it as being from her father. Drawing on her personal experience of communicating with the dead, Elisa explains that 'the deceased want to tell us about life after death and sometimes, to forgive or be forgiven'.

Elisa's narrative thus introduces a therapist-actant who comes to act as a coordinator of uncanny encounters, helping people gain control over, manage and make further use of experiences that previously seemed unexplainable and 'out of place'. Through the sessions led by Elisa, the uncanny comes to affect people's understandings of themselves and the world in a new way. The uncanny then transforms from something strange and possibly disturbing into a therapeutic actant that provides a 'peace of mind'. Furthermore, such occasions affect and transform the therapist's professional path and mode of expertise. For example, when massage therapy customers wish to discuss spiritual matters, her professional act transforms by the adding of a spiritual layer into this treatment.

We might then go on to argue that therapeutic instances are not necessarily about people discovering some already existing truth or 'inner' self, an idea considered emblematic of New Age spirituality (Heelas, 1996: 18). Instead, truths about the self are established in collaborations between the therapist, her customers, the uncanny, material settings and other actants assembling in practices or 'improvising acts' of spiritual entrepreneurship (Hulkkonen, 2017: 5). Group sessions and treatments can be seen as events in a sense that through these gatherings, actants like customers, the therapist and the uncanny come to affect each other and transform; for example in the aforementioned example of channelling a message from a dead father Elisa's skill as a healer is actualised, as is the continuing existence of a loved one – and perhaps for example forgiveness – for the customer. This is how the therapeutic assemblage, involving the uncanny, 'hangs together'.

Elisa's narrative also highlights an effort to transform society on a wider scale, which traces back to experiences of stigmatisation she has endured in her social environment due to her sensitivity. She believes that she was misunderstood by her family, and says she had felt a deeper connection to her childhood spiritual friend than to her actual siblings. In fact, her spiritual friend provided her with mental support during feelings of loneliness that seemingly had to do with her special sensitivity. She eventually had to ask her spiritual friend to keep their distance since her parents had started to worry about her mental health.

Through such experiences of distinctness and loneliness, Elisa has come to recognise uncanny experiences as very alienating and widely misunderstood in a technoscientific society that tends to treat them as pathological. For herself, a series of particular uncanny encounters has led to a lifetime of work trying to normalise these experiences and help other experiencers come to terms with their special character. As she herself sees it,

> People experience and sense many kinds of incidents. Before, they used to tell me about spiritual matters, fearing being labelled as crazy, and they asked me, like, in secret if they could talk to me about such things. I avoid using the term supernatural because to me, these things are natural things and events that belong in the circle of life. [...] Many people simply sense more finely, but they would not need medication but a down-to-earth approach to spiritual matters. Sure, there are also those who do need help from doctors and medication for their problems. Some people react in a defiant manner when somebody talks about "supernatural" things, spirits, or the deceased. This causes the most sensitive ones to question their own mental health and feel anxious about their uniqueness. My concern about how supernatural things are conceived in society and how alone highly sensitive people are, fearing stigmatisation, keeps me going [in therapeutic work].

The stigmatising character of uncanny experiences then comes to act as Elisa's primary motivation in carrying on her work with other experiencers (see also Koski, 2016). She emphasises the normality of such experiences; for example, she explicitly problematises the notion of 'supernatural', as do many other writers of the archive's letters. By narrating uncanny experiences as natural and intrinsic to some people, Elisa seeks to challenge and transform dominant pathologising discourses that have been influential in not only the sphere of modern medicine, but also everyday life. Elisa makes a critical remark about how people with uncanny experiences can needlessly be put on medication, but also admits that some people benefit from medical expertise. Thus, she does not try to prove medicine wrong, but rather suggests a widening of perspectives on human mind/body to cover spiritual matters, that is, she proposes the inclusion of uncanny actants in our conceptions of humanity, health and well-being.

Narrating personal experiences to representatives of institutionalised science can be understood as an effort to socially normalise uncanny experiences since these narratives are directed at people who are supposed to have the power to affect the social construction of knowledge and thus change the prevailing social structures that insistently seek to pathologise the individual experiencer. Through a (narrative of) lifelong experience of uncanny encounters, Elisa's knowledge has become experiential expertise. Elisa writes about how she has learned to talk about the uncanny in a generally understandable way, and she also invites the researchers to participate in one of her sessions. These actions can be understood as practices that seek to change the social perceptions of the uncanny experiences as deviant and/or matters of belief and thus not real. Writing to the researchers can be seen as a 'therapeutic event' in a sense that it seeks to establish new 'truths' about the world, although the outcomes and repercussions of such acts cannot be controlled by the writer and might be unexpected (cf. Latour, 1999).

In summary, the dominant scientific-rational worldview along with accompanying scientific discourses emerge in Elisa's narrative as actants that affect the perceptions of uncanny experiences and experiencers in society. In this context, active work on others and society by helping others and writing to researchers give shape to therapeutic assemblages which seek to provide people with comfort and peace of mind, as well as act upon dominant discourses and transform scientific and cultural ways of perceiving uncanny encounters.

While the main focus has been on Elisa's work on others and society, her narrative points to how uncanny encounters may involve active work on one's social relationships, work that transgresses the boundary between life and death. We now move on to investigate this particular aspect of uncanny experiences. In the next section we will illustrate how the uncanny comes to play a part in maintaining and nurturing continuous bonds.

The uncanny and work on social relations

Maija is a mother of three adult children. She is academically trained as an economist and has worked as a teacher and entrepreneur. Although retired, she is still in charge of a family-owned firm. Her father was a pilot in the Second World War and died in a plane crash when she was only five months old, yet Maija is convinced of her father's continuing presence and protection. After her mother's new marriage, Maija had a good life with her stepfather and siblings. She writes of her uncanny experiences, ranging from telepathic abilities to an ability to communicate with the deceased, and mentions her family's benevolent attitudes towards them. Most of the uncanny experiences she writes about are intertwined with social practices that seek to strengthen the social bonds between one's closest. Importantly, she does not draw a practical distinction between life and death, that is, this world and 'otherworld' in terms of social relationships. In this narrative the 'otherworld' does not denote a distinct 'place', but rather a continuum of human existence and care relations, and the fact that 'everything is well and goes on'. The 'otherworld' appears as an actant that arranges one's social assemblage in a way that is simultaneously old and new, as Maija's social relations persist, albeit mediated through a novel arrangement of actants.

Maija, like Joonas, describes the uncanny as an intrinsic part of her life, and like Elisa, she has both gone through uncanny experiences and made use of them to benefit other people. Through the uncanny Maija has gained a powerful sense of trust and gratitude towards continuous care relations which she seeks to turn into hope and comfort for others by volunteering in the local church and hospital. However, in contrast to Elisa, Maija's therapeutic assemblage is not so much about changing society as it is about preserving and stabilising one's personal social circle. As an actant, she resembles both a caretaker and the one who is being cared for; both a subject and object of the practice of care. Making no distinction between care of the living and the dead, she vividly describes her contacts with friends, relatives and neighbours and the signs they send her from 'afterlife'. These signs convince Maija of the well-being of her deceased loved ones who nevertheless remain very important actants in her life. For her, uncanny experiences have thus been empowering and positive, convincing her of the continuity of her most important social relationships.

Maija recounts examples about two friends whom she supported when they were dying. An important moment was when she got a guarantee of their status after death by receiving a sign. Reflecting the tendency of the uncanny to intertwine with the material context of human life and technology, the sign was mediated by candles that became lit. This can be seen as another 'therapeutic event' through which the transgressive and continuous social relation is actualised:

> I was standing on her grave and the candle had gone out. I had that candle in my left hand and I was putting my right hand in my pocket to find the matches when the candle suddenly lit. 'Wonderful, Hilda, wonderful!' was my immediate reaction. I succeeded in putting the burning candle in the lantern, and for a while I was jumping, excited.

In another story, she speaks of feeling 'bottomless happiness' after receiving a sign from a deceased neighbour whose spouse had passed away before. In this story too the candle was decisive as an actant that propagated a hope that the neighbours would be able again 'to enjoy togetherness' in the afterlife.

Most of the signs of the uncanny actants which convince her of the well-being of her loved ones are visual. In these occurrences the lights can also turn on and off without perceptible cause. Moreover, she speaks of getting other visual signs that have warned her of a danger or threat to herself or others. For example, Maija writes that a flickering of lights, for which she had no explanation at the time of occurrence, turned out to be a sign of skin cancer that was consequently diagnosed early and healed. In this way, Maija's story resembles Joonas' account about the uncanny as work on oneself, as she has come to consider herself as 'loved and protected' as part of a larger bundle of relations that transcends the boundaries between material and non-material, human and non-human, life and death.

> Last spring I was sitting in my study and solving sudokus and the tabletop lamp went off by itself. I thought it was a blackout but other lamps were working. After a while the lamp turned on by itself. The same thing the next day. And the next. And the next. I got nervous. And I said that I know something is wrong, but I don't know what it is, so stop that. I realised that I was receiving a message [...] At some point my husband was washing my back

and said that I have a strange mole. It was black. I called a dermatologist. Melanoma. It was removed and it had not spread. The doctors said that never before had they found a melanoma at such an early stage. [...] I am thankful every day for being truly loved [...] I am convinced that my loved ones take care of me even after death, and most likely I will carry on the tradition.

Maija, like Elisa and Joonas, also acknowledges the stigmatising character of uncanny experiences, and in her own way is also politicised to change social perceptions of such experiences. However, we interpret her narrative also as reflecting a need of continuous confirmation of the 'truth' of the uncanny. Maija meticulously reports on how the candles work, in which situations they light up and in which they don't, and in general about the profoundly powerful and unexpected nature of uncanny occurrences, as evident in the previous description of the unlikely event of just one lamp going off repeatedly. In this way she 'validates' signs from the afterlife. This can be seen as further therapeutic work that seeks to actualise the existence of life after death and nurture the social relations that she finds dear to herself. Furthermore, in addition to feeling 'protected' in this life, Maija expresses a wish to herself keep looking after loved ones after her own death as well. This reflects the reciprocal character of care in Maija's personal circle, as she expresses a will to continue her care work and the maintenance of social relationships after her own death.

Maija's narrative also highlights the embodiment of the uncanny as part of therapeutic assemblages: how the presence of the uncanny, and thus the existence of the social relation, is confirmed through the body, by way of emotions and sensuous experiences rather than direct communication and interaction with uncanny beings. Maija recounts the way in which she recognised the presence – and well-being – of her deceased stepfather in her body. After receiving word of her [step]father's death

> I was crying a lot and was very anxious. On Saturday night I was crying and turning around and around in my bed, it was as if I had an iron belt around my chest. Just a horrible feeling. And then, suddenly, the feeling started from my head and moved down gradually, and I was gasping for breath like a fish on dry land, out of relief and happiness. I am sure that my dad wanted to tell me that self-pity and a heavy conscience are futile, that he was pleased with me and he was doing well.

Here Maija felt the presence of the deceased in her body in much the same way the traditional healers describe iconoclastic elements in the healing process (Taussig, 1993, see Bowman and Valk, 2012). The healers explain how they were able to make a 'diagnosis' by recognising and feeling the other's ailment in their own body and how they are able to take over the patient's pain while healing. This is also what happens in healing ceremonies with ancestral possession rituals (see Schmidt and Hutchinson, 2010), where the ritual subject is able to speak – and know the world – through the ancestor's often powerful voice. It is by mimesis[4] and replication that the healer is able to cure.

In summary, we interpret Maija's story being about the strengthening of social bonds beyond the binaries present in everyday perceptions of the world. Maija's dealings with the uncanny extend the reciprocal care relations into the domain of the 'otherworldly'. Making social bonds – instead of 'working them out by grief work' – is a theme that has recently been vividly studied and discussed (see Walter, 1999, 2007). People's ties with the deceased are interpersonal and multifaceted. As Maija's narrative demonstrates, they also manifest in bodily acts in addition to emotions and memories. Generally, by forging such ties, grieving persons construct a durable biography that enables them to integrate the memory of the dead into their ongoing lives. According to Walter (1999), the process by which this is achieved is principally considered a conversation between the living and the dead. Rather than being abandoned, the relationships with the deceased are renegotiated and sustained in one way or another. They can be a salient aspect of everyday life. In his phenomenological research of the mind, Ratcliffe (2017: 205–206) points out that the grieving process can include several embodied ways of experiencing and relating to the dead. Walter emphasises that the grief process hinges on talk more than feeling; and the purpose of grief includes moving on with, as well as without, the deceased. However, what is unique in Maija's narrative is the content and reciprocity of her way of relating to the dead, that of sustaining social relations.

Conclusion: uncanny experiences as therapeutic events

We have presented three autobiographical narratives of uncanny experiences and demonstrated not only how uncanny experiences are thoroughly social practices but how uncanny actants can become an integral part of people's therapeutic assemblages. The analysis of Joonas' narrative shows how uncanny experiences shape one's self-understanding and how they relate to self-care in the face of personal and political, local and global, (dis)continuities. Elisa's narrative focuses on how uncanny experiences have promoted actions of helping others, as well as politicised her to conduct transformative work on society. Maija's narrative is about working on personal social relations that transgress the impenetrable boundary between life and death. In many respects these narratives overlap, yet also reveal distinct ways of 'assembling' the uncanny into one's life and further into social discourses.

We argue that uncanny experiences can thus be understood as 'therapeutic events' that propagate social knowledge production; that is, new and/or old 'truths' in relation to oneself, the world and one's social relations. Importantly, we do not see uncanny experiences as *a priori* positive phenomena or being *in essence* about healing. In certain assemblages and situations they become productive of anxiety and chaos rather than healing and stability, yet even as such they can be 'worked with' in order to self-care and/or change society. Through an understanding of uncanny things as contingent 'actants' within people's therapeutic assemblages in everyday life – as they appear in the narratives above – we may seek to look beyond the question on the objective reality of such events and better focus on the role that such experiences play in the social shaping of reality and lifeworlds. After all, the uncanny vividly produces effects and materialises in the language, bodies, technologies and practices of human culture.

Acknowledgements

The authors would like to acknowledge support from the following projects: *Mind and the Other*, Academy of Finland, grant number 266573; *Tracking the Therapeutic*, Academy of Finland, grant number 289004; *Crossing Borders for Health and Wellbeing*, Kone Foundation and the Finnish Cultural Foundation. The authors specifically wish to thank Ülo Valk and Jon Mitchell and all our colleagues who have been involved in working on this edited book for sharing their thoughts and insights on earlier versions of this chapter.

Notes

1 In this work we want to avoid the term 'supernatural' due to its normative bias. The term 'uncanny' originates from Freud (1919), for whom it refers to ambiguous experiences that are simultaneously familiar and frightening. Despite its Freudian baggage, we think that the uncanny is the most suitable analytic concept for our work.
2 Peter Lamont (2007) has made a critical notion that in cognitive psychology uncanny experiences are typically reduced to 'paranormal beliefs' and/or explained as errors or anomalies in mental functions (see Rancken, 2017). In an evolutionary sense, in the cognitive theory of religion, the uncanny may be seen, for example, as an anomaly that stems from the human mind's tendency to anthropomorphize and animate its surroundings for adaptive purposes (Guthrie, 1993: 3–6; see also Boyer, 2001: 145–147).
3 According to Latour (2005, 72) things as actants 'affect' the world in a variety of ways: 'Things may authorize, allow, afford, encourage, permit, suggest, influence, block, render possible, forbid, and so on'.
4 Mimesis is an old healing technique by which threat and danger are warded off by means of imitating and consequently taming them.

References

Blanke, O. and Arzy, S. 2005. The out-of-body experience: Disturbed self-processing at the temporo-parietal junction. *Neuroscientist 11*, 16–24.

Bowman, M. and Valk, U. 2012. *Vernacular Religion in Everyday Life*. Oxon and New York: Routledge.

Boyer, P. 2001. *Religion Explained: The Evolutionary Foundations of Religious Belief*. New York: Basic Books.

Bury, M. 1982. Chronic illness as biographical disruption. *Sociology of Health and Illness 4*:2, 167–182.

Bury, M. 2001. Illness narratives: Fact or fiction? *Sociology of Health and Illness 23*:3, 263–285.

Dein, S. 2012. Mental health and the paranormal. *International Journal of Transpersonal Studies 31*:1, 61–74.

Descola, P. 2013. *The Ecology of Others*. Chicago: Pricky Paradigm Press.

Eliade, M. 1964. *Shamanism; Archaic Techniques of Ecstasy*. London: Arkada.

Freud, S. 1919. The 'Uncanny'. In English Translation: *The Standard Edition of the Complete Psychological Works of Sigmund Freud*, Volume XVII (1917–1919), edited by S. Freud. Harmondsword: Penguin Classics.

Guthrie, S. 1993. *Faces in the Clouds: A New Theory of Religion*. New York: Oxford University Press.

Heelas, P. 1996. *The New Age Movement: The Celebration of the Self and the Sacralisation of Modernity*. Oxford: Blackwell.

Heelas, P. and Woodhead, L. 2005. *The Spiritual Revolution: Why Religion Is Giving Way to Spirituality?* Oxford: Blackwell.

Honkasalo, M. 2017a. Hipaisuja ja ryminää – aineellisten ja aineettomien toimijoiden jäljillä. In *Mielen rajoilla. Arjen kummat kokemukset*, edited by M. Honkasalo and K. Koski. Helsinki: Suomalaisen Kirjallisuuden Seura, 196–234.

Honkasalo, M. 2017b. Neither real nor true. In *Extending Experience through the Arts. Proceedings of Artistic Research in Performing Arts*, edited by L. Rouhiainen. Helsinki: University of the Arts. https://nivel.teak.fi/carpa5/marja-liisa-honkasalo-neither-real-nor-true-sharing-voices-in-the-intersubjective-space-and-beyond

Honko, L. 1960. Varhaiskantaiset taudinselitykset ja parantamisnäytelmä. In *Jumin keko*, edited by J. Hautala. Helsinki: Suomalaisen Kirjallisuuden Seura, 43–111.

Hulkkonen, K. 2017. Kanavointi ja jakautunut yrittäjyys – *new age* -henkisyyden ja yrittäjyyden yhdistämisen rajat ja mahdollisuudet. *Elore 24*:1, 1–20.

Josephson-Storm, J. 2017. *The Myth of Disenchantment: Magic, Modernity and the Birth of Human Sciences*. Chicago: University of Chicago Press.

Kapferer, B. 2002. *Beyond Rationalism: Rethinking Magic, Witchcraft and Sorcery*. New York: Berghahn Books.

Koski, K. 2016. Discussing the supernatural in contemporary finland: Discourses, genres, and forums. *Folklore: Electronic Journal of Folklore 65*, 11–36. https://www.folklore.ee/folklore/vol65/koski.pdf.

Lamont, P. 2007. Paranormal belief and the avowal of prior scepticism. *Theory & Psychology 17*:5, 681–696.

Latour, B. 1992. Where are the missing masses? The sociology of a few mundane artifacts. In *Shaping Technology-Building Society: Studies in Sociotechnical Change*, edited by W. Bijker and J. Law. Cambridge: MIT Press, 225–259.

Latour, B. 1993. *We Have Never Been Modern*. Cambridge: Harvard University Press.

Latour, B. 1999. *Pandora's Hope: Essays on the Reality of Science Studies*. Cambridge and London: Harvard University Press.

Latour, B. 2005. *Reassembling the Social – An Introduction to Actor-Network-Theory*. Oxford: Oxford University Press.

Levi-Strauss, C. 1968. *The Savage Mind*. Chicago: University of Chicago Press.

Luhrmann, T. 2018. The sound of madness. *Harper's Magazine*, June, 45–54.

Mauss, M. 1902/2001. *A General Theory of Magic*. London: Routledge.

Mauss, M. 1909/2003. *On Prayer*. Oxford and New York: Berghahn.

Mobbs, D. and Watt, C. 2011. There is nothing paranormal about near-death experiences. *Trends Cognitive Sciences 15*:10, 447–449.

Mol, A. 2002. *The Body Multiple: Ontology in Medical Practice*. Durham: Duke University Press.

Raij, T., Valkonen-Korhonen, M., Holi, M., Therman, S., Lehtonen, L. and Hari, R. 2009. Reality of auditory verbal hallucinations. *Brain 132*:11, 2994–3001.

Rancken, J. 2017. *Yliluonnollinen kokemus*. Tampere: Vastapaino.

Ratcliff, M. 2017. *Real Hallucinations*. Boston: MIT Press.

Sansi, R. 2013. The latour event: History, symmetry and diplomacy. *Social Anthropology* *21*:4, 448–461.

Schmidt, B. 2016. *The Study of Religious Experience: Approaches and Methodologies*. Bristol: Equinox.

Schmidt, B. and Hutchinson, L. (eds.) 2010. *Spirit Possession and Trance, New Interdisciplinary Perspectives*. London and New York: Bloomsbury.

Siikala, A.-L. 1978. *The Rite Technique of the Sibirian Shamans*. Folklore Fellows Communications 220. Helsinki: Academia Scientiarum Fennica.

Silvanto, J. 2015. Why is "blindsight" blind? A new perspective on primary visual cortex, recurrent activity and visual awareness. *Consciousness and Cognition 32*:2, 15–32.

Taussig, M. 1993. *Mimesis and Alterity*. New York: Routledge.

Tucker, J. 2004. New age healers and the therapeutic culture. In *Therapeutic Culture: Triumph and Defeat*, edited by J. Imber. New Brunswick and London: Transaction, 153–169.

Turner, V. 1968. *Drums of Affliction*. Oxford: Clarendon Press.

Viveiros de Castro, E. 2004. Perspectival anthropology and the method of controlled equivocation. *Tipiti: Journal of the Society for Anthropology of Lowland South America* *2*:1, 1–22.

Walter, T. 1999. *On Bereavement. The Culture of Grief*. Berkshire: Open University Press.

Walter, T. 2007. Modern grief, postmodern grief. *International Review of Sociology 17*:1, 123–134.

Weber, M. 1922/1967. *Essays in Sociology*. New York and London: Routledge & Kegan Paul.

Afterword
Life of psy

Elaine Swan

I call this afterword life of psy, partly to make a bad joke but more importantly, to highlight the way *Assembling Therapeutics* breathes new life into studies of therapeutics. In no insignificant way, this is because *Assembling Therapeutics* rigorously examines how the therapeutic lives are lived in different political, historical and national contexts, and professional and everyday lives. Reading the chapters in this ground-breaking book, *Assembling Therapeutics* made me excited as the authors in each chapter strip away the congealed taken-for-granteds about therapeutic culture, practitioners, participants and practices. As Ariel Yankellevich puts it in his chapter, citing Aubry and Travis, a 'canonical critique of therapeutic culture' has emerged over the past 30 years, mostly from Anglo-American writers (2015: 10). In this view, therapeutic culture depoliticises, individualises, self-responsibilises and privatises. The effect of this proliferating critique has been to flatten differences across geographical and therapeutic contexts and approaches; erase the collectivism of therapeutic events; ignore the progressive potential of therapeutic politics; pathologise consumers and practitioners, most often women; denigrate culturally feminised practices; and evacuate people of any agency or critical insight.

This monolithic thinking arises because critiques rarely undertake ethnographic research and often neglect feminist studies of therapeutic culture. Research has tended to focus on the bird's eye, macro view of therapy culture. As a result, the distinctiveness and contextual specificities of therapeutic practices get blurred, and newly emerging versions invisibilised. Thankfully, *Assembling Therapeutics* departs from these methodologies and offers a rich and stimulating collection of chapters which live up to the editors' aim of decentring the US centric, deterministic and attenuated view of therapeutic culture and politics. A vital element in this insightful volume is the provision of close-ups of practitioners and participants, and their lived meanings, practices and motivations. Accordingly, many authors inhabit a position of what Steven Stanley and Ilmari Kortelainen in their chapter call the 'sympathetic-critic' in their analyses. Significantly too, chapters by Marjo Kolehmainen and Inna Perheentupa bring feminist perspectives, and histories to the fore, challenging the citational practices and taken-for-granted genealogies of therapeutic culture scholarship, and the assumed gender- and class-neutrality of therapeutics. Accordingly, the book

Assembling Therapeutics challenges what Tatiana Tiaynen-Qadir describes appositely as the 'totalizing effects and normalizing power of a singular therapeutic culture', and propels a fascinating and prescient study of therapeutic practices.

Epistemologies of the therapeutic

The book makes an urgent and significant contribution by developing practices of inquiry, methodologies and methods that go beyond the macro or the purely textual and provide new lines of empirical inquiry. To some extent, self-help books have become the poster-child for critiques of therapy culture, a gloss for the whole of therapy practices. In mobilising ethnographic, participant-observation and multi-method approaches, the book shifts the types of research questions being asked, moves forward empirical studies of geographical and therapeutic contexts, and lays out new research trajectories to the field. These methodological, empirical and theoretical developments matter as therapeutic approaches and power relations vary with histories, geographies, institutions and contexts, as Bondi and Fewell (2003) stressed over 15 years ago, and the introduction to this volume explains. Through these approaches, *Assembling Therapeutics* takes the field in genuinely new directions.

Tiaynen-Qadir notes in her chapter that ethnographic methods demand commitment, reflexivity and immersion, and we should note resources such as time and funding are not readily available in the accelerated university. But such engagement enables researchers to pay attention to verbal, emotional, affective and bodily reactions which underpin therapeutic events and experiences – what Tiaynen-Qadir calls an 'ethnography of the tacit'. Accordingly, chapters deftly illustrate how the so-called 'talking cure' relies on affects, emotions and bodies, and as Kolehmainen gives a vibrant sense of, the bodies are not always human nor fleshy (see Kolehmainen, Stanley and Kortelainen and Peteri in this book). All of which raises incisive questions about what kinds of data we will need to trace therapeutic assemblages across other geographical contexts not included in the collection and those which coerce affects, emotions and bodies.

The book is enriched by the ways in which authors take the time to listen to and learn from practitioners of and participants in therapeutic practices. This is an important counter to the field because in spite of various calls to find out about practitioners' meanings, motivations and methods, we still know very little as noted by the editors (see also Swan, 2008). But the sensibility in *Assembling Therapeutics* means we meet a panoply of practitioners: coaches, employed counselling professionals, psychotherapists, couple counsellors, mindfulness practitioners, and alternative medicine and new age practitioners working across different national and institutional contexts. In a similar vein, participants in therapeutic practices are often ignored, painted with a condescending broad brush, or represented by self-help book readers but one of the strengths of this book is that authors introduce us to the thoughts, feelings and experiences of choir attendees, feminist trauma activists, migrant Christians, people suffering from depression and even academics!

An oft-trotted out aphorism is that the therapeutic industry is proliferating, but rarely do studies research the events, spaces and organising practices, through which the industry is proliferating. In contrast, *Assembling Therapeutics* gives a deep insight into therapeutic industry events such as seminars, lectures, training courses, conferences and workshops taking place in libraries, fairs, hotels and workplaces. Moreover, the authors' openness to what constitutes the therapeutic means we learn about new therapeutic spaces, such as churches, feminist trauma activism and uncanny experiences, which produce therapeutic effects less by design and more as 'by-products' (Tiaynen-Qadir, this book). In doing so, the book offers a rich and stimulating glimpse of 'actually-existing' therapeutic practices and leads the way in suggesting future therapeutic event ethnographies.

This book makes a welcome contribution to studies of mediated and textual therapeutics and how they produce investment, affect and identification. A most surprising textual archive comes in the chapter by Kia Andell, Harley Bergroth and Marja-Liisa Honkasalo, which analyses unsolicited letters about uncanny experiences sent to the researchers. Their rich chapter reminds us to consider the unexpected in our empirical work. Thus, Harley Bergroth and Ilpo Helén and Felix Freigang vividly trace 'therapeutic imaginaries' through promotional materials for digital therapeutic devices. In their auspicious chapters, Bergroth and Helén, Freigang and Perheentupa bring a much-needed analysis of digital and social media, underlining how technological affordances mediate therapeutic experiences. All of the chapters in the book profile the contradictions that undergird the therapeutic assemblages they analyse and in his analysis of social media, Freigang shows how a commercial digital device company produced social media through which unexpected therapeutic activism took place as consumers challenged mental health stereotypes and lack of funding of support services. Through these approaches, the chapters go beyond current studies of mediated therapeutics, often dominated by analyses of US television programmes, to highlight how new media promulgate cultural imaginaries, politics and versions of self-care. Such analyses offer a springboard for developing research on the technological affordances and mediated specificities of digital therapeutics.

Another contribution of the book is the presentation of data. Thus, many authors present fulsome verbatim quotations from their respondents and vivid, detailed field notes so that we can see the light and shade in people's meanings and practices in ways which break open rigid categories often found in critiques. Thus, in her chapter on the rise of corporate fun initiatives, Virve Peteri provides rich excerpts representing people's mixed experiences of fun spaces and practices. Kolehmainen underlines embodied knowledge production in her writing up regarding her ambivalence participating in relationship counselling events, in what she wonderfully describes as her 'sour' field notes. Drawing on interviews, Julia Lerner gives space in her chapter to let her respondents speak in some depth about their experiences of well-being and religion. In a similar vein, Andell, Bergroth and Honkasalo purposefully present one interviewee at a time in their chapter to illuminate their individual stories and experiences of uncanny processes. Through these analytical practices, the book shows what is at stake in how we represent those who participate in therapy practices and how we can illuminate the processual and emergent in our studies.

The book raises timely insights about how to study therapeutic events, and raises fundamental questions about organising practices and who organises what type of events for which audiences through what kinds of practices and under what conditions. This is central to understanding the politics of therapeutics and hierarchisations of authority, expertise, resources and in the language of the book, assemblages of gender, race and class.

Category of the therapeutic

Another major contribution of the collection is that it expands our understanding of the category of the therapeutic, its ideals and teloi because authors unpack what therapeutic means to the people they interviewed, and processes, people and objects they observed rather than deciding a priori. As the chapters in the book detail, the canonical critique characterises the therapeutic as emotivist and confessional, typically viewed as degraded ways to perform the self; Foucauldian commentators differentiate the therapeutic through its discourses of autonomy, independence, detachment and self-improvement; feminists focus on its rhetoric of healing and coping; and many theorists posit self-transformation as a central leitmotif; while studies of mediated therapy see catharsis as the opus operandi (see Swan, 2010 for more discussion on definitions of the therapeutic). Some chapters in the collection build on these definitions as a point of departure from which they extend our understandings, while others directly challenge such depictions. A guiding premise of the collection, as the editors note in their introduction, is that it insists on the 'multiplicity of the therapeutic, and how "the meaning of 'the therapeutic" itself shifts with shifting assemblages'.

In this regard, one of the strengths of the book is the analysis of how therapeutics emerge from non-secular practices (Stanley and Kortelainen, Lerner and Tiaynen-Qadir). In her chapter, Lerner defines the therapeutic through psychoanalytically informed leitmotifs: 'the narrative of identifying problems, probing the unconscious, making connections with past events or even one's childhood, and summoning the self onto a path of healing and the elimination of suffering'. But she shows that her interviewees co-mingle these ways of thinking with their religious commitments. Thus, in the context of their immigration to Israel, her Russian speaking interviewees merge what she refers to as a contradictory but meaningful, neoliberal religious-therapeutic subjectivity. The data in Tiaynen-Qadir's chapter also shows how the therapeutic draws on the religious. In this case, research participants interlace religion, contemporary therapeutics and *therapeia* – old traditions of health of the soul and body in Finnish Orthodox Christianity. As part of her analysis, Tiaynen-Qadir insists on multiplicity – 'various cultural therapeutics' – some of which 'challenge *secular* psychological narratives of the self' and 'reach out to the divine, within and beyond the self' rather than reproducing notions of self-optimisation. Her respondents are not simply assimilating psychology into Orthodox theology, but re-vivifying *therapeia*, which has resonances with self-help and New Age. Insightfully, she stresses that the term 'therapeutic' means distinct things to her respondents, some use it to refer to a secular sense of emotional well-being, while others, the effect of 'sacred' singing.

Life management practices become the focus of other fascinating chapters in the collection. Andell, Bergroth and Honkasalo understand the uncanny experiences of their letter-writers as therapeutic events because they form part of people's existential repertoire, and are shot through with what they see as therapeutic ideas of comfort, care and healing. The uncanny experiences and their narration provide people with resources to make sense of human existence, and work as forms of self-care and care for others. Moving towards a very different kind of existential project, Bergroth and Helén's chapter incisively shows how the therapeutic becomes a data-driven practice in digital self-tracking devices. Our therapeutic practices of knowing, transforming and improving oneself are re-shaped through metrics and quantification-based haptic and visual data. In this way, datafied life management conjoins somewhat contradictorily with a therapeutic ethos. They stress that the data devices are not just epistemic but ontological tools, inflecting relations of the self to the self, and enacting the self through self-tracking.

Freigang shows how *DepressApp*, a mood-tracking app for people suffering from depression in Germany, reinvents self-disclosure, a classic practice of therapy culture. The app replaces the traditional pen and paper therapeutic tools with digital journals – as he puts it, 'swiping instead of writing'– and reconfigures emotion management as people monitor, quantify, and visualise their mood shifts. The quantification of emotion has been part of the history of therapy culture but these chapters underscore how the digital transforms what constitutes emotion management (Shackhak, 2017). But a vital point made by Freigang is that the digital device produces its own affects, which place its user in a hopeful relation with the device but also in a wider economy of emotions and digital quantifications and images.

In a very different context, Perheentupa shows how feminist trauma activism against violence in Russia, at a time of regressive policies, combines therapeutic and political ideas. Charting the complex history of feminism and popular psychology in Russia, she underscores the importance of psychology as an epistemic resource for women who have survived violence and trauma and find it difficult to get professional therapy or support elsewhere. Furthermore, the feminists incorporate therapeutic elements such as testimony, witnessing and proactivity in their performances, bringing feminist principles in dialogue with therapeutic practices, in what she describes as 'collective therapy'.

Selfhoods

The chapters contest another shibboleth of studies of therapy culture: selfhood. As the authors in the collection argue, therapeutic practices foreground notions of subjectivity and personhood and provide resources for self-formation. For critics, the focus on the self leads to narcissism and atomistic individualism. The project in many of the chapters is to reconfigure how we understand therapeutic selfhood by foregrounding how non-humans live in therapeutic relations and de-centre the human self. The non-humans brought to our attention throughout the book vary in kind, order and capacity. In their chapter, Bergroth and Helén reveal how self-tracking takes shape through congeries of non-human and human bodies, digital and quantitative data, technological objects and the ideas of self-care. Deploying Deleuze's concept of 'dividualisation', they argue that self-tracking devices complicate traditional notions of holistic therapeutic selfhood in what they call 'fragmentary holism'. In this way, the self becomes a data assemblage and process. Their rigorous analyses add to debates about how psychological interiorities are being reconfigured from notions of depth and past memories to futures and anticipation. Freigang shows us how the non-human mobile and mood-tracking app he researched became a 'therapeutic companion' for people with mental illnesses and depression, physically *living* with his respondents to bus-stops, restaurants and waiting rooms. Indeed, marketers portray the app as a 'pocket therapist'. Its non-human affordance of portability means that it becomes an embodied part of the self, easily assimilated into everyday habits and spaces. But it is not just the app that makes up the therapeutic assemblage but also the diverse elements of the hardware of the mobile, the software programme, the data, social networks, media outlets and startup entrepreneurs.

Other chapters focus on the importance of affect and space. For instance, Kolehmainen describes how therapeutic practices of relationship counselling work through non-human bodies and impersonal flows of affect. As she writes, reconfiguring understandings of the therapeutic, 'a non-human-centred concept of atmosphere ... does not start with an 'I' but invites us to pay attention to the transpersonal, the intercorporeal and the more-than-only-human'. In their chapter on mindfulness, Stanley and Kortelainen foreground the concatenation of the body-mind of the mindfulness practitioner, lighting, seating and the space of meditation practice. Peteri underlines the significance of space in her discussion of corporate fun culture in designing so-called positive emotions through the set-up of office spaces, their décor and the provision of toys, bean-bags, slogans and TV references.

The book encourages us to think of the lives of non-humans, objects, spaces, representations and ideas and how they make therapeutics? How might access to such non-humans be unevenly distributed and with what effects? When might atmospheres not just turn sour but be unwelcoming or violent and for whom? How might spaces, seating and lighting assemble inequalities and oppression in enforced therapeutics for minoritised groups in prisons, hospitals, courtrooms and schools?

Assembling the therapeutic assemblage

This brings us to the exciting conceptual contribution of the book: its analytical lens of assemblage. Although, Rose (1998) mentions assemblages in his influential book, *Inventing Our Selves* on the 'psy-complex', few scholars have taken up the cudgel until now (also see Tiaynen-Qadir and Salmenniemi, 2017). In the introduction the editors explain that assemblage thinking means understanding the therapeutic as a multifaceted collection of 'ideas, practices, spaces, objects and bodies yielding multiple, contextually specific and sometimes contradictory effects', which work processually, relationally and emergently to challenge universalistic, monolithic, static understandings of therapy culture. The chapters attend to these elements in different ways. It's refreshing that authors are not doctrinaire Deleuze and Guattarian assemblage thinkers but mobilise different understandings of assemblage theorising from geographers, feminists and anthropologists, albeit influenced by Deleuze and Guttari's notion of *agencement*, and put these in dialogue with other concepts such as affect. Through their detailed analyses, authors reveal different scales of assembling, and some show the linkages and exchanges between and across broader assemblages.

In conceiving of therapeutics as an assemblage of atmospheres, Kolehmainen highlights 'connectivities' and blockages between situational and material practices, affects, objects and bodies – non-human, non-organic, imaginary. She draws on assemblage thinking to underline how therapeutic events are not just 'top down governance' but 'lived, networked, relational and embodied experiences' that generate collective connections. Felling a number of taken-for-granteds, she informs us that this shifts the focus from 'the self to the collective, from advice-giving to experience, and from governmentality to lived experience' and in so doing, challenges many of the shibboleths in the canonical critique.

Freigang reminds us that assemblages demand the active labour of humans and non-humans and several chapters focus on this, including that of Stanley and Kortelainen who reveal that mindfulness practitioners pull on various resources to make mindful-bodies and spaces. Suvi Salmenniemi, Johanna Nurmi and Joni Jaakola also attend to practitioners but about how they assemble what the authors call 'personalised self-care packages', a bricolage from elements from the New Age movement, alternative medicine, self-help, lifestyle, alternative health and new spirituality. These personalised assemblages help them to mediate the injuries of contemporary neoliberal work. Andell, Bergroth and Honkasalo focus on individual therapeutic assembling, not that of practitioners but of people who have experienced uncanny events, the narrations of which comingle uncanny and other actants as 'ways of "assembling" one's life'. Lerner reveals how new migrants mobilise a 'therapeutic-religious assemblage' as a salve against their immigrant experience in the post-Soviet cultural context. Importantly, she stresses that they do this in situated, flexible constellations alongside neoliberalism.

Other chapters emphasise how therapeutics are assembled across cultural and social institutions, histories and transnational geographies. As a result, studies are grounded in specificities at the level of the therapeutic practices, national contexts and histories in ways which de-centre US theories and practices. Tiaynen-Qadir conceives of a 'glocalized therapeutic assemblage', bringing analytic attention to how the global and the local merge in embedded, historically situated interactions of human and non-human actors, which in her chapter includes the specificities of religion and psychology in Russia. In so doing, she vividly challenges the repeated motif in the canonical critique of the relationship between US Protestantism and therapeutics. Stanley and Kortelainen argue that it is the 'sheer multiplicity of the assemblage of mindfulness' that accounts for its proliferation across so many social and cultural domains. Importantly, they remind us of the importance of histories to therapeutic assemblages highlighting how both early twentieth century British colonial expansion in Southeast Asia and the 1960s counter-cultural movement influenced the transnational appropriations of mindfulness ideas and practices. They ask us to think about the situated and the broader milieu.

Lerner coins the term 'emotional socialism' in direct opposition to Illouz' (2007) EuroAmerican theorisation of emotional capitalism. She does this to underscore a different historical relation to psychology in Russia and the Soviet Union and foreground what she calls the Russian emotional style and its socialist inflecting. Central to her project is showing how 'the global therapeutic language' works alongside local discourses and ideals to shape newly emerging post-Soviet Russian versions of selfhood, emotions and personal relations. The chapter by Yankellevich asks us to reflect on how therapeutic practices are not just about assembling lives but about assembling a nation, asking us to reflect on the scales of assemblages. Writing specifically about coaching in Israel, he tells us that self-improvement discourses and practices play a critical part in the construction of national identities in the aftermath of neoliberalist reform.

Emergence and relational connectivity are two characteristics of assemblages which chapters bring out in their discussion. Freigang shows how affective intensities help the socio-material elements of mood-tracking apps assemble or disassemble as people invest hope in them. At the same time, this hope intensifies the affective flows that form part of an app's assemblage. Peteri argues that the assemblages of corporate fun culture construct contradictions are always productive of new behaviours, expressions, actors and realities. Bergroth and Helén show that 'the self', the 'therapeutic' and the practice of 'self-tracking' are constantly being assembled from diverse elements. Rather than understanding self-tracking as therapeutic, they use assemblage thinking to show how self-tracking 'becomes' therapeutic in relation to the sociotechnical and political context in which it is practised. Importantly, Bergroth and Helén's chapter underlines how therapeutic assemblages are related to other assemblages, in their example, personalised health care but provoking researchers of therapeutic to map other interconnected assemblages. For example, how does the state assemble therapeutics and through which other assemblages, institutions, representations and objects?

Therapeutic assemblage politics

How then to think about the politics of therapeutics? If we want to move away from the idea that therapeutics stop people from having critical thoughts, nuanced reflexivities and political inclinations, then how might we need to rethink therapeutics and politics? A popular vein of thinking insists that therapeutic practices deplete social critique, collectivism, critical capacities and possibilities for social change. The book roundly challenges this view. This is not to say that authors are cheer-leaders for all aspects of therapeutic culture but rather that they plumb the nuances, contradictions and multiplicities of people's engagement with therapeutic ideas and practices. Moreover, if non-humans have agency then what does this mean for understanding the political? How do policies, reports, powerpoints, social media, psychological tests, therapeutic exercises, games, chairs, rooms and flipcharts capacitate and inhibit? How do bodily encounters make race, heteronormativity, class and gender? And as chapters deftly illuminate, through their stimulating analyses of self-care, embodied care, collective care, care for others, how can we reflect on the politics of care, when care and the labours of care are unevenly distributed by race, class and gender.

Some chapters offer clearer possibilities for more progressive politics than is often imagined in popular and theroetical critiques of therapy culture. Not all though. For instance, in the chapters on digital devices, and workplace fun cultures, authors point to oppressive effects. Although, as Freigang shows in his example of people with depression using social media to speak out against the structural constraints of psychotherapeutic care, these are not cut and dried. Indeed, all of the chapters stress the significance of contradiction and ambivalence.

A common critique of the depoliticising capacities of therapeutics is that they encourage people to take on a neoliberal subjectivity but Salmenniemi, Nurmi and Jaakola disrupt this view. After speaking with practitioners who mobilise therapeutic practices against alienation from work, the authors insist that they 'may also be mobilized to critique, contest and disengage from the destructive and exploitative effects of neoliberalism'. Their interviewees curate 'a package' of self-care practices, not simply to self-optimise, but to critique work and imagine alternatives. An important tool in their analytics is their holding onto contradiction and the possibilities of both and, as they make clear, therapeutic practices can reinforce neoliberal subjectivities *and* enable resistance, and this depends on how practices are assembled.

While Salmenniemi, Nurmi and Jaakola's chapter examines the politics of individual self-care and resistance, others question whether therapeutic practices generate social change. Thus, Yankellevich challenges 'the dichotomous view' that opposes 'the therapeutic ethos to a model of civic virtue or political engagement' (Illouz, 2008). He argues that the coaching enacted by middle-class Ashkenazim Jews does not always lead to a lack of political disengagement. His interviewees see individual self-development and social engagement as mutually reinforcing. He insists that coaching can promote a collectivist ethos to act for the common good when therapeutic neoliberal rationality works dialectically with local discourses of the self.

Feminist activism can be supported by therapeutic practices as Perheentupa shows in her chapter on trauma culture. Mobilising the term 'therapeutic politics' to challenge head on the idea that therapeutic practices are always politically denuded, she argues that it is the feminist agenda that promotes collective and societal responsibility and makes trauma therapy a collective radical politics. Indeed, her respondents see psychology as a useful form of knowledge to help them with experiences of violence and to initiate social change.

These chapters and others point to the collective experiencing and sociality of therapeutic events. Indeed, several chapters underline how collectivism and sociality are important to therapeutic practices, in contrast to the idea that therapy culture encourages an emotional detachment from others (Hochschild, 1994; Rimke, 2000). Even when individualistic discourses are mobilised, as Kolehmainen argues, therapeutic events can facilitate collective experience and connections.

Future research agendas: therapeutic lives

This collection of chapters stimulates us to reflect on other questions about politics. As someone who writes on gender, race, class and therapy culture, I was very pleased to read feminist-inspired reflections about social differentiation and inequalities. I would argue that one of the questions the book leaves us with is why women numerically dominate therapeutic practices, as practitioners and participants, as Salmenniemi, Nurmi and Jaakola note in their chapter.

Feminist theorists provide us with some useful pathways to follow. As I argue elsewhere (Swan, 2008, 2017a, b) women participate in therapeutic practices because they offer resources to cope with the impossible demands and costs of performing 'successful femininity'; 'propping up' postfeminism; and undertaking the self-work to become the never-ending, self-improving, independent subject (Baker, 2010; Ringrose and Walkerdine, 2008). As chapters in this book suggest, therapeutic practices offer connections and sociality and, as has been argued, intimacy, friendship and emotional sustenance that was once met by friends and family (George, 2013; Swan, 2010). Indeed, in thinking about assemblages, it can be argued that psychological practices help people to paper over the cracks caused by the 'fracturing and fragmentation of neo-liberal and globalised economies which are no longer willing to provide long-term forms of support' (Walkerdine and Ringrose, 2008: 35).

Women looking for feminist support in their everyday lives can find elements in popular psychology. As chapters in the book suggest, feminism and psychology have long assembled, disassembled and re-assembled and have 'rhetorical continuities', for example, in notions about self-reflexivity and the family as sites of change (Illouz, 2008; Peck, 1995; Moskowitz, 2001). It has been argued that self-help is a proto-political form of feminism given its principles of self-determination and fulfilment and 'might be tapped for a progressive, even a radical, agenda' (McGee, 2005: 24; Crowley, 2011; Simonds, 1992). Feminists also insist that women readers of self-help books are critical of some of their ideas but value the personal disclosure and experiential knowledge of the authors, and how the books offer new gendered behaviours (Grodin, 1995; Knudson, 2013; McGee, 2005; Simonds, 1992).

In addition to the numerical feminisation of therapeutics, cultural feminisation of therapeutic culture needs interrogation. For instance, feminist researchers insist counselling and coaching draw on symbolically feminine styles of discourse. Such discourse encompasses sharing feelings and personal problems, being facilitative, empathetic and supportive, all modes of talking culturally associated with women's intimate private friendships (George, 2013; Graf and Pawelczyk, 2014; Pawelzyk and Graf, 2011; McLeod and Wright, 2009; Swan, 2006, 2008, 2017a, b). While chapters in the book don't discuss feminine styles of talk, they point to other culturally gendered elements in therapeutic assemblages. For instance, Salmenniemi, Nurmi and Jaakola show that the feminised fragile vulnerable self, promulgated in neoliberal therapeutic practices and much critiqued in the canonical critique, challenges the go-getting, productive masculinised ideal worker in affirming ways. Kolehmainen notes the 'firm reliance' on gendered stereotypes and heteronormative values in the relationship counselling she studied. Peteri reveals how organisational fun culture in spite of its apparent associations with feminised aesthetics and emotions encourages masculinist forms of embodiment and laddish culture, reproducing old hierarchies. Putting it baldly, she writes that one man's fun culture is another woman's #metoo campaign.

But as some authors in the collection allude to and others, including me, have pointed out, therapy culture also has classed and racialised implications (Frantsman-Spector and Shoshana, 2018; Sa'ar, 2016; Swan, 2008, 2017a, b). Because of the book's focus on everyday lives, less attention is given to the ways in which racially minoritised and white working-class people are forced by state institutions and other assemblages to participate in therapeutic practices and reproduce themselves through therapeutic vocabularies and subjectivities (Lawler, 2005; Skeggs, 2004; Steedman, 2002). As Bergroth and Helén note en passant in their chapter, some people are 'obliged' to use self-tracking devices. In contrast, the middle-classes often take up therapeutic practices voluntarily. They have the time and income to be able to purchase self-improvement services (Swan, 2017a). Indeed, as I and others argue, middle-class, white women are culturally constructed as the ideal, self-transforming subject, having 'psychological capital' to effect self-work and self-transformation (Swan, 2017a, b; Baker, 2010; Blackman, 2004, 2005, 2007; Pfister, 1997). Seen as having this 'proper subjectivity', middle-class white women are positioned in opposition to racially minoritised and working white women, who are depicted as less willing, and less able to reinvent themselves, possessing shallow and more defective 'psychologies' (Lawler, 2005; Skeggs, 2002, 2004; Steedman, 2002). Therapeutic culture valorises the psychological and emotional styles of white middle-classness (Illouz, 1997; Lawler, 2005; Skeggs, 2009). Moreover, many tips and techniques point to problems and solutions that do not characterise the social situations or difficulties that are faced by racialised and white working-class women (Swan, 2017a).

In this vein, Salmenniemi and Adamson (2015) argue that popular psychology creates symbolic hierarchies by attaching value to middle-class women who are able to reproduce self-help tropes and narratives and thus construct Others as lacking value. Indeed, Mäkinen (2014) stresses that coaching aimed at people who are unemployed promotes the ideal subject of neoliberal individualism: someone who is autonomous, full of capacities and limitless power, who 'makes their own future'. But coaches need to acknowledge subjects' failures in order to sell their services and imply that no one's individuality is quite good enough.

Therefore, coaching for people who are unemployed exacerbates feelings of insecurity and precarity, feeding off failure and fear. And as Perheentupa points out in her chapter in this book, class affects who gets to access critical knowledge and professional help in trauma culture, noting that women from working-class backgrounds are at greater risk of gendered violence.

At the same time, as the book highlights so carefully, therapeutic practices throw up complexities and contradictions. Thus, Frantsman-Spector and Shoshana (2018) show how women married to prisoners manage to reject what they know is a white, middle-class therapeutic subjectivity into which social workers attempt to inveigle them. Sa'ar (2016) reveals that working-class Israeli women who taught middle-class emotional skills in an entrepreneur workshop enjoyed the opportunity to garner middle-class capital and collective sociality with each other.

In my own work, I have tried to explore the racialisation of therapeutic practices, especially the whiteness of psychological and emotional capital promoted by coaching in a British context. In particular, I draw on studies of digital whiteness and critical white critiques of psychological notions of emotional control, positive thinking and feeling and enterprise (Swan, 2017a, b). Indeed, in their chapter, Stanley and Kortelainen highlight the limits of diversity in the mindfulness practices they study, with mindfulness seen as race, gender and class neutral and universally accessible and inclusive.

I leave this afterword with a few lines of inquiry enlivened by this wonderful book and its welcome contributions to help us follow the lives of psy as it moves and emerges in new contexts, bodies, media and practices. How do racialisation, ethnicisation and whiteness play out in therapeutic assemblages and their politics in Finland, Israel, Russia and other national contexts (Hervik, 2018; Zakharov, 2013)? How might assemblage thinking trace how gender, race and class are assembled through connectivities and elements that make up therapeutics? What other kinds of non-humans – representations, documents, technologies, objects, bodies and spaces – comingle to produce progressive and oppressive therapeutic politics? What kinds of labours are involved, by whom and what? How do minoritised groups harness assemblages to resist and reject? How are lives enabled, supported, inhibited and repressed through congeries of therapeutic affects, atmospheres, socialities, spaces and events?

References

Aubry, T. and T. Travis (Eds.) 2015. *Rethinking Therapeutic Culture*. Chicago: University of Chicago Press.

Baker, J. 2010. Claiming volition and evading victimhood: Post-feminist obligations for young women. *Feminism & Psychology 20*(2), 186–204.

Blackman, L. 2004. Self-help, media cultures and the production of female psychopathology. *European Journal of Cultural Studies 7*(2), 219–236.

Blackman, L. 2005. The dialogical self, flexibility and the cultural production of psychopathology. *Theory and Psychology 15*(12), 183–206.

Blackman, L. 2007. Inventing the psychological. In J. Curran and D. Morley (Eds.) *Media and Cultural Theory*. London: Routledge, 209–220.

Bondi, L. and J. Fewell. 2003. 'Unlocking the cage door': The spatiality of counselling. *Social & Cultural Geography 4*(4), 527–547.

Crowley, K. 2011. *Feminism's New Age: Gender, Appropriation and the Afterlife of Essentialism.* New York: SUNY.

Frantsman-Spector, A. and A. Shoshana. 2018. Shameless accounts: Against psychological subjectivity and vulnerable femininity among prisoners' wives in Israel. *Qualitative Sociology 41*(3), 381–398.

George, M. 2013. Seeking legitimacy: The professionalization of life coaching. *Sociological Inquiry 83*(2), 179–208.

Graf, E. M. and J. Pawelczyk. 2014. The interactional accomplishment of feelings-talk in psychotherapy and executive coaching. In E. M. Graf, M. Sator, and T. Spranz-Fogasy (Eds.) *Discourses of Helping Professions* (Vol. 252). Amsterdam: John Benjamins Publishing Company, 59–89.

Grodin, D. 1995. Women reading self-help: Themes of separation and connection. *Women's Studies in Communication 18*(2), 123–134.

Hervik, P. 2018. *Racialization, Racism, and Anti-Racism in the Nordic Countries.* New York: Palgrave MacMillan.

Hochschild, A. R. 1994. The commercial spirit of intimate life and the abduction of feminism: Signs from women's advice books. *Theory Culture and Society 11*(2), 1–23.

Illouz, E. 1997. Who will care for the caretaker's daughter? Toward a sociology of happiness in the era of reflexive modernity. *Theory, Culture and Society 14*(4), 31–66.

Illouz, E. 2007. *Cold Intimacies: The Making of Emotional Capitalism.* Cambridge: Polity.

Illouz, E. 2008. *Saving the Modern Soul: Therapy, Emotions, and the Culture of Self-Help.* New York: University of California Press.

Knudson, S. 2013. Crash courses and lifelong journeys: Modes of reading non-fiction advice in a North American audience. *Poetics 41*(3), 211–235.

Lawler, S. 2005. Disgusted subjects: The making of middle-class identities. *The Sociological Review 53*(3), 429–446.

Mäkinen, K. 2014. The individualization of class: A case of working life coaching. *The Sociological Review 62*(4), 821–842.

McGee, M. 2005. *Self-Help, Inc.: Makeover Culture in American Life.* Oxford: Oxford University Press.

McLeod, J. and K. Wright. 2009. The talking cure in everyday life: Gender, generations and friendship. *Sociology 43*:1, 122–139.

Moskowitz, E. S. 2001. *In Therapy We Trust: America's Obsession With Self-Fulfillment.* Baltimore, MD: Johns Hopkins University Press.

Pawelczyk, J. and E. M. Graf. 2011. Living in therapeutic culture. In I. Lassen (Ed.) *Living with Patriarchy: Discursive Constructions of Gendered Subjects Across Cultures.* Amsterdam, The Netherlands: John Benjamins Publishing Company, 273–302.

Peck, J. 1995. TV talk shows as therapeutic discourse: The ideological labor of the televised talking cure. *Communication Theory 5*:1, 58–81.

Pfister, J. 1997. Glamorizing the psychological: The politics of the performances of modern psychological identities. In J. Pfister and N. Schnog (Eds.) *Inventing the Psychological: Toward a Cultural History of Emotional Life in America.* New York: Yale University Press, 167–213.

Rimke, H. M. 2000. Governing citizens through self-help literature. *Cultural Studies 14*(1), 61–78.

Ringrose, J. and V. Walkerdine. 2008. Regulating the abject. *Feminist Media Studies 8*(3), 227–246.

Rose, N. 1998. *Inventing Our Selves: Psychology, Power, and Personhood.* Cambridge: Cambridge University Press.

Sa'ar, A. 2016. Emotional performance as work skill: Low-income women in Israel learning to talk the talk. *Ethos 44*(2), 171–185.

Salmenniemi, S. and M. Adamson. 2015. New heroines of labour: Domesticating post-feminism and neoliberal capitalism in Russia. *Soctology 49*(1), 88–105.

Simonds, W. 1992. *Women and Self-Help Culture: Reading Between the Lines.* New Brunswick, NJ: Rutgers University Press.

Shachak, M. 2017. (Ex) changing feelings: On the commodification of emotions in psychotherapy. In E. Illouz (Ed.) *Emotions as Commodities.* London: Routledge, 159–184.

Skeggs, B. 2002. Techniques for telling the reflexive self. In T. May (Ed.) *Qualitative Research in Action.* London: Sage, 349–374.

Skeggs, B. 2004. *Class, Self, Culture.* London: Routledge.

Skeggs, B. 2009. The moral economy of person: The class relations of self-performance on 'reality' television. *The Sociological Review 57*(4), 626–644.

Steedman, C. 2002. Enforced narratives. In T. Coslett, C. Lury, and P. Summerfield (Eds.) *Feminism & Autobiography: Texts, Theories, Methods.* London: Routledge, 25–39.

Swan, E. 2006. Gendered leadership and management development: Therapeutic cultures at work. In D. McTavish and K. Millen (Eds.) *Women in Leadership and Management.* Cheltenham: Edward Elgar, 52–70.

Swan, E. 2008. 'You make me feel like a woman': Therapeutic cultures and the contagion of femininity. *Gender, Work & Organization 15*(1), 88–107.

Swan, E. 2010. *Worked Up Selves: Personal Development Workers, Self-Work and Therapeutic Culture.* Basingstoke: Palgrave.

Swan, E. 2017a. Keep calm and carry on being slinky: Postfeminism, resilience coaching and whiteness. In P. Lewis, Y. Benschop, and R. Simpson (Eds.) *Postfeminism and Organization.* London: Routledge, 57–84.

Swan, E. 2017b. Postfeminist stylistics, work femininities and coaching: A multimodal study of a website. *Gender, Work & Organization 24*(3), 274–296.

Tiaynen-Qadir, T. and S. Salmenniemi. 2017. Self-help as a glocalised therapeutic assemblage. *European Journal of Cultural Studies 20*(4), 381–396.

Zakharov, N. 2013. *Attaining Whiteness: A Sociological Study of Race and Racialization in Russia* (Doctoral dissertation, Acta Universitatis Upsaliensis).

Index

Note: Page numbers in *italics* indicate figures.

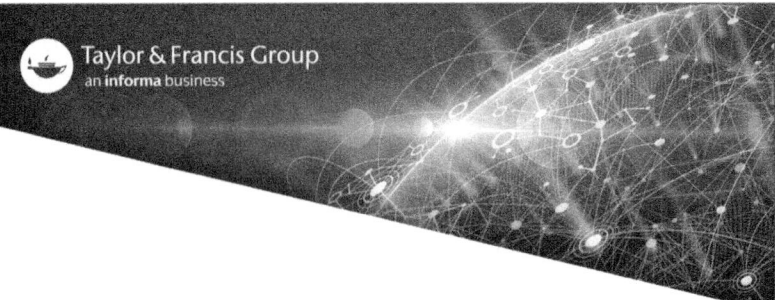
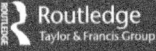
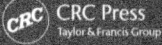